# 2016
# The Year Book of MEDICINE®

Editors
**Kenneth R. DeVault**
**Renee Garrick**
**Michael R. Gold**
**Nancy M. Khardori**
**Derek LeRoith**
**Janet R. Maurer**
**Amanda M. Sammut**

ELSEVIER
MOSBY

ELSEVIER
MOSBY

*Acquisitions Editor:* Jessica McCool
*Developmental Editor:* Kristen Helm



Composition by TNQ Books and Journals Pvt Ltd, India

Editorial Office:
Elsevier
Suite 1800
1600 John F. Kennedy Blvd
Philadelphia, PA 19103-2899

International Standard Serial Number: 0084-3873
International Standard Book Number: 978-0-323-44686-0

# Editorial Board




Contributors

**Richard R. Bayer II, MD**

*Assistant Professor of Medicine and Radiology, Medical University of South Carolina, Charleston, South Carolina*

**Meredith A. Brisco, MD, MSCE, FACC**

*Assistant Professor of Medicine, Heart Failure and Cardiac Transplantation, The Lewis Katz School of Medicine at Temple University, Philadelphia, Pennsylvania*

**Venkata Buddharaju, MD**

*Renal Fellow, New York Medical College, Westchester Medical Center, Valhalla, New York*

**Savneek Singh Chugh, MD, FACP, FASN**

*Assistant Professor of Medicine at New York Medical College; Nephrology Attending in the Department of Medicine at Westchester Medical Center; Nephrology Associates of Westcheter in affliation with Boston Children's Health Physicians and Nephrologist at White Plains Hospital, Hartsdale, New York*

# Table of Contents

# Journals Represented

Journals represented in this YEAR BOOK are listed below.

American Journal of Cardiology
American Journal of Clinical Pathology
American Journal of Gastroenterology
American Journal of Infection Control
American Journal of Kidney Diseases
Annals of the Rheumatic Diseases
Arthritis Care & Research
Arthritis Care & Research (Hoboken)
Arthritis Research & Therapy
Arthritis & Rheumatology
BMC Musculoskeletal Disorders
BMC Nephrology
British Journal of Sports Medicine
Canadian Journal of Cardiology
Cancer Treatment Reviews
Circulation
Clinical Chemistry
Clinical Gastroenterology and Hepatology
Clinical Infectious Diseases
Clinical Journal of the American Society of Nephrology
Current Opinion in Obstetrics and Gynecology
Current Opinion in Oncology
Diabetes Care
Drugs
Endocrine Practice
European Heart Journal
European Journal of Internal Medicine
Gastroenterology
Gut
Intensive Care Medicine
Journal of Bone Mineral Research
Journal of Clinical Microbiology
Journal of Diabetes and its Complications
Journal of Hypertension
Journal of Immunology
Journal of the American College of Cardiology
Journal of the American Heart Association
Journal of the American Medical Association
Journal of the American Medical Association Internal Medicine
Journal of the American Medical Association Neurology
Journal of the American Society of Nephrology
Journal of the European Academy of Dermatology & Venereology
Kidney International
Lancet
Medicine
Nature
Nutrition Journal

New England Journal of Medicine
Obstetrics & Gynecology
Osteoporosis International
Pituitary
Proceedings of the National Academy of Sciences of the United States of America
Science
Surgical Endoscopy
The Journal of Clinical Endocrinology and Metabolism
The Lancet Diabetes & Endocrinology
Thorax
Transfusion

## Standard Abbreviations

The following terms are abbreviated in this edition: acquired immunodeficiency syndrome (AIDS), cardiopulmonary resuscitation (CPR), central nervous system (CNS), cerebrospinal fluid (CSF), computed tomography (CT), deoxyribonucleic acid (DNA), electrocardiography (ECG), health maintenance organization (HMO), human immunodeficiency virus (HIV), intensive care unit (ICU), intramuscular (IM), intravenous (IV), magnetic resonance (MR) imaging (MRI), ribonucleic acid (RNA), and ultrasound (US).

## Note

The Year Book of Medicine is a literature survey service providing abstracts of articles published in the professional literature. Every effort is made to assure the accuracy of the information presented in these pages. Neither the editors nor the publisher of the Year Book of Medicine can be responsible for errors in the original materials. The editors' comments are their own opinions. Mention of specific products within this publication does not constitute endorsement.

To facilitate the use of the Year Book of Medicine as a reference tool, all illustrations and tables included in this publication are now identified as they appear in the original article. This change is meant to help the reader recognize that any illustration or table appearing in the Year Book of Medicine may be only one of many in the original article. For this reason, figure and table numbers will often appear to be out of sequence within the Year Book of Medicine.

PART ONE

# RHEUMATOLOGY

AMANDA M. SAMMUT, MD

# Introduction

Rheumatology is the most intriguing subspecialty in internal medicine. No other field of medicine has as many fascinating and mysterious diseases, which we rheumatologists intellectually entangle ourselves in on a daily basis. It has been a pleasure to help Elsevier with selecting and commenting on the advances in rheumatology over the past year. The majority of articles highlighted in this section were selected specifically to help non-rheumatologist physicians and other healthcare providers learn more about the rheumatic diseases, and to come away with practical, useful clinical pearls that are applicable to everyday practice.

This past year several treatment guidelines, recommendations and classification criteria for certain rheumatic diseases were published. These have been included and I encourage you to be familiar with them as they are clinically useful.

What is a relatively newly discovered autoantibody found in patients with inclusion body myositis? What rheumatic disease can Chikungunya viral arthritis mimic closely? What is known about the role of cannabinoid treatment in rheumatic diseases? The answers to these questions, and more, can be found in this exciting section!

I want to thank all the contributors for their time and effort, Ms. Kristen Helm and the staff at Elsevier for exceptional assistance, patience and the opportunity to contribute to this publication, and Dr. Eric Mariuma, my beloved husband, for all his support and insight.

**Amanda M. Sammut, MD**

# 1 Systemic Lupus Erythematosus

**Factors associated with damage accrual in patients with systemic lupus erythematosus: results from the Systemic Lupus International Collaborating Clinics (SLICC) Inception Cohort**

Bruce IN, O'Keeffe AG, Farewell V, et al (Univ of Manchester, UK; Univ College London, UK; MRC Biostatistics Unit, Cambridge, UK; et al)

*Ann Rheum Dis* 74:1706-1713, 2015

*Background and Aims.*—We studied damage accrual and factors determining development and progression of damage in an international cohort of systemic lupus erythematosus (SLE) patients.

*Methods.*—The Systemic Lupus International Collaborating Clinics (SLICC) Inception Cohort recruited patients within 15 months of developing four or more 1997 American College of Rheumatology (ACR) criteria for SLE; the SLICC/ACR damage index (SDI) was measured annually. We assessed relative rates of transition using maximum likelihood estimation in a multistate model. The Kaplan–Meier method estimated the probabilities for time to first increase in SDI score and Cox regression analysis was used to assess mortality.

*Results.*—We recruited 1722 patients; mean (SD) age 35.0 (13.4) years at cohort entry. Patients with damage at enrolment were more likely to have further worsening of SDI (SDI 0 vs $\geq$1; $p < 0.001$). Age, USA African race/ethnicity, SLEDAI-2K score, steroid use and hypertension were associated with transition from no damage to damage, and increase(s) in pre-existing damage. Male gender (relative transition rates (95% CI) 1.48 (1.06 to 2.08)) and USA Caucasian race/ethnicity (1.63 (1.08 to 2.47)) were associated with SDI 0 to $\geq$1 transitions; Asian race/ethnicity patients had lower rates of new damage (0.60 (0.39 to 0.93)). Antimalarial use was associated with lower rates of increases in pre-existing damage (0.63 (0.44 to 0.89)). Damage was associated with future mortality (HR (95% CI) 1.46 (1.18 to 1.81) per SDI point).

*Conclusions.*—Damage in SLE predicts future damage accrual and mortality. We identified several potentially modifiable risk factors for damage accrual; an integrated strategy to address these may improve long-term outcomes.

▶ The care of patients with systemic lupus erythematosus (SLE) is complex. This paper highlights several concepts that are applicable to the primary care physician. When caring for patients with SLE, it is important to monitor their current disease activity, quality of life, and damage accrual over time. These 3 aspects can be applied to other diseases as well, such as diabetes.

A useful scoring system was developed to monitor the degree of end-organ damage that accrues in patients with SLE, known as the Systemic Lupus Erythematous Disease Index (SDI).[1] The American College of Rheumatology SDI provides a convenient way for physicians to quantitatively measure damage accrual in patients with SLE over time. The SDI represents irreversible damage that has occurred after the diagnosis of SLE, although it also includes damage from other diseases that patients may have (which may or may not be related to the patient's SLE, ie, diabetes, cerebrovascular accidents, cataracts). Higher SDI scores have been associated with older age, chronic disease activity, major lupus flares, steroid exposure, and Hispanic and African ancestry/race.[2-6]

This is a large study from Systemic Lupus International Collaborating Clinics (SLICC) that examines the SDI over time in patients with SLE. The SLICC cohort comprised 31 centers from 11 countries in North America, Latin America, Europe, and Asia. This study showed a steady increase in organ damage over time in SLE patients, with preexisting damage being an important predictor of future damage accrual. It highlighted the importance of controlling hypertension and encouraging the use of antimalarial medication in patients with SLE. The strengths of this study included the large number of SLE patients studied, and the diverse geographic and multiethnic/multiracial cohort.

**A. Sammut, MD**

*References*

1. Gladman D, Ginzler E, Goldsmith C, et al. The development and initial validation of the systemic Lupus International Collaborating Clinics/American College of Rheumatology damage index for systemic lupus erythematosus. *Arthritis Rheum.* 1996;39:363-369.
2. Maddison P, Farewell V, Isenberg D, et al. The rate and pattern of organ damage in late onset systemic lupus erythematosus. *J Rheumatol.* 2002;29:913-917.
3. Becker-Merok A, Nossent HC. Damage accumulation in systemic lupus erythematosus and its relation to disease activity and mortality. *J Rheumatol.* 2006;33:1570-1577.
4. Nossent JC. SLICC/ACR Damage Index in Afro-Caribbean patients with systemic lupus erythematosus: changes in and relationship to disease activity, corticosteroid therapy, and prognosis. *J Rheumatol.* 1998;25:654-659.
5. Stoll T, Seifert B, Isenberg DA. SLICC/ACR Damage Index is valid, and renal and pulmonary organ scores are predictors of severe outcome in patients with systemic lupus erythematosus. *Br J Rheumatol.* 1996;35:248-254.
6. Stoll T, Sutcliffe N, Mach J, Klaghofer R, Isenberg DA. Analysis of the relationship between disease activity and damage in patients with systemic lupus erythematosus—a 5-yr prospective study. *Rheumatology.* 2004;43:1039-1044.

**Racial and Ethnic Differences in Mortality and Cardiovascular Events Among Patients with End-Stage Renal Disease Due to Lupus Nephritis**

Gómez-Puerta JA, Feldman CH, Alarcón GS, et al (Harvard Med School, Boston, MA; Univ of Alabama at Birmingham; et al)

*Arthritis Care Res (Hoboken)* 67:1453-1462, 2015

*Objective.*—To identify racial and ethnic differences in mortality and cardiovascular (CV) risk among patients with end-stage renal disease (ESRD) due to lupus nephritis (LN).

*Methods.*—Within the US ESRD registry (1995–2008), we identified individuals ages >17 years with incident ESRD due to systemic lupus erythematosus. We ascertained demographics, clinical factors, and deaths from registry patient files and CV events (myocardial infarction, heart failure, and hemorrhagic and ischemic strokes) from inpatient Medicare claims. We calculated incidence rates (95% confidence intervals [95% CIs]) per 1,000 person-years for study events, stratified by race and ethnicity. We compared probabilities of the events among racial and ethnic groups using cumulative incidence function curves and multivariable-adjusted subdistribution proportional hazard ratios (HRsd), taking into account the competing events of kidney transplantation and death (for nonfatal CV events).

*Results.*—Of 12,533 patients with LN-associated ESRD, the mean ± SD age was 40.7 ± 14.9 years, 82% were women, and 49% were African American. The overall mortality rate was 98.1/1,000 person-years (95% CI 95.3–100.9). In multivariable models, Asian and Hispanic LN-associated ESRD patients had lower mortality than whites (HRsd 0.70 [95% CI 0.58–0.84] and 0.79 [95% CI 0.71–0.88], respectively), whereas African Americans had higher mortality (HRsd 1.27 [95% CI 1.18–1.36]). African American patients >40 years old had higher mortality than their white counterparts (HRsd 1.67 [95% CI 1.44–1.93]). African Americans were more likely to be admitted for heart failure or hemorrhagic stroke.

*Conclusion.*—Among patients with LN-associated ESRD, Asians and Hispanics experienced lower mortality and CV event risks than whites, and African Americans had higher mortality and CV event risks than whites.

► Cardiovascular disease (CVD) is the leading cause of death among patients with long-standing systemic lupus erythematosus (SLE). Over the past several years, studies have examined racial disparities in CVD in the SLE population. CVD events and CVD-related hospitalizations resulting in death occur at a younger age in all patients with SLE, but more so among black individuals compared with white individuals with SLE. For instance, in a study by Scalzi et al, among 218 women with SLE who died of CVD-related causes during hospitalization, black women were on average 14.3 years younger than white women. Black women in these studies tended to have a higher body mass index, higher blood pressure, and higher levels of C-reactive protein, fibrinogen, and lipoprotein A, as well as a longer history of corticosteroid use, and were more likely to be admitted to the hospital. They were also more likely to have a longer hospital stay.

Lupus nephritis (LN) occurs in 50% to 60% of all patients with SLE. Of those patients with LN, about 30% develop end-stage renal disease (ESRD) within 10 years, despite aggressive therapy.[1-4] As a rheumatologist in Harlem, New York, I care for patients who have ESRD due to LN who are on hemodialysis. I chose this article because ESRD due to LN is an understudied topic. Although this article does a good job providing information on mortality rates and cardiovascular events in patients with ESRD due to LN, there were a few issues with the methodology in this study that are worth noting.

This was a large group of individuals older than 17 years with ESRD due to LN, identified through the US Renal Data System (USRDS), a national registry of patients with ESRD. Data regarding CV events were available for those patients with Medicare coverage, and data regarding death were available for patients regardless of insurance coverage. Patients were categorized as white, African American, Asian American, or Native American, and then a separate category for whether or not they were Hispanic. The patients I care for include patients who are West African, Caribbean, African American, among others, and many patients would not fit into only 1 of those categories. Furthermore, patients who are undocumented in this country were not included in any of these data. This study added to the mounting evidence that African Americans with SLE have higher mortality rates and more cardiovascular events than whites. The new information gleaned from this study is that Asians and Hispanics were found to have better 1, 5, and 10-year survival rates than whites.

The actual rates and numbers do not matter as much as the underlying concept, namely, that there are differences in mortality rates depending on race and ethnicity among patients with ESRD due to LN. Future studies should include more specific information on race and ethnicity; subtypes of Hispanic; include more categories such as Caribbean, West African, and East African; account for patients who have immigrated to the United States; and include information on undocumented individuals.

**A. Sammut, MD**

*References*

1. Huong DL, Papo T, Beaufils H, et al. Renal involvement in systemic lupus erythematosus: a study of 180 patients from a single center. *Medicine (Baltimore)*. 1999;78:148-166.
2. Cervera R, Khamashta MA, Font J, et al. Morbidity and mortality in systemic lupus erythematosus during a 10-year period: a comparison of early and late manifestations in a cohort of 1,000 patients. *Medicine (Baltimore)*. 2003;82:299-308.
3. Adler M, Chambers S, Edwards C, Neild G, Isenberg D. An assessment of renal failure in an SLE cohort with special reference to ethnicity, over a 25-year period. *Rheumatology (Oxford)*. 2006;45:1144-1147.
4. Costenbader KH, Desai A, Alarcon GS, et al. Trends in the incidence, demographics, and outcomes of end-stage renal disease due to lupus nephritis in the US from 1995 to 2006. *Arthritis Rheum*. 2011;63:1681-1688.

**Exposure to Air Pollutants and Disease Activity in Juvenile-Onset Systemic Lupus Erythematosus Patients**

Fernandes EC, Silva CA, Braga AL, et al (Faculdade de Medicina da Universidade de São Paulo, Brazil)

*Arthritis Care Res (Hoboken)* 67:1609-1614, 2015

*Objective.*—To investigate the association between exposure to air pollutants in the Sao Paulo metropolitan area and disease activity in juvenile-onset systemic lupus erythematosus (SLE) patients.

*Methods.*—A longitudinal panel study based on 409 consecutive visits of juvenile-onset SLE patients living in the Sao Paulo metropolitan area was carried out. Disease activity was evaluated in accordance with the Systemic Lupus Erythematosus Disease Activity Index 2000 (SLEDAI-2K), and the patients were divided into 2 groups: those with SLEDAI scores ≤8 and those with SLEDAI scores >8. Daily concentrations of inhaled particulate matter ($PM_{10}$), sulfur dioxide, nitrogen dioxide ($NO_2$), ozone, and carbon monoxide (CO) were evaluated on the 21 days preceding the medical visits. A generalized estimation equation model was used to assess the impact of these measurements on SLEDAI-2K scores, considering the fixed effects for repetitive measurements. The models were adjusted for erythrocyte sedimentation rate, corticosteroid use (daily and cumulative doses), antimalarial use, the use of immunosuppressive agents, the presence of infection 20 days preceding the medical appointment, and the minimum temperature and relative humidity outdoors.

*Results.*—$PM_{10}$, $NO_2$, and CO were risk factors for juvenile-onset SLE disease activity (SLEDAI-2K score >8) approximately 2 weeks after exposure. A 13.4 $\mu g/m^3$ increase in the $PM_{10}$ moving average (from lag 12 to lag 15) was associated with a 34% increase (95% confidence interval 7.0–68.0) in the risk of a SLEDAI-2K score >8.

*Conclusion.*—This is the first study to show that exposure to inhaled pollutants may increase the risk of disease activity in children with juvenile-onset SLE in a large urban center.

► A major public health hazard in large cities is air pollution. Air pollution is composed of a mixture of particles and gases including ozone, sulfur dioxide, nitrates, lead, products of tobacco smoke, carbon monoxide, volatile organic compounds, and particulate matter. Even when traffic-generated pollutants are within legally established limits, this pollution can be harmful to children with autoimmune disease and to children and adults with respiratory conditions, such as asthma. A recent study revealed that exposure to air pollution has been associated with an increased incidence of chronic inflammatory diseases, including autoimmune diseases.[1]

This is an exciting study from Sao Paulo, a metropolitan area in Brazil. It showed that exposure to particulate matter may trigger systemic inflammation, leading to an increased risk of disease activity in children with juvenile-onset systemic lupus erythematosus (SLE). In patients with any autoimmune illness, the goal is to minimize disease activity and to keep the patient in remission or as close to remission as possible. Any factors that may increase disease activity are important to identify, especially if they are potentially modifiable, as is air pollution from particulate matter that arises from vehicle exhaust. There is a paucity of literature on air pollution's association with autoimmune illness, and I applaud the authors for taking on this important topic. This is an area of study that desperately needs to be explored further and is a major public health issue that demands broader recognition.

**A. Sammut, MD**

*Reference*

1. Farhat SC, Silva CA, Orione MA, et al. Air pollution in autoimmune rheumatic disease: a review. *Autoimmune Rev.* 2011;11:14-21.

---

## Vitamin D Supplementation in Adolescents and Young Adults With Juvenile Systemic Lupus Erythematosus for Improvement in Disease Activity and Fatigue Scores: A Randomized, Double-Blind, Placebo-Controlled Trial

Lima GL, Paupitz J, Aikawa NE, et al (Faculdade de Medicina da Universidade de São Paulo, Brazil)

*Arthritis Care Res (Hoboken)* 68:91-98, 2016

---

*Objective.*—Vitamin D has an important immunomodulatory effect, but there are no trials that directly address the boosting of serum levels of 25-hydroxyvitamin D (25[OH]D) in juvenile-onset systemic lupus erythematosus (SLE). The aim of this study was to evaluate the effect of vitamin D supplementation on disease activity and fatigue in juvenile-onset SLE.

*Methods.*—This study was a randomized, double-blind, placebo-controlled, 24-week trial. Forty juvenile-onset SLE patients were randomized (1:1) to receive oral cholecalciferol 50,000 IU/week (juvenile-onset SLE-VitD) or placebo (juvenile-onset SLE-PL). Medications remained stable throughout the study. Serum levels of 25(OH)D were measured using radioimmunoassay. Disease activity was assessed using the Systemic Lupus Erythematosus Disease Activity Index (SLEDAI) and the European Consensus Lupus Activity Measurement (ECLAM). Fatigue was assessed using the Kids Fatigue Severity Scale (K-FSS).

*Results.*—At baseline, groups were similar regarding age, body mass index, organ involvement, glucocorticoid dose, use of immunosuppressive drugs, SLEDAI, ECLAM, K-FSS, and levels of 25(OH)D. After 24 weeks, the mean level of 25(OH)D was higher in the juvenile-onset SLE-VitD group than in the juvenile-onset SLE-PL group ($P < 0.001$). At the end of the intervention, a significant improvement in SLEDAI ($P = 0.010$) and in ECLAM ($P = 0.006$) was observed in the juvenile-onset SLE-VitD group compared to the juvenile-onset SLE-PL group. Regarding fatigue evaluation, a reduction of fatigue related to social life score was found in the juvenile-onset SLE-VitD group compared to the juvenile-onset

SLE-PL group ($P = 0.008$). Cholecalciferol was well tolerated with no serious adverse events.

*Conclusion.*—This study suggests that cholecalciferol supplementation for 24 weeks is effective in decreasing disease activity and improving fatigue in juvenile-onset SLE patients.

▶ A major goal in the management of a patient with systemic lupus erythematosus (SLE) is to reduce and control disease activity. Fatigue is a common symptom in patients with SLE and can occur in patients with otherwise controlled disease activity. In fact, patients commonly report fatigue as one of the worst symptoms of SLE. It has been reported in up to 81% of patients with SLE[1,2] and can be challenging to treat. Vitamin D deficiency in SLE patients has been associated with increased SLE disease activity and an increased risk of SLE flares.[3,4]

This study is the first randomized, double-blinded, placebo-controlled trial to evaluate the effect of cholecalciferol supplementation on disease activity scores and fatigue in juvenile-onset SLE patients. The methodology of this study was strong. All patients and physicians were blinded to whether the patient received placebo or vitamin D supplementation. All patients who were included went through a vitamin D washout 3 months before randomization, and there were assessments to ensure patient compliance.

There were 2 major findings in this study. The first was consistent with previous studies in adult SLE patients—namely, a significant reduction in anti-dsDNA frequency was observed in the juvenile-onset SLE patients who received vitamin D supplementation. The disease activity scores were also significantly improved in the group of patients who received 6 months of vitamin D supplementation. The other major finding in this study was unique and also clinically useful; it showed a reduction in fatigue in the group of patients who received vitamin D supplementation. Improving the quality of life for our patients with SLE includes reducing not only disease activity but also reducing pervasive symptoms, such as fatigue. This study provides strong evidence that vitamin D supplementation can help relieve fatigue in patients with SLE, which is great news for these patients.

**A. Sammut, MD**

*References*

1. Wysenbeek AJ, Leibovici L, Weinberger A, Guedj D. Fatigue in systemic lupus erythematosus: prevalence and relation to disease expression. *Br J Rheumatol.* 1993;32:633-635.
2. Tench CM, McCurdie I, White PD, D'Cruz DP. The prevalence and associations of fatigue in systemic lupus erythematosus. *Rheumatology (Oxford).* 2000;39: 1249-1254.
3. Bonakdar ZS, Jahanshahifar L, Jahanshahifar F, Gholamrezaei A. Vitamin D deficiency and its association with disease activity in new cases of systemic lupus erythematosus. *Lupus.* 2011;20:1155-1160.
4. Cutolo M, Otsa K, Paolino S, Yprus M, Veldi T, Seriolo B. Vitamin D involvement in rheumatoid arthritis and systemic lupus erythematosus. *Ann Rheum Dis.* 2009; 68:446-447 [letter].

**Placebo-controlled randomized clinical trial of fish oil's impact on fatigue, quality of life, and disease activity in Systemic Lupus Erythematosus**

Arriens C, Hynan LS, Lerman RH, et al (Univ of Texas Southwestern Med Ctr, Dallas; et al)

*Nutr J* 14:82, 2015

*Introduction.*—A recent metabolomic screen of sera from patients with Systemic Lupus Erythematosus (SLE) found reduction of antioxidants and substrates for energy generation. These metabolic alterations may underlie one of the most common features of SLE - fatigue. The metabolomic studies also noted reduced omega-3 fatty acids, which are powerful anti- oxidants. This deficiency may be causally related to oxidative stress, inflammation, disease activity, and fatigue in SLE. Supplementation of omega-3 fatty acids using fish oil in SLE has been shown to reduce oxidative stress in other studies. The objective of this study is to evaluate the effect of fish oil supplementation on clinical measures of fatigue, quality of life, and disease activity as part of a randomized clinical trial.

*Methods.*—Fifty SLE patients recruited in outpatient clinics were randomized 1:1 to fish oil supplementation or olive oil placebo, and blinded to their treatment group. At baseline and after 6 months of treatment, RAND Short Form-36 (RAND SF-36), Fatigue Severity Scale (FSS), SLE Disease Activity Index (SLEDAI), and Physician Global Assessment (PGA) were completed; serum was also collected for soluble mediator analysis.

*Results.*—Thirty-two patients completed the study. PGA improved significantly in the fish oil group compared with the placebo group ($p = 0.015$). The RAND SF-36 Energy/fatigue and Emotional well-being scores demonstrated improvement trends ($p = 0.092$ and 0.070). No clear difference was seen in FSS and SLEDAI ($p = 0.350$ and $p = 0.417$). Erythrocyte sedimentation rate and serum IL-12 were reduced ($p = 0.008$ and $p = 0.058$); while serum IL-13 was increased by fish oil supplementation ($p = 0.033$).

*Conclusions.*—In this randomized, placebo-controlled 6-month trial, SLE patients randomized to fish oil supplementation demonstrated improvement in their PGA, RAND SF-36, and some circulating inflammatory markers.

*Trial Registration.*—ClinicalTrials.gov Identifier: NCT02021513 (registered 13 December 2013).

▶ Fatigue is a common and often overlooked symptom in patients with systemic lupus erythematosus (SLE). It occurs in up to 81% to 86% of patients with SLE, even in patients whose SLE is well controlled. There have been several studies of fish oil supplementation in SLE, both in murine models of SLE and in humans. Most of these studies have conflicting results; some have shown improved disease activity,[1,2] and others have not.[3] Patients with SLE have been found to have lower levels of omega-3 fatty acids compared with healthy controls.[4] In studies of depressed elderly patients without autoimmune disease, supplementation of omega-3 fatty acids has been associated with improvement in quality of life and depressive symptoms. Given these studies and other anecdotal evidence, several rheumatologists recommend omega-3 fatty acids to patients with SLE to help with fatigue.

This study was a small randomized clinical trial of omega-3 supplementation versus placebo (the placebo being olive oil in this study), performed over 6 months. It investigated resultant changes in fatigue, emotional and physical functioning, pain, emotional well-being, disease activity of SLE, and inflammatory markers. The design of the study was well thought out, but there were too few patients to draw firm conclusions. There were only 25 patients in each group (omega-3 supplementation and placebo), and of those, only 14 patients in the placebo group and 18 patients in the fish oil group completed the study. There were some positive changes in the fish oil group, including improvement in the physician global assessment, the ESR, and the RAND Short Form-36 (used as a fatigue scale). Although these results were encouraging, there were only 2 time points investigated, and this was over 6 months. Although this was a small study, the results suggested the need for further study of omega-3 supplementation in the SLE population. If fish oil supplementation does indeed help with fatigue in SLE, it would be a great option that is widely available, and with minimal risk.

**A. Sammut, MD**

*References*

1. Wright SA, O'Prey FM, McHenry MT, et al. A randomised interventional trial of omega-3-polyunsaturated fatty acids on endothelial function and disease activity in systemic lupus erythematosus. *Ann Rheum Dis.* 2008;67:841-848.
2. Duffy EM, Meenagh GK, McMillan SA, Strain JJ, Hannigan BM, Bell AL. The clinical effect of dietary supplementation with omega-3 fish oils and/or copper in systemic lupus erythematosus. *J Rheumatol.* 2004;31:1551-1556.
3. Clark WF, Parbtani A, Naylor CD, et al. Fish oil in lupus nephritis: clinical findings and methodological implications. *Kidney Int.* 1993;44:75-86.
4. Wu T, Xie C, Han J, et al. Metabolic disturbances associated with systemic lupus erythematosus. *PLoS One.* 2012;7:e37210.

# 2 Rheumatoid Arthritis

## 2015 American College of Rheumatology Guideline for the Treatment of Rheumatoid Arthritis

Singh JA, Saag KG, Bridges SL Jr, et al (Univ of Alabama at Birmingham; et al)
*Arthritis Care Res* 68:1-25, 2016

*Objective.*—To develop a new evidence-based, pharmacologic treatment guideline for rheumatoid arthritis (RA).

*Methods.*—We conducted systematic reviews to synthesize the evidence for the benefits and harms of various treatment options. We used the Grading of Recommendations Assessment, Development and Evaluation (GRADE) methodology to rate the quality of evidence. We employed a group consensus process to grade the strength of recommendations (either strong or conditional). A strong recommendation indicates that clinicians are certain that the benefits of an intervention far outweigh the harms (or vice versa). A conditional recommendation denotes uncertainty over the balance of benefits and harms and/or more significant variability in patient values and preferences.

*Results.*—The guideline covers the use of traditional disease-modifying antirheumatic drugs (DMARDs), biologic agents, tofacitinib, and glucocorticoids in early (<6 months) and established (≥6 months) RA. In addition, it provides recommendations on using a treat-to-target approach, tapering and discontinuing medications, and the use of biologic agents and DMARDs in patients with hepatitis, congestive heart failure, malignancy, and serious infections. The guideline addresses the use of vaccines in patients starting/receiving DMARDs or biologic agents, screening for tuberculosis in patients starting/receiving biologic agents or tofacitinib, and laboratory monitoring for traditional DMARDs. The guideline includes 74 recommendations: 23% are strong and 77% are conditional.

*Conclusion.*—This RA guideline should serve as a tool for clinicians and patients (our two target audiences) for pharmacologic treatment decisions in commonly encountered clinical situations. These recommendations are not prescriptive, and the treatment decisions should be made by physicians and patients through a shared decision-making process taking into account patients' values, preferences, and comorbidities. These recommendations should not be used to limit or deny access to therapies.

▶ The American College of Rheumatology (ACR) has recently published updated guidelines on the treatment of rheumatoid arthritis (RA). These guidelines are integral not only for all rheumatologists but for any physician caring for patients with RA, given that they provide structured algorithms and address several specific patient scenarios. They also build on the 2008 and 2012 published guidelines for RA management.

The "treat to target" approach continues to be the focus of therapy across all forms of RA, early and established. The principles of treat to target include creating an agreed-on treatment plan between the patient and the physician, setting goals to maximize long-term health-related quality of life and monitoring disease activity with adjustment of treatments if indicated.[1] In terms of medication therapy, it is strongly recommended to start disease-modifying antirheumatic drug (DMARD) monotherapy in any DMARD-naive patient with low disease activity with the preferred agent still being methotrexate. What is different in the 2015 guideline is the additional option for the treating physician to incorporate the non–tumor necrosis factor (TNF) biologics earlier in the treatment algorithm of active rheumatoid arthritis. The expert panel of physicians specifically points out that there is no recommendation on ranking of the various treatment options given that there is limited comparative evidence between the potential therapies. Potential treatment options in patients with active RA despite DMARD monotherapy includes combination DMARD therapy or TNF inhibitor biologic or non-TNF inhibitor biologic therapy (all choices with or without methotrexate, in no particular order of preference).

Something that is slowly making its way into the recommendations is the new concept of tapering therapy once disease control is achieved. There is a fair amount of evidence for continuation of DMARD and biologic therapy rather than discontinuation despite low disease activity based on clinical observations and physician experience. If the patient's disease is in remission, the recommendation of the expert panel is also not to discontinue all RA therapies despite very low quality evidence to support this. I predict that this will continue to be a topic of high interest in the future as more therapies become available and more patients are achieving low disease activity and eventual remission.

Additional highlights of this article include recommendations on immunosuppressive therapy in patients with hepatitis B, hepatitis C, congestive heart failure, prior malignancy, and serious infections. In terms of immunizations, the take-home message is that whenever possible, vaccines should be given before receiving immunosuppressive therapy. One new addition to the vaccination recommendations was that physicians should be aware that responses to certain killed vaccines may be reduced after rituximab therapy and possibly after therapy with methotrexate.

Overall, the 2015 ACR guideline for management of rheumatoid arthritis is an essential read, and I recommend the article highly. Important issues that are still yet to be addressed include the role of biosimilars and recommendations for therapy during the period of conception, pregnancy, and lactation, as well as biomarker testing in RA.

**B. Fradlis, MD**

*Reference*

1. Smolen JS, Aletaha D, Bijlsma JWJ, et al. Treating rheumatoid arthritis to target: recommendations of an international task force. *Ann Rheum Dis*. 2010;69:631-637.

**Rheumatoid Arthritis and Mortality Among Women During 36 Years of Prospective Follow Up: Results From the Nurses' Health Study**

Sparks JA, Chang S-C, Liao KP, et al (Brigham and Women's Hosp and Harvard Med School, Boston, MA)

*Arthritis Care Res* 68:753-762, 2016

*Objective.*—To evaluate rheumatoid arthritis (RA) and mortality risk among women followed prospectively in the Nurses' Health Study (NHS).

*Methods.*—We analyzed 119,209 women in the NHS who reported no connective tissue disease at enrollment in 1976. Comorbidity and lifestyle data were collected through biennial questionnaires. Incident RA cases were validated by medical records review. Cause of death was determined by death certificate and medical records review. Cox regression models estimated hazard ratios (HRs) and 95% confidence intervals (95% CIs) for all-cause, cardiovascular disease (CVD), cancer, and respiratory disease mortality for women with RA compared to those without RA.

*Results.*—We validated 964 incident RA cases and identified 28,808 deaths during 36 years of prospective follow-up. Of 307 deaths among women with RA, 80 (26%) were from cancer, 70 (23%) were from CVD, and 44 (14%) were from respiratory causes. Women with RA had increased total mortality (HR 1.40, 95% CI 1.25−1.57) compared to those without RA, independent of mortality risk factors, including smoking. RA was associated with significantly increased respiratory disease mortality (HR 2.06, 95% CI 1.51−2.80) and cardiovascular disease mortality (HR 1.45, 95% CI 1.14−1.83), but not cancer mortality (HR 0.93, 95% CI 0.74−1.15). For women with seropositive RA, respiratory disease mortality was nearly 3-fold higher than among non-RA women (HR 2.67, 95% CI 1.89−3.77).

*Conclusion.*—Women with RA had significantly increased mortality compared to those without RA. Respiratory disease and cardiovascular disease mortality were both significantly elevated for women with RA. The nearly 3-fold increased relative risk of respiratory disease mortality was observed only for those with seropositive RA.

▶ Rheumatoid arthritis (RA) is a systemic, chronic autoimmune inflammatory disease that affects approximately 1% of the population. It has been associated with an increased mortality compared with the general population,[1,2] and it is well known that patients with RA have an increased risk of cardiovascular disease. Several studies have hypothesized that accelerated cardiovascular disease in patients with RA may be a result of chronic inflammation causing accelerated atherosclerosis.[3-5]

This is a large study from the Nurses' Health Study that investigated RA and mortality in 119 209 women aged 30 to 55 years without RA at baseline, who were followed from 1976 until 2012. The authors evaluated 964 women in the Nurses' Health Study who developed RA and compared their mortality rates to women in the study who did not develop RA. The team controlled for other risk factors, including smoking (a known cause of worse respiratory and cardiovascular mortality) as well as age, body mass index, physical activity, and diet.

The study provides a long duration of prospective follow-up of women with and without RA and a detailed assessment of cause-specific mortality. On the basis of this study, women diagnosed with RA during the 36 years of prospective follow-up had a 40% increase in total mortality risk compared with women without RA. Notably, this increased mortality risk was only seen in patients with seropositive RA. Similar to the results of previous studies, there was an increased risk of cardiovascular disease—related mortality (hazard ratio [HR] 1.4) in patients with seropositive RA. A key finding in this study was that the patients with seropositive RA also had an increased risk of respiratory disease—related mortality (HR 2.06), even when controlled for risk factors such as smoking.

The generalizability of these results may be somewhat limited because of the population studied; the Nurses' Health Study consists mainly of white women who are well educated and were high-level nurses at study inception. Although the generalizability maybe limited, this study nonetheless sheds light on the importance of assessing pulmonary status in patients with RA. Clinicians should be aware that patients with RA are at increased risk of not only cardiovascular disease—related mortality but also respiratory disease—related mortality.

**A. Sammut, MD**

*References*


1. Solomon DH, Karlson EW, Rimm EB, et al. Cardiovascular morbidity and mortality in women diagnosed with rheumatoid arthritis. *Circulation.* 2003;107: 1303-1307.
2. Gonzalez A, Maradit Kremers H, Crowson CS, et al. The widening mortality gap between rheumatoid arthritis patients and the general population. *Arthritis Rheum.* 2007;56:3583-3587.
3. Bergstrom U, Jacobsson LT, Turesson C. Cardiovascular morbidity and mortality remain similar in two cohorts of patients with long-standing rheumatoid arthritis seen in 1978 and 1995 in Malmo, Sweden. *Rheumatology (Oxford).* 2009;48: 1600-1605.
4. Young A, Koduri G, Batley M, et al. Mortality in rheumatoid arthritis: increased in the early course of disease, in ischaemic heart disease and in pulmonary fibrosis. *Rheumatology (Oxford).* 2007;46:350-357.
5. Gonzalez A, Icen M, Kremers HM, et al. Mortality trends in rheumatoid arthritis: the role of rheumatoid factor. *J Rheumatol.* 2008;35:1009-1014.


## Impact of Bariatric Surgery on Patients With Rheumatoid Arthritis

Sparks JA, Halperin F, Karlson JC, et al (Brigham and Women's Hosp and Harvard Med School, Boston, MA)
*Arthritis Care Res* 67:1619-1626, 2015

*Objective.*—To investigate the effect of weight loss after bariatric surgery among patients with rheumatoid arthritis (RA).

*Methods.*—We conducted a retrospective cohort study of RA patients who underwent bariatric surgery (Roux-en-Y gastric bypass, laparoscopic adjustable gastric banding, or sleeve gastrectomy) at 2 medical centers. We obtained information on anthropometrics, laboratory values, RA disease activity, and medication use at baseline (prior to surgery), at 6 and 12 months following surgery, and at the most recent followup visits. RA disease activity was determined by clinical or validated measures. At each postsurgical visit, characteristics were compared to baseline.

*Results.*—We identified 53 RA patients who underwent bariatric surgery. At baseline prior to surgery, mean ± SD body mass index was 47.8 ± 7.7 $kg/m^2$, mean ± SD weight was 128.2 ± 24.1 kg, and 57% had moderate to high RA disease activity. Twelve months following surgery, subjects lost a mean ± SD weight of 41.0 ± 17.3 kg, mean ± SD 70% ± 24% excess weight ($P < 0.001$). RA disease activity significantly improved at postsurgical visits ($P < 0.001$). At 12 months following surgery, 6% had moderate to high disease activity, compared to 57% at baseline ($P < 0.001$). At the most recent followup (mean ± SD 5.8 ± 3.2 years after surgery), 74% were in remission, compared to 26% at baseline ($P < 0.001$). Subjects had significantly lower erythrocyte sedimentation rate, C-reactive protein level, and RA-related medication use at followup visits compared to baseline ($P < 0.05$).

*Conclusion.*—After substantial weight loss from bariatric surgery, RA patients had lower disease activity, decreased serum inflammatory markers, and less RA-related medication use. Weight loss may be an important nonpharmacologic strategy to reduce RA disease activity. However, other factors, such as improved efficacy of medications, improved physical activity, and metabolic changes, may also have contributed to these postsurgical improvements.

► The observation that obesity has been associated with an increased state of systemic inflammation has been a topic of great interest in the rheumatology community. There have been suggestions that obesity is associated with a higher risk of developing rheumatoid arthritis (RA) and that pro-inflammatory cytokines that are produced by adipocytes contribute to persistent inflammation, worse RA outcomes, and less response to disease-modifying antirheumatic drug (DMARD) therapy. This article was novel in its aim to determine the effect of dramatic weight loss after bariatric surgery on RA disease activity, serum markers of inflammation, as well as DMARD and glucocorticoid use. Twelve months after bariatric surgery, patients with RA lost on average 41 kg (70% mean excess weight) and demonstrated a dramatic improvement in disease activity with many more patients being in remission at the end of the study than before surgery. In addition, significant decreases in C-reactive protein and erythrocyte sedimentation rate were noted that were beyond what was expected from weight loss alone. Fewer patients were on DMARD therapy and cumulative glucocorticoid and nonsteroidal antiinflammatory drug use was also lower. These findings are encouraging and put forth the importance of nonpharmacologic treatments such as dietary changes, physical activity, and weight loss in the management of RA. Also, this study makes the physician more aware of the benefits of weight loss surgery for the patient not just in terms of improved mobility with less excess weight on board but also in terms of decrease in the overall inflammatory burden.

**B. Fradlis, MD**

**Cervical spine involvement in rheumatoid arthritis over time: results from a meta-analysis**

Zhang T, Pope J (Western Univ of Canada, London, Ontario)

*Arthritis Res Ther* 17:148, 2015

*Introduction.*—Complications in rheumatoid arthritis (RA) seem less common than they were years ago. The prevalence and progression of anterior atlantoaxial subluxations (aAASs), vertical subluxations (VSs), subaxial subluxations (SASs), and associated cervical myelopathy in RA over the past 50 years were determined.

*Methods.*—A literature search was performed by using Medline-OVID/EMBASE, PubMed, and Scopus (from 1960 to June 21, 2014). Prevalence studies were included if the sample size was at least 100 or the prevalence/progression of cervical subluxations was reported. Study quality was assessed by using the Strengthening the Reporting of Observational Studies in Epidemiology (STROBE) checklist. Prevalence of cervical subluxations was calculated for each study. Student's *t* test and meta-regression were used to evaluate for significance.

*Results.*—In total, 12,249 citations were identified and 59 studies were included. The prevalence of aAAS decreased from 36% (95% confidence interval (CI) 30% to 42%) before the 1980s to 24% (95% CI 13% to 36%) in the 2000s ($P = 0.04$). The overall prevalence rates were 11% (95% CI 10% to 19%) for VS, 13% (95% CI 12% to 20%) for SAS, and 5% (95% CI 3% to 9%) for cervical myelopathy, and there were no significant temporal changes. Rates of progression of aAAS, VS, and SAS were 4, 6, and 3 lesions per 100 patients per year, respectively. The incidence of new or progressive cervical myelopathy was 2 cases per 100 patients with known cervical subluxations per year.

*Conclusions.*—Since the 1960s, only aAAS has decreased dramatically. It is still more than twice as common as VS or SAS. No temporal changes in the development of cervical myelopathy in affected patients with RA were noted. The progression rates of cervical subluxations and myelopathy were unchanged over time.

▶ With advances in therapy of rheumatoid arthritis (RA), complications such as corneal melts and vasculitis are being seen less frequently now than our predecessors did 50 years ago. Cervical spine involvement in rheumatoid arthritis takes on many forms. This meta-analysis aims to quantify the changes in prevalence and progression of various cervical complications of rheumatoid arthritis, specifically atlantoaxial subluxation (AAS) and cervical myelopathy. Given the high mortality of myelopathy (as high as 50% 1-year mortality if untreated), it is important to be aware of these complications. The most common subtype of AAS is the anterior AAS with the other common subtypes being ventral subluxation and subaxial subluxation. After analysis of multiple studies, the authors came to a conclusion that there has been a significant reduction in the prevalence of anterior AAS; however, that there is no significant decline in the prevalence of the other subtypes of subluxation. What I found to be extremely important in this article was that many of the patients with radiographic abnormalities consistent with subluxation were clinically asymptomatic. Others complained of neck pain, but few actually had documented neurologic deficits. In terms of cervical myelopathy, the authors noted that there was no change in prevalence of neurologic findings; however, these are rare to begin with and continued to have low overall prevalence rate (5%). Currently, cervical spine imaging is recommended for all patients with RA scheduled to undergo surgery requiring manipulation of the neck for either anesthesia or surgery, but there is no specific guideline within the rheumatologic community regarding baseline cervical spine imaging studies. I agree with the authors that disease-modifying antirheumatic drug (DMARD) therapy plays an important role in disease control and contributes to change in the overall epidemiology of RA. The long-term impact on cervical spine involvement in patients with RA on DMARD therapy should be addressed in future longitudinal studies.

**B. Fradlis, MD**

# 3 Seronegative Spondyloarthropathies

**American College of Rheumatology/Spondylitis Association of America/Spondyloarthritis Research and Treatment Network 2015 Recommendations for the Treatment of Ankylosing Spondylitis and Nonradiographic Axial Spondyloarthritis**

Ward MM, Deodhar A, Akl EA, et al (Natl Inst of Arthritis and Musculoskeletal and Skin Diseases, Bethesda, MD; Oregon Health & Science Univ, Portland; American Univ of Beirut, Lebanon; et al)

*Arthritis Rheumatol* 68:282-298, 2016

*Objective.*—To provide evidence-based recommendations for the treatment of patients with ankylosing spondylitis (AS) and nonradiographic axial spondyloarthritis (SpA).

*Methods.*—A core group led the development of the recommendations, starting with the treatment questions. A literature review group conducted systematic literature reviews of studies that addressed 57 specific treatment questions, based on searches conducted in OVID Medline (1946–2014), PubMed (1966–2014), and the Cochrane Library. We assessed the quality of evidence using the Grading of Recommendations, Assessment, Development and Evaluation (GRADE) method. A separate voting group reviewed the evidence and voted on recommendations for each question using the GRADE framework.

*Results.*—In patients with active AS, the strong recommendations included use of nonsteroidal antiinflammatory drugs (NSAIDs), use of tumor necrosis factor inhibitors (TNFi) when activity persists despite NSAID treatment, not to use systemic glucocorticoids, use of physical therapy, and use of hip arthroplasty for patients with advanced hip arthritis. Among the conditional recommendations was that no particular TNFi was preferred except in patients with concomitant inflammatory bowel disease or recurrent iritis, in whom TNFi monoclonal antibodies should be used. In patients with active nonradiographic axial SpA despite treatment with NSAIDs, we conditionally recommend treatment with TNFi. Other recommendations for patients with nonradiographic axial SpA were based on indirect evidence and were the same as for patients with AS.

*Conclusion.*—These recommendations provide guidance for the management of common clinical questions in AS and nonradiographic axial SpA. Additional research on optimal medication management over time,

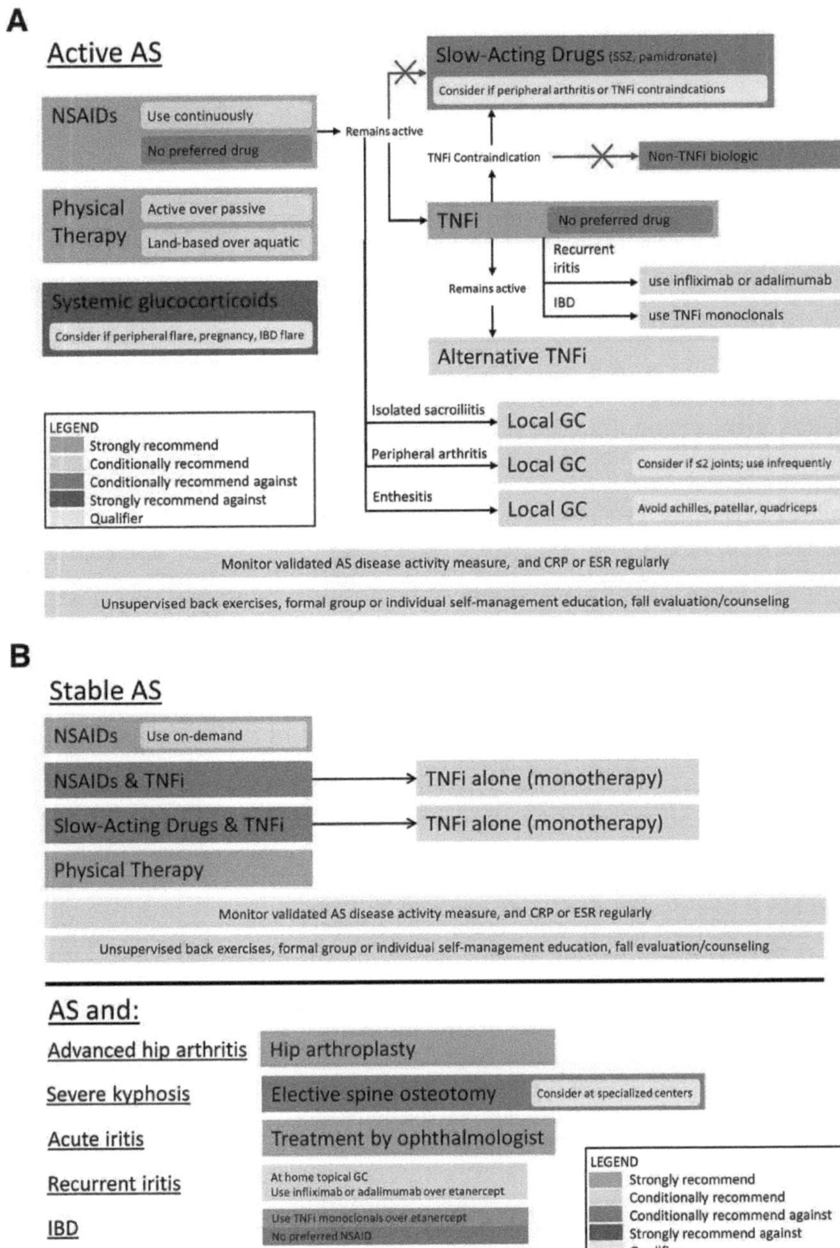


FIGURE 3.—Summary of the main recommendations for the treatment of patients with active ankylosing spondylitis (AS) (A) or stable AS (B). NSAIDs=nonsteroidal antiinflammatory drugs; SSZ=sulfasalazine; TNFi=tumor necrosis factor inhibitors; IBD=inflammatory bowel disease; GC=glucocorticoid; CRP=C-reactive protein; ESR=erythrocyte sedimentation rate. (Reprinted from Ward MM, Deodhar A, Akl EA, et al. American College of Rheumatology/Spondylitis Association of America/ Spondyloarthritis Research and Treatment Network 2015 recommendations for the treatment of ankylosing spondylitis and nonradiographic axial spondyloarthritis. *Arthritis Rheumatol.* 2016;68:282-298, with permission from American College of Rheumatology.)

disease monitoring, and preventive care is needed to help establish best practices in these areas (Fig 3).

▶ The 2015 American College of Rheumatology/Spondylitis Association of America/Spondyloarthritis Research and Treatment Network guideline was developed using the rigorous Grading of Recommendations, Assessment, Development and Evaluation methodology. It provides optimal advice for management of ankylosing spondylitis (AS) and nonradiographic axial spondyloarthritis (SpA) not only to rheumatology providers, but also to primary care physicians, physiatrists, and physical therapists. Nonsteroidal antiinflammatory drugs (NSAIDs) were recommended as first-line treatment for AS, and tumor necrosis factor inhibitors (TNFi) as second-line therapy for NSAID nonresponders. Physical therapy was considered a key component in management of AS. The authors strongly recommended against use of systemic steroid. In addition, treatment recommendations in certain patient populations were discussed. For example, in patients with AS and inflammatory bowel disease, TNFi monoclonal antibodies were preferred over etanercept; in patients with advanced hip arthritis, total hip arthroplasty was recommended. Given the controversy on nonradiographic axial SpA, the authors separated it from AS and conditionally recommended use of TNFi in NSAIDs nonresponders. A quick reference guide that summarized the main recommendations was provided in the article (Fig 3).

**R. Wang, MD, MHS**

---

**Secukinumab, a human anti-interleukin-17A monoclonal antibody, in patients with psoriatic arthritis (FUTURE 2): a randomised, double-blind, placebo-controlled, phase 3 trial**

McInnes IB, on behalf of the FUTURE 2 Study Group (Univ of Glasgow, UK; et al)

*Lancet* 386:1137-1146, 2015

---

*Background.*—Interleukin 17A is a proinflammatory cytokine that is implicated in the pathogenesis of psoriatic arthritis. We assessed the efficacy and safety of subcutaneous secukinumab, a human anti-interleukin-17A monoclonal antibody, in patients with psoriatic arthritis.

*Methods.*—In this phase 3, double-blind, placebo-controlled study undertaken at 76 centres in Asia, Australia, Canada, Europe, and the USA, adults (aged ≥18 years old) with active psoriatic arthritis were randomly allocated in a 1:1:1:1 ratio with computer-generated blocks to receive subcutaneous placebo or secukinumab 300 mg, 150 mg, or 75 mg once a week from baseline and then every 4 weeks from week 4. Patients and investigators were masked to treatment assignment. The primary endpoint was the proportion of patients achieving at least 20% improvement in the American College of Rheumatology response criteria (ACR20) at week 24. Analysis was by intention to treat. This study is registered with ClinicalTrials.gov, number NCT01752634.

*Findings.*—Between April 14, and Nov 25, 2013, 397 patients were randomly assigned to receive secukinumab 300 mg (n = 100), 150 mg (n = 100), 75 mg (n = 99), or placebo (n = 98). A significantly higher proportion of patients achieved an ACR20 at week 24 with secukinumab 300 mg (54 [54%] patients; odds ratio versus placebo 681, 95% CI 342–1356; $p < 0{\cdot}0001$), 150 mg (51 [51%] patients; 652, 325–1308; $p < 0{\cdot}0001$), and 75 mg (29 [29%] patients; 232, 1·14–473; $p = 0{\cdot}0399$) versus placebo (15 [15%] patients). Up to week 16, the most common adverse events were upper respiratory tract infections (four [4%], eight [8%], ten [10%], and seven [7%] with secukinumab 300 mg, 150 mg, 75 mg, and placebo, respectively) and nasopharyngitis (six [6%], four [4%], six [6%], and eight [8%], respectively). Serious adverse events were reported by five (5%), one (1%), and four (4%) patients in the secukinumab 300 mg, 150 mg, and 75 mg groups, respectively, compared with two (2%) in the placebo group. No deaths were reported.

*Interpretation.*—Subcutaneous secukinumab 300 mg and 150 mg improved the signs and symptoms of psoriatic arthritis, suggesting that secukinumab is a potential future treatment option for patients with this disorder.

▶ Interleukin-17 (IL-17) is a key cytokine in the pathogenesis of psoriatic arthritis (PsA). Inhibition of IL-17A receptor with secukinumab, a monoclonal antibody that binds to IL-17A receptor, was shown to improve signs and symptoms in patients with PsA. The FUTURE 2 trial was a phase III, double-blind, placebo-controlled study in patients with active PsA. Three hundred ninety-seven patients were randomized to receive placebo or secukinumab 300 mg, 150 mg, or 75 mg once a week from baseline and then every 4 weeks from week 4 until week 24. The primary end point was American College of Rheumatology 20 (ACR20), meaning 20% improvement in tender or swollen joints and 3 of 5 other domains. At 24 weeks, the response rates were 54%, 51%, and 29% in secukinumab 300-, 150-, and 75-mg groups respectively, versus 15% in placebo group. Together with the FUTURE 1 trial, this has led to US Food and Drug Administration approval of secukinumab use in PsA.

**R. Wang, MD, MHS**

---

**Effect of tight control of inflammation in early psoriatic arthritis (TICOPA): a UK multicentre, open-label, randomised controlled trial**

Coates LC, Moverley AR, McParland L, et al (Univ of Leeds, UK)

*Lancet* 386:2489-2498, 2015

---

*Background.*—Early intervention and tight control of inflammation optimise outcomes in rheumatoid arthritis but these approaches have not yet been studied in psoriatic arthritis. We aimed to assess the effect of tight control on early psoriatic arthritis using a treat-to-target approach.

*Methods.*—For this open-label multicentre randomised controlled trial, adult patients (aged ≥18 years) with early psoriatic arthritis (<24 months symptom duration), who had not previously received treatment with any disease-modifying anti-rheumatic drugs, were enrolled from eight secondary care rheumatology centres in the UK. Enrolled patients were randomly assigned in a 1:1 ratio to receive either tight control (with review every 4 weeks and with escalation of treatment if minimal disease activity criteria not met) or standard care (standard therapy according to the treating clinician, with review every 12 weeks) for 48 weeks. Randomisation was done by minimisation incorporating a random element, to ensure treatment groups were balanced for randomising centre and pattern of arthritis (oligoarticular *vs* polyarticular). The randomisation procedure was done through a central 24-h automated telephone system based at the Leeds Institute of Clinical Trials Research (Leeds, UK). This was an open-label study in which patients and clinicians were aware of treatment group assignment. Clinical outcomes were recorded by a masked assessor every 12 weeks. The primary outcome was the proportion of patients achieving an American College of Rheumatology (ACR) 20% (ACR20) response at 48 weeks, analysed by intention to treat with multiple imputation for missing ACR components. Cost-effectiveness was also assessed. This trial is registered with ClinicalTrials.gov, number NCT01106079, and the ISCRCTN registry, number ISCRCTN30147736.

*Findings.*—Between May 28, 2008, and March 21, 2012, 206 eligible patients were enrolled and randomly assigned to receive tight control (n = 101) or standard care (n = 105). In the intention-to-treat patient population, the odds of achieving an ACR20 response at 48 weeks were higher in the tight control group than in the standard care group (odds ratio 1·91, 95% CI 1·03–3·55; $p = 0{\cdot}0392$). Serious adverse events were reported by 20 (10%) patients (25 events in 14 [14%] patients in the tight control group and eight events in six [6%] patients in the standard care group) during the course of the study. No unexpected serious adverse events or deaths occurred.

*Interpretation.*—Tight control of psoriatic arthritis disease activity through a treat-to-target approach significantly improves joint outcomes for newly diagnosed patients, with no unexpected serious adverse events reported.

▶ In the past 20 years, the development of traditional and biological disease modifying antirheumatic drugs (DMARDs) has changed the management of inflammatory arthritis. The concept of "treat-to-target" (TTT) was brought up first in rheumatoid arthritis and then in psoriatic arthritis (PsA). TTT was defined as "a treatment strategy in which the clinician treats the patient aggressively enough to reach and maintain explicitly specified and sequentially measured goals, such as remission or low disease activity."[1] This proactive treatment strategy needs careful evaluation by clinical trials. In TICOPA study, 206 patients with early PsA who had not previously received DMARDs were randomized into a tight control group and a standard care group. After 48 weeks, the odds of achieving ACR20 were higher in the tight control group. Despite an open-label study, it proved, for the first time in patients with PsA, that the TTT approach significantly improved joint outcomes.

**R. Wang, MD, MHS**

*Reference*

1. Solomon DH, Bitton A, Katz JN, Radner H, Brown E, Fraenkel L. Treat to target in rheumatoid arthritis: fact, fiction or hypothesis? *Arthritis Rheumatol.* 2014;66: 775-782.

# 4 Osteoarthritis

**Synovitis in knee osteoarthritis: a precursor of disease?**

Atukorala I, Kwoh CK, Guermazi A, et al (Univ of Sydney, New South Wales, Australia; Univ of Arizona, Tucson; Boston Univ School of Medicine, MA; et al)

*Ann Rheum Dis* 75:390-395, 2016

*Objectives.*—It is unknown whether joint inflammation precedes other articular tissue damage in osteoarthritis. Therefore, this study aims to determine if synovitis precedes the development of radiographic knee osteoarthritis (ROA).

*Methods.*—The participants in this nested case–control study were selected from persons in the Osteoarthritis Initiative with knees that had a Kellgren Lawrence grading (KLG)=0 at baseline (BL). These knees were evaluated annually with radiography and non-contrastenhanced MRI over 4 years. MRIs were assessed for effusion-synovitis and Hoffa-synovitis. Case knees were defined by ROA (KLG ≥ 2) on the postero-anterior knee radiographs at any assessment after BL. Radiographs were assessed at P0 (time of onset of ROA), 1 year prior to P0 (P-1) and at BL. Controls were participants who did not develop incident ROA (iROA) from BL to 48 months).

*Results.*—133 knees of 120 persons with ROA (83 women) were matched to 133 control knees (83 women). ORs for occurrence of iROA associated with the presence of effusion-synovitis at BL, P-1 and P0 were 1.56 (95% CI 0.86 to 2.81), 3.23 (1.72 to 6.06) and 4.7 (1.10 to 2.95), respectively. The ORs for the occurrence of iROA associated with the presence of Hoffa-synovitis at BL, P-1 and P0 were 1.80 (1.1 to 2.95), 2.47 (1.45 to 4.23) and 2.40 (1.43 to 4.04), respectively.

*Conclusions.*—Effusion-synovitis and Hoffa-synovitis strongly predicted the development of iROA.

► In osteoarthritis, it is unclear whether joint inflammation is a precursor to cartilage damage. A nested case-control study was performed on patients from the Osteoarthritis Initiative. In the study, 133 knees of 120 patients were matched to 133 control knees. The knees were evaluated annually over 4 years with radiographs and non—contrast enhanced magnetic resonance imaging (MRI) with a Kellgren Lawrence grading (KLG) of 0 at baseline. MRIs assessed for effusion-synovitis and Hoffa synovitis. The odds ratio for incident radiographic knee osteoarthritis (iROA) associated with effusion-synovitis at baseline (BL), 1 year before onset of iROA (P-1), and time of onset of iROA (P0) were 1.56 (95% confidence interval [CI] 0.86-2.81), 3.23 (1.72-6.06), and 4.7

(1.10-2.95), respectively. The odds ratio associated with the presence of Hoffa synovitis at BL, P-1, and P0 were 1.80 (95% CI 1.1-2.95), 2.47 (1.45-4.23), and 2.40 (1.43-4.04), respectively, for the occurrence of iROA. In this study, effusion synovitis and Hoffa synovitis were strongly correlated with the development of radiographic knee osteoarthritis.

**T. Kapoor, MD**

**Synovial tissue volume: a treatment target in knee osteoarthritis (OA)**

O'Neill TW, Parkes MJ, Maricar N, et al (Univ of Manchester, UK; et al)

*Ann Rheum Dis* 75:84-90, 2016

*Background.*—Synovitis occurring frequently in osteoarthritis (OA) may be a targeted outcome. There are no data examining whether synovitis changes following intra-articular intervention.

*Methods.*—Persons aged 40 years and older with painful knee OA participated in an open label trial of intraarticular steroid therapy. At all time points they completed the Knee Injury and Osteoarthritis Outcome Score (KOOS) questionnaire. They had a contrast-enhanced (CE) MRI immediately prior to an intraarticular steroid injection with a repeat scan within 20 days. Response status was assessed using the Osteoarthritis Research Society International (OARSI) response criteria. OARSI responders were followed until their pain relapsed either within 20% of baseline or 6 months, shortly after which a third MRI was performed. Synovial tissue volume (STV) was measured on postcontrast knee images. We looked at changes in the STV and in pain, and their association.

*Results.*—120 subjects with preinjection and postinjection CE MRI were followed. Their mean age was 62.3 years (SD=10.3) and 62 (52%) were women. The median time between injection and follow-up scan was 8 days (IQR 7–14 days). 85/120 (71%) were OARSI responders. Pain decreased (mean change in KOOS = +23.9; 95% CI 20.1 to 27.8, $p < 0.001$) following steroid injection, as did mean STV (mean change = $-1071$ mm$^3$; 95% CI $-1839$ mm$^3$ to $-303$ mm$^3$, $p = 0.01$). Of the 80 who returned for a third MRI, pain relapsed in 57, and in the 48 of those with MRI data, STV increased between follow-up and final visit (+1220 mm$^3$; 95% CI 25 mm$^3$ to 2414 mm$^3$, $p = 0.05$). 23 were persistent responders at 6 months and, in these, STV did not increase (mean change = $-202$ mm$^3$; 95% CI $-2008$ mm$^3$ to 1604 mm$^3$, $p = 0.83$). Controlling for variation over time, there was a significant association between synovitis volume and KOOS pain (b coefficient—change in KOOS pain score per 1000 mm$^3$ change in STV = $-1.13$; 95% CI $-1.87$ to $-0.39$, $p = 0.003$), although STV accounted for only a small proportion of the variance in change in pain.

*Conclusions.*—Synovial tissue volume in knee OA shrinks following steroid therapy, and rebounds in those whose pain relapses. It can be considered a treatment target in symptomatic knee OA.

*Trial Registration Number.*—ISRCTN07329370.

▶ Studies have shown that synovial thickening on MRI correlates with histological synovitis and pain in patients with knee osteoarthritis (OA). This study assessed whether synovial tissue volume (STV) on MRI can be used as a treatment target in knee OA. One hundred twenty adults with painful knee OA participated in an open-label trial of intraarticular steroid therapy. A contrast-enhanced MRI was done before and after a steroid-injection within a 20-day period, measuring STV on MRI. A Knee Injury and Osteoarthritis Outcome Score (KOOS) questionnaire was also used to assess pain outcomes. Seventy-one percent (85 of 120) met the response criteria. There was a significant decrease in pain (mean change in KOOS = +23.9; 95% confidence interval [CI] 20.1-27.8, $P < .001$) following steroid injection, as well as a significant decrease in mean STV (mean change −1071 $mm^3$; 95% CI −1839 $mm^3$ to −303 $mm^3$, $P = .01$). Of the 80 patients who returned for third MRI, pain relapsed in 57 patients, and 48 of those patients showed an increase in STV between the follow-up visit and final visit (+1220 $mm^3$; 95% CI 25-2414 $mm^3$, $P = .05$). There was no increase in STV in persistent responders. In conclusion, synovial tissue volume correlates with pain in knee OA and may be considered a treatment target.

**T. Kapoor, MD**

---

**Which determinants predict tibiofemoral and patellofemoral osteoarthritis after anterior cruciate ligament injury? A systematic review**

van Meer BL, Meuffels DE, van Eijsden WA, et al (Univ Med Centre Rotterdam, The Netherlands)

*Br J Sports Med* 49:975-983, 2015

---

*Background.*—Anterior cruciate ligament (ACL) injury is an important risk factor for development of knee osteoarthritis (OA). To identify those ACL injured patients at increased risk for knee OA, it is necessary to understand risk factors for OA.

*Aim.*—To summarise the evidence for determinants of (1) tibiofemoral OA and (2) patellofemoral OA in ACL injured patients.

*Methods.*—MEDLINE, EMBASE, Web of Science and CINAHL databases were searched up to 20 December 2013. Additionally, reference lists of eligible studies were manually and independently screened by two reviewers. 2348 studies were assessed for the following main inclusion criteria: ≥20 patients; ACL injured patients treated operatively or non-operatively; reporting OA as outcome; description of relationship between OA outcome and determinants; and a follow-up period ≥2 years. Two reviewers extracted the data, assessed the risk of bias and performed a best-evidence synthesis.

*Results.*—Sixty-four publications were included and assessed for quality. Two studies were classified as low risk of bias. Medial meniscal injury/meniscectomy showed moderate evidence for influencing OA development (tibiofemoral OA and compartment unspecified). Lateral meniscal injury/meniscectomy showed moderate evidence for no relationship (compartment unspecified), as did time between injury and reconstruction (tibiofemoral and patellofemoral OA).

*Conclusions.*—Medial meniscal injury/meniscectomy after ACL rupture increased the risk of OA development. In contrast, it seems that lateral meniscal injury/meniscectomy has no relationship with OA development. Our results suggest that time between injury and reconstruction does not influence patellofemoral and tibiofemoral OA development. Many determinants showed conflicting and limited evidence and no determinant showed strong evidence.

▶ Anterior cruciate ligament (ACL) injury is a common injury in sports. The prevalence of knee osteoarthritis (OA) at 10 to 20 years postinjury is very variable (10%–90%). This is a systematic review to identify the risk factors for knee OA in patients with anterior cruciate ligament (ACL) injury. MEDLINE, EMBASE, Web of Science, and CINAHL databases were searched up to December 20, 2013, and 2348 studies were assessed. Sixty-four publications were included, and 2 were classified as low risk of bias. Medial meniscal injury and medial meniscectomy showed a moderate evidence for OA development. There was no relationship between lateral meniscal injury/meniscectomy and OA development (moderate evidence). There was no relationship between time between injury and reconstruction and OA development (moderate evidence).

**T. Kapoor, MD**

---

**A dose response analysis of a specific bone marrow concentrate treatment protocol for knee osteoarthritis**

Centeno CJ, Al-Sayegh H, Bashir J, et al (Centeno-Schultz Clinic, Broomfield, CO; et al)

*BMC Musculoskelet Disord* 16:258, 2015

---

*Background.*—Prior studies describing the treatment of symptomatic knee osteoarthritis with injections of bone marrow concentrate have provided encouraging results. The relationship between the cellular dose contained within the bone marrow concentrate and efficacy of the treatment, however, is unclear. In the present study we describe clinical outcomes for symptomatic knee osteoarthritis in relation to higher and lower cell concentrations contained within a bone marrow concentrate treatment protocol.

*Methods.*—Data from an ongoing patient registry was culled to identify 373 patients that received bone marrow concentrate injections for the treatment of 424 osteoarthritic knee joints. The clinical scales for these patients were assessed at baseline and then tracked post-procedure at 1, 3, 6 and 12 months, and annually thereafter. Tracked outcomes included the numeric pain scale; a lower extremity functional questionnaire; an

International Knee Documentation Committee scale; and a subjective improvement rating scale. Using pain and functional outcome measures, a receiver operating characteristic analysis was used to define an optimal clinical outcome threshold at which bone marrow nucleated cell count could be divided into either a lower or higher cell count group within a treatment protocol.

*Results.*—The lower and higher cell count groups were defined using a threshold of $4 \times 10^8$ cells. There were 224 and 185 knee joints treated in the lower ($\leq 4 \times 10^8$) and higher ($>4 \times 10^8$) cell count groups respectively. Most joints were diagnosed with early stage knee osteoarthritis. Both the lower and higher cell count groups demonstrated significant positive results with the treatment for all of the pain and functional metrics. The higher cell count group reported lower post treatment numeric pain scale values, in comparison with the lower cell count group (1.6 vs. 3.2; $P < 0.001$). No significant differences were detected for the other metrics, however.

*Conclusions.*—Improved function and reduced pain was observed in patients treated with a bone marrow concentrate protocol regardless of cellular dose; however, patients receiving a higher concentration of cells reported a better pain outcome in comparison with the lower dose group. These preliminary findings suggest that cell dose may be an important factor governing clinical outcomes in autologous bone marrow concentrate treatment of knee osteoarthritis. Further studies using a larger patient population may help elucidate these findings.

▶ Previous studies with bone-marrow nucleated cell (BMNC) injections have shown improved pain and function in knee osteoarthritis. Cells are isolated from bone marrow (BM) aspirates and injected into an osteoarthritic joint. Animal studies have shown BMNC injections improve cartilage healing by providing a mediation of catabolic immune responses using a variety of nucleated cells, including mesenchymal stem cells (MSC), hematopoietic stem cells, and white blood cells. The relationship between the cellular dose within the BM concentration and its efficacy of treatment remains unclear.

In this study, 373 patients were identified in an osteoarthritis (OA) registry that received BMNC injections to 424 osteoarthritic knee joints, with most as early-stage knee OA joints. A threshold of $4 \times 10^8$ cells divided the groups into lower or higher cell counts. There were 224 knee joints treated with low cell count ($\leq 4 \times 10^8$ cells) BMNC injections and 185 knee joints treated with high cell count ($> 4 \times 10^8$ cells) BMNC injections.

Both groups demonstrated significant improvement in pain and functional outcome measures, with the higher cell count group having greater improvements in numeric pain scales compared with the lower cell count group (1.6 vs 3.2; $P < .001$). Although the results are promising, further studies with a randomized placebo-controlled trial are needed to validate these findings.

**T. Kapoor, MD**

# 5 Gout

**2015 Gout Classification Criteria: An American College of Rheumatology/ European League Against Rheumatism Collaborative Initiative**

Neogi T, Jansen TLTA, Dalbeth N, et al (Boston Univ School of Medicine, MA; Radboud Univ Med Ctr, Nijmegen, The Netherlands; Univ of Auckland, New Zealand; et al)

*Arthritis Rheumatol* 67:2557-2568, 2015

*Objective.*—Existing criteria for the classification of gout have suboptimal sensitivity and/or specificity, and were developed at a time when advanced imaging was not available. The current effort was undertaken to develop new classification criteria for gout.

*Methods.*—An international group of investigators, supported by the American College of Rheumatology and the European League Against Rheumatism, conducted a systematic review of the literature on advanced imaging of gout, a diagnostic study in which the presence of monosodium urate monohydrate (MSU) crystals in synovial fluid or tophus was the gold standard, a ranking exercise of paper patient cases, and a multicriterion decision analysis exercise. These data formed the basis for developing the classification criteria, which were tested in an independent data set.

*Results.*—The entry criterion for the new classification criteria requires the occurrence of at least 1 episode of peripheral joint or bursal swelling, pain, or tenderness. The presence of MSU crystals in a symptomatic joint/ bursa (i.e., synovial fluid) or in a tophus is a sufficient criterion for classification of the subject as having gout, and does not require further scoring. The domains of the new classification criteria include clinical (pattern of joint/ bursa involvement, characteristics and time course of symptomatic episodes), laboratory (serum urate, MSU-negative synovial fluid aspirate), and imaging (double-contour sign on ultrasound or urate on dual-energy computed tomography, radiographic gout-related erosion). The sensitivity and specificity of the criteria are high (92% and 89%, respectively).

*Conclusion.*—The new classification criteria, developed using a data-driven and decision analytic approach, have excellent performance characteristics and incorporate current state-of-the-art evidence regarding gout.

► The 2015 Gout Classification Criteria were developed and approved by the American College of Rheumatology (ACR) and the European League Against Rheumatism (EULAR). In general, classification criteria are mainly used for enrollment of patients into clinical studies. However, these new criteria for gout are also useful for practicing clinicians because they can help guide clinicians who are considering the diagnosis of gout in a patient, particularly when the patient may not be having an acute attack but when a history of gout is suspected.

Gout is characterized by deposition of monosodium urate monohydrate (MSU) crystals in synovial fluid and tissues and is the most common form of inflammatory arthritis. Unlike many other rheumatologic diseases, gout is a disease that has a gold standard method of diagnosis: demonstration of MSU crystals in the synovial fluid or tissues of the affected joint. Although this is still considered the gold standard method of diagnosis, it may not be possible to diagnose someone with gout who is not actively having a gouty flare. For instance, in clinical practice, I commonly see patients who have had episodes that sound like they may have been gout, but by the time they are seen in consultation, their symptoms have resolved, and their joint examinations may be normal. In cases such as these, when there is no acute flare of gout, diagnostic arthrocentesis would not typically be performed. These classification criteria account for such situations, which occur frequently. The criteria allow for consideration of gout when it is not confirmed by the presence of MSU crystals. It includes a scoring system and takes into account patterns of joint/bursa involvement, characteristics of symptomatic episode(s), time course of episode(s), evidence of tophus on examination, serum urate levels, negative synovial fluid for MSU crystals, and imaging. Of note, these new classification criteria include imaging evidence demonstrable by ultrasound, which has not been included in previous criteria.

There is even an online calculator to help with scoring, which can be found on the ACR's and the EULAR's websites. Overall this is a great article to review gout's clinical symptomatology and characteristics. It describes helpful nuances in the recognition of gout, observed by experts, that may not be taught in medical school or found in textbooks.

**A. Sammut, MD**

---

**Physical Function, Hyperuricemia, and Gout in Older Adults**

Burke BT, Köttgen A, Law A, et al (Johns Hopkins Univ, Baltimore, MD; et al)

*Arthritis Care Res (Hoboken)* 67:1730-1738, 2015

---

*Objective.*—Gout prevalence is high in older adults and those affected are at risk of physical disability, yet it is unclear whether they have worse physical function.

*Methods.*—We studied gout, hyperuricemia, and physical function in 5,819 older adults (age ≥65 years) attending the 2011–2013 Atherosclerosis Risk in Communities Study visit, a prospective US population-based cohort. Differences in lower extremity function (Short Physical Performance Battery [SPPB] and 4-meter walking speed) and upper extremity function (grip strength) by gout status and by hyperuricemia prevalence were estimated in adjusted ordinal logistic regression (SPPB) and linear regression (walking speed and grip strength) models. Lower scores or times signify worse function. The prevalence of poor physical performance (first quartile) by gout and hyperuricemia was estimated using adjusted modified Poisson regression.

*Results.*—Ten percent of participants reported a history of gout and 21% had hyperuricemia. There was no difference in grip strength by history of gout ($P = 0.77$). Participants with gout performed worse on the SPPB test; they had 0.77 times (95% confidence interval [95% CI] 0.65, 0.90, $P = 0.001$) the prevalence odds of a 1-unit increase in SPPB score and were 1.18 times (95% CI 1.07, 1.32, $P = 0.002$) more likely to have poor SPPB performance. Participants with a history of gout had slower walking speed (mean difference −0.03; 95% CI −0.05, −0.01, $P < 0.001$) and were 1.19 times (95% CI 1.06, 1.34, $P = 0.003$) more likely to have poor walking speed. Similarly, SPPB score and walking speed, but not grip strength, were worse in participants with hyperuricemia.

*Conclusion.*—Older adults with gout and hyperuricemia are more likely to have worse lower extremity, but not upper extremity, function.

▶ Gout is one of the most common diagnoses seen in many arthritis clinics. Gout patients are cared for by primary care physicians, family medicine physicians, and rheumatologists. It is a common form of inflammatory arthritis, and its prevalence increases in the older population. Gout is characterized by painful attacks of swelling, burning, and stiffness in joints, the initial attack most commonly involving the first metatarsophalangeal joint. Distal joints are more often affected than proximal joints. Patients with gout have elevated uric acid, or hyperuricemia, although it is possible (and also common) to have hyperuricemia without having gout. Over the past few years, hyperuricemia without gout has been studied more and more as a risk factor for cardiovascular disease and other diseases.

This study is a prospective US population-based cohort that included 5819 individuals 65 years old or older and looked at gout, hyperuricemia, and physical function. It found that patients with gout, as well as patients with hyperuricemia but without gout, were more likely to have poor lower extremity function compared with patients without either of these conditions. Furthermore, it identified a subgroup of gout patients who were more likely to have poor lower extremity physical function. This subgroup included patients who are older, are African American, those with a history of stroke, diabetes, osteoarthritis, and patients with higher body mass indexes.

Although gout is quite common, it is important to remember that it is a serious disease. It may start out as just pain in the big toe, but without treatment, it can lead to disability, especially if there are tophi. This study highlights the association of both gout and asymptomatic hyperuricemia with poor lower extremity function. Asymptomatic hyperuricemia in association with poor lower extremity function is especially concerning because this is not a condition that is generally treated. Hyperuricemia and its associated risks need to be studied further to help clarify which patients with asymptomatic hyperuricemia would benefit from treatment.

**A. Sammut, MD**

# 6 Scleroderma

**Risk of Pulmonary Embolism and Deep Venous Thrombosis in Systemic Sclerosis: A General Population-Based Study**

Schoenfeld SR, Choi HK, Sayre EC, et al (Massachusetts General Hosp and Harvard Med School, Boston; Arthritis Res Canada, Vancouver, British Columbia; et al)

*Arthritis Care Res (Hoboken)* 68:246-253, 2016

*Objective.*—To determine the risk of venous thromboembolism (VTE) (pulmonary embolism [PE] and deep vein thrombosis [DVT]) in individuals with incident systemic sclerosis (SSc; scleroderma) in the general population.

*Methods.*—Using a population database that includes all residents of British Columbia, Canada, we conducted a cohort study of all patients with incident SSc and up to 10 age-, sex-, and entry time–matched individuals from the general population. We compared incidence rates of PE, DVT, and VTE between the 2 groups according to SSc disease duration. We calculated hazard ratios (HRs), adjusting for confounders.

*Results.*—Among 1,245 individuals with SSc (83% female, mean age 56 years), the incidence rates of PE, DVT, and VTE were 3.47, 3.48, and 6.56 per 1,000 person-years, respectively, whereas the corresponding rates were 0.78, 0.76, and 1.37 per 1,000 person-years among 12,670 non-SSc individuals. Compared with non-SSc individuals, the multivariable HRs among SSc patients were 3.73 (95% confidence interval [95% CI] 1.98–7.04), 2.96 (95% CI 1.54–5.69), and 3.47 (95% CI 2.14–5.64) for PE, DVT, and VTE, respectively. The age-, sex-, and entry time–matched HRs for PE, DVT, and VTE were highest during the first year after SSc diagnosis (32.77 [95% CI 6.60–162.75], 8.50 [95% CI 3.13–23.04], and 12.03 [95% CI 5.27–27.45], respectively).

*Conclusion.*—These findings provide population-based evidence that SSc patients are at a substantially increased risk of VTE, especially within the first year after SSc diagnosis. Increased monitoring for this potentially fatal outcome and its modifiable risk factors is warranted in this patient population.

► Patients with inflammatory autoimmune diseases have been reported to have an increased risk of venous thromboembolism (VTE), deep vein thrombosis (DVT), and pulmonary embolism (PE). In my practice, I have cared for patients with rheumatoid arthritis, systemic lupus erythematosus, granulomatosis with polyangiitis, and Behcet disease who have had DVTs, PEs, or other VTEs.

The increased risk of VTEs in these diseases has been well described.[1-3] This study compares the risk of PEs and DVTs in patients with systemic sclerosis (SSc) to patients who do not have an autoimmune illness. It uses the data from a comprehensive Canadian database of all patients with SSc. Although patients with additional rheumatologic autoimmune illnesses are excluded, the type of scleroderma is not specified, that is, whether the patients have limited or systemic scleroderma. Nonetheless, the number of patients studied for such a rare disease is quite large at 1245 individuals and the nonscleroderma control patient population used was also large at 12 670 individuals. Hazard ratios were calculated for PEs, DVTs, and VTEs in both the SSc and non-SSc groups. The SSc group was found to be at substantially higher risk for the development of PEs, DVTs, or VTEs than the non-SSc group. The risk was highest in the first year after the diagnosis of SSc.

I selected this article because it reminds us that autoimmune diseases are associated with inflammation, which may increase the risk of venous thromboembolic conditions. Patients with SSc also suffer from endothelial dysfunction, which also may increase the risk of blood clot formation. SSc patients frequently have Raynaud syndrome, edema in their hands, and/or pulmonary artery hypertension, all of which are additional manifestations of endothelial dysfunction. When caring for a patient with SSc, it is important to be aware of this increased risk and to monitor closely for signs of a PE, DVT, or VTE.

**A. Sammut, MD**

*References*

1. Zoller B, Li X, Sundquist J, Sundquist K. Risk of pulmonary embolism in patients with autoimmune disorders: a nation- wide follow-up study from Sweden. *Lancet.* 2012;379:244-249.
2. Merkel PA, Lo GH, Holbrook JT, et al. Brief communication: high incidence of venous thrombotic events among patients with Wegener granulomatosis: the Wegener's Clinical Occurrence of Thrombosis (WeCLOT) Study. *Ann Intern Med.* 2005;142:620-626.
3. Choi HK, Rho YH, Zhu Y, Cea-Soriano L, Avina-Zubieta JA, Zhang Y. The risk of pulmonary embolism and deep vein thrombosis in rheumatoid arthritis: a UK population-based outpatient cohort study. *Ann Rheum Dis.* 2013;72:1182-1187.

# 7 Sjogren's Syndrome

**Rheumatoid Factor and Disease Activity Are Independent Predictors of Lymphoma in Primary Sjögren's Syndrome**

Nocturne G, Virone A, Ng W-F, et al (Université Paris-Sud, Le Kremlin-Bicêtre, France; Hôpitaux Universitaires Paris-Sud, Le Kremlin-Bicêtre, France; Newcastle Univ, Newcastle-upon-Tyne, UK; et al)

*Arthritis Rheumatol* 68:977-985, 2016

*Objective.*—To define parameters predictive of lymphoma development in patients with primary Sjögren's syndrome (SS).

*Methods.*—A multicenter case–control survey was performed to identify predictors of lymphoma. Cases were patients who developed lymphoma after diagnosis of primary SS and were mainly recruited through the Club Rhumatismes et Inflammation network. For each case, 2 controls (matched for disease duration and age) were randomly selected among patients with primary SS and without lymphoma. Cases and controls were compared using univariate analysis and then using multivariate analysis to identify independent predictors of lymphoma.

*Results.*—One hundred one patients with primary SS and lymphoma were included. Eighty-seven patients were women (86.1%), and the mean ± SD age at lymphoma diagnosis was 57.4 ± 12.6 years. The most frequent histologic type was B cell non-Hodgkin's lymphoma (NHL) in 99 of 101 patients, with marginalzone lymphoma in 76 of the 99 patients (76.8%) including 58 (58.6%) with lymphoma of the mucosa-associated lymphoid tissue type. Lymphomas were most frequently located in the salivary glands (43 patients). A specific treatment was initiated at diagnosis in 87 patients with B cell NHL, and 61 patients (61.6%) achieved complete sustained remission after the first line of treatment. In the multivariate analysis, salivary gland enlargement, the presence of rheumatoid factor (RF), low C4, cryoglobulinemia, lymphopenia, and disease activity according to the European League Against Rheumatism Sjögrens Syndrome Disease Activity Index (excluding the lymphoma domain) were found to be predictors of lymphoma. No previous treatment for primary SS was associated with any effect on lymphoma occurrence.

*Conclusion.*—In addition to previously known factors predictive of lymphoma occurrence, the independent roles of RF and disease activity were demonstrated in this case–control study of primary SS–associated

**lymphoma. Our findings highlight the roles of chronic antigenic stimulation and disease activity in the development of this severe complication.**

▶ Sjogren syndrome is a chronic, inflammatory autoimmune disease that primarily attacks salivary and lacrimal glands. The symptom severity in patients can range from mild to severe and can be disabling. Primary Sjogren syndrome is not associated with other autoimmune illnesses, whereas secondary Sjogren syndrome typically does occur in the presence of other autoimmune illnesses, such as rheumatoid arthritis and systemic lupus erythematosus. Primary Sjogren syndrome patients can develop systemic manifestations affecting the kidneys, nervous system, lungs, and joints.

One of the challenges in the long-term care of Sjogren patients is that these patients have a high risk of developing lymphoma compared with the general population,[1-3] and identification of lymphoma in these patients can be difficult. In Primary Sjogren syndrome, about 5% to 10% of patients will develop lymphoma.[4] In my practice, one of my major concerns when seeing a patient who has Sjogren is whether he or she has or will develop lymphoma. It is important to educate these patients on the risk of lymphoma and to make the patient aware that if he or she notices new symptoms, especially night sweats, weight loss, or fevers, these need to be reported to the rheumatologist or the physician taking care of them. Unfortunately, not all patients with lymphoma will have these "B" symptoms. When caring for patients with Sjogren, it is important to know what studies have shown to be clinical and laboratory findings associated with a higher risk of lymphoma.

This study looked at a large series of patients with primary SS who developed lymphoma. It was performed to further study the classical clinical and biological predictors that increase the risk of lymphoma in primary SS. Clinical predictors of those at high risk for the development of lymphoma include permanent swelling of the salivary glands, splenomegaly, lymphadenopathies, and palpable purpura. Laboratory predictors include lymphopenia, cryoglobulinemia, low complement levels, and a monoclonal component in the serum or urine.[5,6] This study has added to these predictors that the presence of rheumatoid factor, as well as Sjogren disease activity, are also associated with higher rates of lymphoma. I found the table of characteristics of the 101 patients studied particularly helpful. In these patients with lymphoma and Sjogren syndrome, the histologic type of lymphoma, the localization of the lymphoma and the outcomes were detailed. Notable findings include that the majority of these patients had low-grade B-cell non-Hodgkin lymphomas and that patients with diffuse large B-cell lymphoma (DLBCL) had a worse prognosis.

The take-home message is that patients with Sjogren syndrome are at high risk for lymphoma, and that there are certain clinical and lab findings that can help determine that risk when these patients are evaluated.

**A. Sammut, MD**

*References*

1. Fallah M, Liu X, Ji J, Forsti A, Sundquist K, Hemminki K. Autoimmune diseases associated with non-Hodgkin lymphoma: a nationwide cohort study. *Ann Oncol.* 2014;25:2025-2030.
2. Johnsen SJ, Brun JG, Goransson LG, et al. Risk of non-Hodgkin's lymphoma in primary Sjögren's syndrome: a population-based study. *Arthritis Care Res (Hoboken).* 2013;65:816-821.
3. Smedby KE, Hjalgrim H, Askling J, et al. Autoimmune and chronic inflammatory disorders and risk of non-Hodgkin lymphoma by subtype. *J Natl Cancer Inst.* 2006;98:51-60.
4. Zintzaras E, Voulgarelis M, Moutsopoulos HM. The risk of lymphoma development in autoimmune diseases: a meta-analysis. *Arch Intern Med.* 2005;165: 2337-2344.
5. Solans-Laque R, Lopez-Hernandez A, Bosch-Gil JA, Palacios A, Campillo M, Vilardell-Tarres M. Risk, predictors, and clinical characteristics of lymphoma development in primary Sjögren's syndrome. *Semin Arthritis Rheum.* 2011;41: 415-423.
6. Tzioufas AG, Boumba DS, Skopouli FN, Moutsopoulos HM. Mixed monoclonal cryoglobulinemia and monoclonal rheumatoid factor cross-reactive idiotypes as predictive factors for the development of lymphoma in primary Sjögren's syndrome. *Arthritis Rheum.* 1996;39:767-772.

# 8 Vasculitis

**Diffuse Alveolar Hemorrhage Secondary to Antineutrophil Cytoplasmic Antibody–Associated Vasculitis: Predictors of Respiratory Failure and Clinical Outcomes**

Cartin-Ceba R, Diaz-Caballero L, Al-Qadi MO, et al (Mayo Clinic, Rochester, MN; Macon Lung Ctr, Macon, GA; Brown Univ, Providence, RI; et al)

*Arthritis Rheumatol* 68:1467-1476, 2016

*Objective.*—To identify predictors of respiratory failure and to evaluate the therapeutic efficacy of plasma exchange (PE) and of rituximab versus cyclophosphamide in a cohort of patients with diffuse alveolar hemorrhage (DAH) secondary to antineutrophil cytoplasmic antibody–associated vasculitis (AAV) with or without respiratory failure.

*Methods.*—We performed a single-center historical cohort study of all consecutive patients with AAV associated DAH who were evaluated over a 16-year period. Logistic regression models were developed to examine the predictive role of the baseline clinical characteristics for the development of respiratory failure, and for the effect of PE and remission induction therapy on the main outcome (complete remission at 6 months).

*Results.*—Seventy-three patients with DAH were identified, and 34 of them experienced respiratory failure. The degree of hypoxemia upon initial presentation, a higher percentage of neutrophils in the bronchoalveolar lavage fluid cell count, and higher C-reactive protein levels were independently associated with the development of respiratory failure. PE was not associated with achieving complete remission at 6 months, with an odds ratio (OR) of 0.49 (95% confidence interval [95% CI] 0.12–1.95) ($P = 0.32$). Rituximab treatment was independently associated with achieving complete remission at 6 months (OR 6.45 [95% CI 1.78–29], $P = 0.003$).

*Conclusion.*—Our findings indicate that the most important predictor of respiratory failure in patients with DAH secondary to AAV is the degree of hypoxemia upon presentation. No clear benefit of the addition of PE to standard remission induction therapy was demonstrated. Complete remission by 6 months was achieved at a higher rate with rituximab than with cyclophosphamide in patients with DAH secondary to AAV, including those needing mechanical ventilation.

▶ Diffuse alveolar hemorrhage (DAH) can be a complication of several rheumatologic and nonrheumatologic diseases. DAH is one of the rheumatologic emergencies seen in patients who have antineutrophil cytoplasmic antibody

(ANCA)-associated vasculitis (AAV), anti-phospholipid antibody syndrome (APS), Behcet's syndrome, cryoglobulinemia, scleroderma, systemic lupus erythematosus, and pulmonary-renal syndromes. Patients with DAH usually present with progressive dyspnea, hypoxemia, hemoptysis, anemia, and a radiographic appearance of alveolar or interstitial infiltrates. Urgent bronchoscopy is usually needed to support the diagnosis. Active bleeding in the bronchoalveolar lavage (BAL) or the presence of hemosiderin-laden macrophages help confirm the diagnosis of DAH. DAH is a severe life-threatening condition that has a high mortality if not treated early and aggressively. These patients are some of the most critically ill patients I have cared for.

This is a study of DAH in patients with known ANCA-associated vasculitis (AAV). The patients in this study had either granulomatosis with polyangiitis (GPA, formerly known as Wegener's) or microscopic polyangiitis (MPA). This study excluded patients with eosinophilic granulomatosus with polyangiitis (EGPA). One of the reasons I selected this article is because of its methods. The authors went to great lengths to prove the diagnosis of DAH as true DAH and not another diagnosis. Unlike several previous studies, the majority of patients in this study had extensive testing on their BAL specimen (including cytologic analysis, cell count with differential count, determination of hemosiderin-laden macrophage percentage, Gram stain and bacterial cultures, acid-fast stain and mycobacterial culture, fungal stains and cultures, legionella culture, *Nocardia* stain, and viral culture), and sufficient clinical evidence for a diagnosis of DAH. Although these data are retrospective, each case is from the same cohort, and the majority of patients were cared for by the same 5 physicians. There were several key findings in this study. It found that patients treated with rituximab achieved remission at 6 months at a higher rate than those patients treated with cyclophosphamide. Patients who developed respiratory failure had worse oxygenation at initial presentation compared with those who did not develop respiratory failure. Higher BAL cell counts and higher serum CRPs were also observed in the group of patients who experienced respiratory failure. This study also looked at patients who received plasma exchange (PE), but the number of patients who received PE was small and typically the most severely ill, making it difficult to draw conclusions.

DAH needs to be recognized early on for the patient to be treated successfully. It has a high mortality; even in this study in which patients were cared for by vasculitis experts, 11% of the patients died (although this is a lower rate of death compared with most studies). In summary, in a patient who is having pulmonary hemorrhage, DAH and the ANCA-associated vasculitides should be considered. Early bronchoscopy helps with the diagnosis of DAH. Aggressive immunosuppression is required to treat patients with DAH associated with AAV.

**A. Sammut, MD**

**Rituximab for the treatment of eosinophilic granulomatosis with polyangiitis (Churg–Strauss)**

Mohammad AJ, Hot A, Arndt F, et al (Addenbrooke's Hosp, Cambridge, UK; Hôpital Edouard Herriot, Lyon, France; Univ Hosp Schleswig-Holstein, Bad Bramstedt, Germany; et al)

*Ann Rheum Dis* 75:396-401, 2016

*Background.*—Conventional treatment of eosinophilic granulomatosis with polyangiitis (EGPA) (Churg–Strauss) with glucocorticoids, with or without additional immunosuppressive drugs, is limited by partial efficacy, frequent toxicity and a high relapse rate. Rituximab is a licensed treatment for granulomatosis with polyangiitis and microscopic polyangiitis and is of potential benefit to patients with EGPA.

*Methods.*—Patients with EGPA who received rituximab as single or repeated courses were identified from four vasculitis centres. Standardised data collection was performed, including disease activity status and adverse events, at the time of initial treatment and after 6 and 12 months. Remission was defined as a Birmingham Vasculitis Activity Score (BVAS) of 0 and partial response as a ≥50% reduction in BVAS compared with baseline.

*Results.*—41 patients (21 women) with EGPA treated with rituximab between 2003 and 2013 were identified. 15 (37%) had refractory, 21 (51%) relapsing and 5 (12%) new onset disease. 19 received a single course and 22 received repeat-dose rituximab to prevent relapse. By 6 months, 83% improved with remission in 34% and partial response in 49%, and by 12 months 49% were in remission and 39% had a partial response. Prednisolone doses decreased in all patients by 6 and 12 months. Antineutrophil cytoplasmic antibody positivity at baseline was associated with a higher remission rate at 12 months. Adverse events included 15 infections (6 were severe).

*Conclusions.*—The treatment of EGPA with rituximab resulted in high rates of improvement and reduced requirement of prednisolone. Rituximab may be considered for the treatment of EGPA.

▶ Eosinophilic granulomatosis with polyangiitis (EGPA), formerly known as Churg-Strauss syndrome, is a rare antineutrophil cytoplasmic antibody (ANCA)-associated vasculitis. It occurs in about 3 to 11 people per million. This disease is characterized by asthma, elevated eosinophils in the blood, eosinophil infiltration of tissues, necrotizing granulomatous inflammation, and vasculitis. The vasculitis typically affects small to medium-sized arteries and can attack any organ in the body, but most commonly attacks the lungs, skin, sinuses, cardiovascular system, kidneys, peripheral nervous system, and joints.[1-3] Recommended treatments for severe cases of EGPA include a combination of glucocorticoids and intravenous cyclophosphamide. The course and prognosis of EGPA depends on the extent of organ involvement, with patients who have mainly ear, nose, and throat involvement having a better prognosis.

Rituximab has been studied in clinical trials as a treatment for granulomatosis with polyangiitis (GPA) and for microscopic polyangiitis (MPA) and was found to be noninferior to treatment with cyclophosphamide.[4,5] This study looked retrospectively at 41 patients with EGPA who were treated with rituximab. It found that rituximab, indeed, was effective in the treatment of EGPA. Although most of the patients had disease that was refractory to other immunosuppressants, the majority of patients treated with rituximab had either a partial response or went into full remission within 6 to 12 months of treatment. In terms of steroid dosing, at 12 months, steroids were still used by most EGPA patients, meaning that rituximab would not be used as a monotherapy, steroid-sparing agent. This may be because the majority of patients have asthma and that long-term steroids may be necessary to control asthma, despite other EGPA activity.

EGPA should be considered in the differential diagnosis of a patient with a history of asthma, sinus issues, and blood hypereosinophilia. In patients with severe EGPA, necrotizing granulomas can infiltrate the lungs and lead to hemoptysis. This study shows that rituximab can be used successfully to decrease EGPA disease activity. The results of this study will hopefully open doors for future research on rituximab in this disease.

**A. Sammut, MD**

*References*

1. Jennette JC, Falk RJ, Bacon PA, et al. 2012 revised international Chapel Hill consensus conference nomenclature of vasculitides. *Arthritis Rheum.* 2013;65:1-11.
2. Sinico RA, Di Toma L, Maggiore U, et al. Prevalence and clinical significance of antineutrophil cytoplasmic antibodies in Churg-Strauss syndrome. *Arthritis Rheum.* 2005;52:2926-2935.
3. Churg J, Strauss L. Allergic granulomatosis, allergic angiitis, and periarteritis nodosa. *Am J Pathol.* 1951;27:277-301.
4. Stone JH, Merkel PA, Spiera R, et al. Rituximab versus cyclophosphamide for ANCA-associated vasculitis. *N Engl J Med.* 2010;363:221-232.
5. Jones RB, Tervaert JW, Hauser T, et al. Rituximab versus cyclophosphamide in ANCA-associated renal vasculitis. *N Engl J Med.* 2010;363:211-220.

# 9 Idiopathic Inflammatory Myopathy

**Disease specificity of autoantibodies to cytosolic 5′-nucleotidase 1A in sporadic inclusion body myositis versus known autoimmune diseases**

Herbert MK, Stammen-Vogelzangs J, Verbeek MM, et al (Radboud Univ, Nijmegen, The Netherlands)

*Ann Rheum Dis* 75:696-701, 2016

*Objectives.*—The diagnosis of inclusion body myositis (IBM) can be challenging as it can be difficult to clinically distinguish from other forms of myositis, particularly polymyositis (PM). Recent studies have shown frequent presence of autoantibodies directed against cytosolic 5'-nucleotidase 1A (cN-1A) in patients with IBM. We therefore, examined the autoantigenicity and disease specificity of major epitopes of cN-1A in patients with sporadic IBM compared with healthy and disease controls.

*Methods.*—Serum samples obtained from patients with IBM (n = 238), PM and dermatomyositis (DM) (n = 185), other autoimmune diseases (n = 246), other neuromuscular diseases (n = 93) and healthy controls (n = 35) were analysed for the presence of autoantibodies using immunodominant cN-1A peptide ELISAs.

*Results.*—Autoantibodies directed against major epitopes of cN-1A were frequent in patients with IBM (37%) but not in PM, DM or non-autoimmune neuromuscular diseases (<5%). Anti-cN-1A reactivity was also observed in some other autoimmune diseases, particularly Sjögren's syndrome (SjS; 36%) and systemic lupus erythematosus (SLE; 20%).

*Conclusions.*—In summary, we found frequent anti-cN-1A autoantibodies in sera from patients with IBM. Heterogeneity in reactivity with the three immunodominant epitopes indicates that serological assays should not be limited to a distinct epitope region. The similar reactivities observed for SjS and SLE demonstrate the need to further investigate whether distinct IBM-specific epitopes exist.

► An autoantibody (anti-Mup44) against cytosolic 5′-nucleotidase 1A (cN-1a) has been recently discovered in the sera of patients with inclusion body myositis (IBM).[1,2] IBM is 1 of the 3 idiopathic inflammatory myopathies.

Unlike dermatomyositis (DM) and polymyositis (PM), IBM affects distal as well as proximal muscles and tends to affect people older than 50. IBM is a sporadic disorder with a male-to-female ratio of 3:1; it is uncommon in African Americans and other non-Caucasians. Serum creatine kinase is not as elevated in IBM compared with DM and PM. Pathologic features of IBM include rimmed vacuoles and abnormal protein accumulation. IBM is the most difficult to treat of the idiopathic inflammatory myopathies. It does not respond well to immunosuppression, unlike DM and PM. It has even been debated whether IBM is more of a degenerative myopathy with secondary inflammation as opposed to a primary autoimmune disease.[3]

Anti-cN-1a is a recently discovered biomarker for IBM. This study further characterized anti-cN-1a antibodies by comparing sera from patients with IBM to sera from patients with other autoimmune diseases, including systemic lupus erythematosus (SLE), Sjögren syndrome, and patients with no diagnosed autoimmune disease. A strength of this study is the number of IBM patients. IBM has a prevalence of only 4 to 9 cases per million, depending on the population.[4] This study included 238 IBM patients, which is a relatively high number for this disease. Of the 238 patients with IBM, 37% had anti-cN-1a autoantibodies. Interestingly, 36% of the 22 Sjögren syndrome patients and 20% of the 44 SLE patients also had anti-cN-1A autoantibodies. Anti-cN-1A antibody testing can be useful in patients who are being worked up for possible IBM. More studies are needed to determine whether having these antibodies is associated with a better or worse prognosis and whether there are certain clinical features of IBM seen more commonly in patients exhibiting the anti-cN-1A antibodies. A great point made by the authors of this article is that although these antibodies were also seen in patients with SLE and Sjögren syndrome, clinically these diagnoses are easy to distinguish. In other words, as is a common epithet in our rheumatology world, when it comes to rheumatologic diseases, diagnosis is based on history, physical exam findings, and laboratory findings; the autoantibody by itself does not make the diagnosis.

**A. Sammut, MD**

*References*

1. Pluk H, van Hoeve BJA, van Dooren SHJ, et al. Autoantibodies to cytosolic 50-nucleotidase 1A in inclusion body myositis. *Ann Neurol.* 2013;73:397-407.
2. Larman HB, Salajegheh M, Nazareno R, et al. Cytosolic 50-nucleotidase 1A autoimmunity in sporadic inclusion body myositis. *Ann Neurol.* 2013;73:408-418.
3. Hengstman GJD, Brouwer R, Vree Egberts WTM, et al. Clinical and serological characteristics of 125 Dutch myositis patients. *J Neurol.* 2002;249:69-75.
4. Dimachkie MM, Barohn RJ. Inclusion body myositis. *Semin Neurol.* 2012;32: 237-245.

# 10 Polymyalgia Rheumatica

**2015 Recommendations for the Management of Polymyalgia Rheumatica: A European League Against Rheumatism/American College of Rheumatology Collaborative Initiative**

Dejaco C, Singh YP, Perel P, et al (Southend Univ Hosp, Essex, UK; London School of Hygiene and Tropical Medicine, London, UK; et al)

*Arthritis Rheumatol* 67:2569-2580, 2015

Therapy for polymyalgia rheumatica (PMR) varies widely in clinical practice as international recommendations for PMR treatment are not currently available. In this paper, we report the 2015 European League Against Rheumatism (EULAR)/American College of Rheumatology (ACR) recommendations for the management of PMR. We used the Grading of Recommendations, Assessment, Development and Evaluation (GRADE) methodology as a framework for the project. Accordingly, the direction and strength of the recommendations are based on the quality of evidence, the balance between desirable and undesirable effects, patients' and clinicians' values and preferences, and resource use. Eight overarching principles and nine specific recommendations were developed covering several aspects of PMR, including basic and follow-up investigations of patients under treatment, risk factor assessment, medical access for patients and specialist referral, treatment strategies such as initial glucocorticoid (GC) doses and subsequent tapering regimens, use of intramuscular GCs and disease modifying antirheumatic drugs (DMARDs), as well as the roles of non-steroidal anti-rheumatic drugs and non-pharmacological interventions. These recommendations will inform primary, secondary and tertiary care physicians about an international consensus on the management of PMR. These recommendations should serve to inform clinicians about best practices in the care of patients with PMR.

► Polymyalgia rheumatic (PMR) is an inflammatory disorder that causes muscle pain and stiffness, especially in the shoulders. It affects people older than 50 years, and the majority of patients with PMR are older than 65 years. The care of a patient with PMR is often complex. Unfortunately, I have often seen patients whose steroids had been tapered too rapidly, as well as those whose steroid dose was too high. The management of PMR is usually initiated by primary care physicians and general internists, and there may not always be a rheumatologist available to manage these patients.

In October 2015, the American College of Rheumatology (ACR) and the European League Against Rheumatism (EULAR) published recommendations for the management of PMR. These recommendations are targeted at general practitioners, specialists in internal medicine, and rheumatologists. The recommendations emphasize that each patient's care depends on her or his own circumstances. These management guidelines help with everything from the initial diagnosis of PMR, including what workup should be performed to exclude other diagnoses and comorbidities, to the care of a patient with long-term PMR. It also stresses the importance of engaging the patient in decision making and management planning. Recommendations are given on steroid dosing and tapering, and when to consider other agents, such as methotrexate. Steroid dosing can be challenging even for those with experience managing inflammatory diseases, and guidelines such as these can help tailor dosing to the needs of the individual patient. Levels of support by evidence are clearly defined for their recommendations. The recommendations conclude with a set of questions that need to be defined further by future studies in PMR.

**A. Sammut, MD**

# 11 Chronic Juvenile Arthritis

---

**2016 Classification Criteria for Macrophage Activation Syndrome Complicating Systemic Juvenile Idiopathic Arthritis: A European League Against Rheumatism/American College of Rheumatology/Paediatric Rheumatology International Trials Organisation Collaborative Initiative**

Ravelli A, on behalf of the Paediatric Rheumatology International Trials Organisation, the Childhood Arthritis and Rheumatology Research Alliance, the Pediatric Rheumatology Collaborative Study Group, and the Histiocyte Society (Università degli Studi di Genova and Istituto Giannina Gaslini, Italy; et al)

*Ann Rheum Dis* 75:481-489, 2016

---

To develop criteria for the classification of macrophage activation syndrome (MAS) in patients with systemic juvenile idiopathic arthritis (JIA). A multistep process, based on a combination of expert consensus and analysis of real patient data, was conducted. A panel of 28 experts was first asked to classify 428 patient profiles as having or not having MAS, based on clinical and laboratory features at the time of disease onset. The 428 profiles comprised 161 patients with systemic JIA—associated MAS and 267 patients with a condition that could potentially be confused with MAS (active systemic JIA without evidence of MAS, or systemic infection). Next, the ability of candidate criteria to classify individual patients as having MAS or not having MAS was assessed by evaluating the agreement between the classification yielded using the criteria and the consensus classification of the experts. The final criteria were selected in a consensus conference. Experts achieved consensus on the classification of 391 of the 428 patient profiles (91.4%). A total of 982 candidate criteria were tested statistically. The 37 best-performing criteria and 8 criteria obtained from the literature were evaluated at the consensus conference. During the conference, 82% consensus among experts was reached on the final MAS classification criteria. In validation analyses, these criteria had a sensitivity of 0.73 and a specificity of 0.99. Agreement between the classification (MAS or not MAS) obtained using the criteria and the original diagnosis made by the treating physician was high ($\kappa = 0.76$). We have developed a set of classification criteria for MAS complicating systemic JIA and provided preliminary evidence of its validity. Use of these criteria will potentially improve understanding of MAS in systemic

JIA and enhance efforts to discover effective therapies, by ensuring appropriate patient enrollment in studies.

▶ Macrophage activation syndrome (MAS) is a life-threatening complication seen mostly in patients with systemic juvenile idiopathic arthritis (SJIA) and adult-onset Still disease (AOSD). MAS is a syndrome of activation, expansion, and uncontrolled proliferation of T lymphocytes and well-differentiated macrophages that leads to widespread cytokine release and a massive systemic inflammatory response. Patients with this condition frequently have fevers, hepatomegaly, splenomegaly, lymphadenopathy, cytopenia, coagulopathy, and liver function abnormalities. Early recognition is critical because mortality rates reach 20% to 30%, and if the diagnosis is unrecognized or the treatment is delayed, the mortality is even higher.

Although MAS is most commonly seen as a complication in patients with SJIA and AOSD, it may also occur in patients with other autoimmune diseases such as systemic lupus erythematosus (SLE) and Kawasaki disease. MAS may also be triggered by infections or certain medications; in these cases, it is termed "reactive hemophagocytic lymphohistiocytosis."

I selected this article because awareness of MAS and knowledge of its presentation and treatment may save a patient's life. It is not uncommon for patients with MAS to be in critical condition in the intensive care unit, and it is up to the clinicians to keep this diagnosis on their differential. The criteria presented in this article originate from a combination of the best literature on MAS and on exert opinion. Note that although these criteria are used to qualify patients for studies of MAS, they are not strict diagnostic criteria used in the clinical setting. Rather, what's important to learn from this article is recognition of the symptoms and the lab findings associated with this condition. If a patient has an unexplained fever and an elevated ferritin, it is already enough to consider the diagnosis of MAS.

**A. Sammut, MD**

# 12 Fibromyalgia

**Differences in Sedentary Time and Physical Activity Between Female Patients With Fibromyalgia and Healthy Controls: The al-Ándalus Project**

Segura-Jiménez V, Álvarez-Gallardo IC, Estévez-López F, et al (Univ of Granada, Spain; et al)

*Arthritis Rheumatol* 67:3047-3057, 2015

*Objective.*—To characterize the levels of objectively measured time spent in sedentary activities (sedentary time) and physical activities in female patients with fibromyalgia and compare them with the levels in age-matched healthy control women.

*Methods.*—The study comprised 413 female patients with fibromyalgia (mean ± SD age 51.9 ± 7.4 years) and 188 female control subjects (age 50.9 ± 7.5 years). Sedentary time, the amount of time spent engaged in physical activity, and step counts were measured using triaxial accelerometry. The amounts of time (minutes/day) during which the participants were engaged in sedentary behaviors as well as in physical activity of different intensities (light, moderate, and moderate-to-vigorous) and the step counts were calculated.

*Results.*—The amount of time spent in sedentary behavior was longer in patients with fibromyalgia compared with controls (estimated mean ± SEM difference 39 ± 8 minutes/day; $P < 0.001$). The patients with fibromyalgia spent less time than controls engaged in light physical activity (mean ± SEM difference −21 ± 7 minutes/ day; $P = 0.005$), moderate physical activity (mean ± SEM difference −17 ± 3 minutes/day; $P < 0.001$), and moderate- to-vigorous physical activity (mean ± SEM difference −19 ± 3 minutes/day; $P < 0.001$). The patients with fibromyalgia took fewer steps/day compared with the control subjects (mean ± SEM difference −1,881 ± 262 steps/ day; $P < 0.001$). Only 20.6% of the patients with fibromyalgia and 46.3% of the control subjects fulfilled the recommendation for 150 minutes/week of moderate-to-vigorous physical activity in bouts of at least 10 minutes/bout ($\chi^2 = 41.8$, $P < 0.001$). Similarly, only 16.0% of the patients fulfilled the recommendation for ≥10,000 steps/ day compared with 44.7% of the control subjects ($\chi^2 = 56.8$, $P < 0.001$). Both the patients and the control subjects were more active (physical activity of all intensities and numbers of steps) on weekdays than on weekend days (all $P \leq 0.001$).

*Conclusion.*—Female patients with fibromyalgia spent more time in sedentary behaviors and were less physically active than age-matched controls. The low proportions of female patients with fibromyalgia and control subjects who met the physical activity and step count recommendations is worrisome.

▶ Fibromyalgia is a disorder characterized by chronic widespread musculoskeletal pain, fatigue, sleep disturbance or poor sleep quality, and memory or mood issues. Patients with fibromyalgia suffer from amplification of pain sensation due to poorly understood brain processes. The prevalence of fibromyalgia is about 3% to 5% in women and 0.5% to 1.6% in men, defined by the 1990 American College of Rheumatology (ACR) classification criteria.[1]

Optimal management of fibromyalgia involves both nonmedical and medical approaches. In terms of nonmedical approaches, lifestyle changes, including improving sleep quality and increasing exercise, will often help reduce pain. In patients with fibromyalgia, sedentary behaviors are associated with impaired pain regulation. This study shows that people with fibromyalgia engage in less physical activity and more sedentary time than healthy control subjects. It is a cross-sectional study, and its strengths include the large number of patients with fibromyalgia and the methods of how activity was measured. One issue I would like to point out is that the 1990 fibromyalgia criteria were used, which relied on "tender points." Today, "tender points" have fallen out of favor in the diagnosis of patients with fibromyalgia. Patients may not have the number of tender points or may have certain areas that are more tender than others and still have fibromyalgia. In 2010, the ACR published new diagnostic criteria for fibromyalgia that included a symptom severity index. This included fatigue, cognitive impairment, and sleep disturbance in the evaluation of patients with suspected fibromyalgia because it is known that these factors play a role.[2] One of the interesting points this article illustrates is that for both the people with fibromyalgia and the healthy controls, there was less physical activity on weekends than on weekdays. This should encourage us to counsel patients to increase activity on weekends. Furthermore, in both groups, the number of steps per day reached >10 000 in very few patients.

**A. Sammut, MD**

*References*

1. Wolfe F, Smythe HA, Yunus MB, et al. The American College of Rheumatology 1990 criteria for the classification of fibromyalgia. report of the multicenter criteria committee. *Arthritis Rheum.* 1990;33:160-172.
2. Wolfe F, Clauw DJ, Fitzcharles MA, et al. The American College of Rheumatology preliminary diagnostic criteria for fibromyalgia and measurement of symptom severity. *Arthritis Care Res (Hoboken).* 2010;62:600-610.

# 13 Drug Toxicity

**The EULAR points to consider for use of antirheumatic drugs before pregnancy, and during pregnancy and lactation**

Götestam Skorpen C, Hoeltzenbein M, Tincani A, et al (Trondheim Univ Hosp, Norway; Charité-Universitätsmedizin Berlin, Germany; Spedali Civili and Univ of Brescia, Italy; et al)

*Ann Rheum Dis* 75:795-810, 2016

A European League Against Rheumatism (EULAR) task force was established to define points to consider on use of antirheumatic drugs before pregnancy, and during pregnancy and lactation. Based on a systematic literature review and pregnancy exposure data from several registries, statements on the compatibility of antirheumatic drugs during pregnancy and lactation were developed. The level of agreement among experts in regard to statements and propositions of use in clinical practice was established by Delphi voting. The task force defined 4 overarching principles and 11 points to consider for use of antirheumatic drugs during pregnancy and lactation. Compatibility with pregnancy and lactation was found for antimalarials, sulfasalazine, azathioprine, ciclosporin, tacrolimus, colchicine, intravenous immunoglobulin and glucocorticoids. Methotrexate, mycophenolate mofetil and cyclophosphamide require discontinuation before conception due to proven teratogenicity. Insufficient documentation in regard to fetal safety implies the discontinuation of leflunomide, tofacitinib as well as abatacept, rituximab, belimumab, tocilizumab, ustekinumab and anakinra before a planned pregnancy. Among biologics tumour necrosis factor inhibitors are best studied and appear reasonably safe with first and second trimester use. Restrictions in use apply for the few proven teratogenic drugs and the large proportion of medications for which insufficient safety data for the fetus/child are available. Effective drug treatment of active inflammatory rheumatic disease is possible with reasonable safety for the fetus/child during pregnancy and lactation. The dissemination of the data to health professionals and patients as well as their implementation into clinical practice may help to improve the management of pregnant and lactating patients with rheumatic disease.

► Rheumatic diseases (RDs) frequently attack women of childbearing age. This is especially true of systemic lupus erythematosus (SLE) and rheumatoid arthritis (RA) but applies to many other RDs. Certain medications used to treat SLE or other RDs need to be stopped before even planning to become pregnant. For instance, leflunomide requires a washout period before the patient attempts to conceive. The points raised in this article by the European League Against Rheumatism's task force are based on best available evidence from a systemic literature review, registry data, and expert opinion. This article addresses considerations regarding antirheumatic drug use before pregnancy, during pregnancy, and during lactation. It is an update from 2008 and now includes more information on biologic agent use during pregnancy. Medications such as hydroxychloroquine, sulfasalazine, azathioprine, ciclosporin, tacrolimus, and colchicine are considered safe to maintain remission or to treat a disease flare in pregnancy. Medications such as methotrexate, mycophenolate mofetil, and cyclophosphamide are teratogenic and should be withdrawn before pregnancy.

This article is useful to rheumatologists and also to primary care physicians and other health care providers who may be caring for patients with RD who are pregnant. It is helpful to be able to counsel patients on what studies have shown for each of the medications used in RD. For each medication, the type of study and number of publications are clearly defined. Furthermore, numbers of total pregnancies on the medications, comments on miscarriages and/or congenital malformations, and the strength of the evidence are also provided. Of note, there is a paucity of data on medication safety in lactation, but what is known is provided in this article.

When caring for a pregnant patient with a RD, it is important to weigh the risks and benefits of the medications and involve the patient in the decision-making process. This article lumps together RDs, but in reality, SLE is very different from RA, and whether to continue medications or which medication to use really depends on the individual patient's disease activity and severity. There are colored pie charts used to describe the expert opinion use of the drug in clinical practice. These were interesting because they clearly show that despite the experts agreeing with the basic consensus statements, they may or may not give the drug depending on the disease severity.

**A. Sammut, MD**

---

## Efficacy, Tolerability, and Safety of Cannabinoid Treatments in the Rheumatic Diseases: A Systematic Review of Randomized Controlled Trials

Fitzcharles M-A, Ste-Marie PA, Häuser W, et al (McGill Univ Health Centre, Montreal, Quebec, Canada; Technische Universität München, Germany; et al)
*Arthritis Care Res* 68:681-688, 2016

---

*Objective.*—To assess the efficacy, tolerability, and safety of cannabinoids (phyto- and syntheto-) in the management of rheumatic diseases.

*Methods.*—Multiple databases, including Medline, Embase, and CENTRAL, were searched. Randomized controlled trials with outcomes of pain, sleep, quality of life, tolerability (dropouts due to adverse events), and safety (serious adverse events), with comparison of cannabinoids with any type of control, were included. Study methodology quality was evaluated with the Cochrane risk of bias tool.

*Results.*—In 4 short-term studies comprising 203 patients (58 with rheumatoid arthritis, 71 with fibromyalgia, and 74 with osteoarthritis [OA]), cannabinoids had a statistically significant effect on pain in 2, sleep in 2, and improved quality of life in 1, with the OA study prematurely terminated due to futility. The risk of bias was high for all 3 completed studies. Dizziness, cognitive problems, and drowsiness, as well as nausea, were reported for almost half of the patients. No serious adverse events were reported for cannabinoids during the study duration. No studies of herbal cannabis were identified.

*Conclusion.*—Extremely small sample sizes, short study duration, heterogeneity of rheumatic conditions and products, and absence of studies of herbal cannabis allow for only limited conclusions for the effects of cannabinoids in rheumatic conditions. Pain relief and effect on sleep may have some potential therapeutic benefit, but with considerable mild to moderate adverse events. There is currently insufficient evidence to recommend cannabinoid treatments for management of rheumatic diseases pending further study.

▶ A patient of mine with rheumatoid arthritis (RA) reported using marijuana on a daily basis and stated that it helped with her pain. She did not want to take any of the traditional disease modifying antirheumatic drugs (DMARDs) or any of the biologic medications. She asked whether medical marijuana could be prescribed for her once it becomes legal. This is a typical question that I am asked by a number of patients with RA, as well as patients with other rheumatologic disorders, including osteoarthritis (OA), fibromyalgia (FM), and systemic lupus erythematosus (SLE).

The authors of this article performed a comprehensive literature review on cannabinoids in rheumatic diseases. Unfortunately, the studies that are available are scarce. There were 4 controlled studies that included a total of 201 patients with rheumatic diseases; 58 patients had RA, 71 had FM, and 74 were diagnosed with OA. These 4 studies, although controlled, were for the most part of short duration, with study periods ranging from 2 to 8 weeks. Each of the 4 studies is detailed and discussed in this article, but the end result is that there is just not enough information for us to know whether cannabinoids are useful in these conditions. These studies did suggest that cannabinoids may help with sleep and pain in patients with FM. There are no randomized controlled studies or formal studies on herbal cannabis preparations in rheumatic diseases.

My RA patient described above had very active RA, and I advised her that there is not enough evidence to draw conclusions regarding the use of cannabinoids in rheumatic diseases. She eventually agreed to start treatment with DMARDs.

**A. Sammut, MD**

# 14 Miscellaneous Rheumatic Diseases and Therapies

**EULAR recommendations for the management of familial Mediterranean fever**

Ozen S, Demirkaya E, Erer B, et al (Hacettepe Univ, Ankara, Turkey; Gülhane Military Med Academy, Ankara, Turkey; Istanbul Univ, Turkey; et al)

*Ann Rheum Dis* 75:644-651, 2016

Familial Mediterranean fever (FMF) is the most common monogenic autoinflammatory disease, but many rheumatologists are not well acquainted with its management. The objective of this report is to produce evidence-based recommendations to guide rheumatologists and other health professionals in the treatment and follow-up of patients with FMF. A multidisciplinary panel, including rheumatologists, internists, paediatricians, a nurse, a methodologist and a patient representative, was assembled. Panellists came from the Eastern Mediterranean area, Europe and North America. A preliminary systematic literature search on the pharmacological treatment of FMF was performed following which the expert group convened to define aims, scope and users of the guidelines and established the need for additional reviews on controversial topics. In a second meeting, recommendations were discussed and refined in light of available evidence. Finally, agreement with the recommendations was obtained from a larger group of experts through a Delphi survey. The level of evidence (LoE) and grade of recommendation (GR) were then incorporated. The final document comprises 18 recommendations, each presented with its degree of agreement (0–10), LoE, GR and rationale. The degree of agreement was greater than 7/10 in all instances. The more controversial statements were those related to follow-up and dose change, for which supporting evidence is limited. A set of widely accepted recommendations for the treatment and monitoring of FMF is presented, supported by the best available evidence and expert opinion. It is believed that these recommendations will be useful in guiding physicians in the care of patients with FMF.

▶ Familial Mediterranean fever (FMF) is the most common of the autoinflammatory diseases. It is a chronic inflammatory disease that causes recurrent fevers and painful inflammation in the joints, abdomen, lungs, and other areas of the body. FMF mostly occurs in people of Mediterranean origin, including Armenians, Greeks, Jews, Italians, Arabs, and Turks, but it may affect any ethnic group. There is no cure for FMF, but there are treatments that can help reduce disease flares and decrease systemic inflammation. A known complication of untreated FMF is amyloid A amyloidosis and resultant kidney failure.

This set of EULAR management recommendations for FMF is useful to rheumatologists, primary care physicians, and pediatricians, especially for those who may not encounter FMF patients on a regular basis. It is equally important for those physicians who do not care for patients with FMF, so that features of the disease can be recognized early to help reduce delay in diagnosis. Each recommendation is explained in detail, and the article does a great job not only of reviewing FMF but also showing what it would be like to care for someone with FMF, including how to deal with the obstacles of complex management.

Using the best available evidence and consensus of expert opinion, this set of recommendations addresses important aspects of the management of FMF including but not limited to the goals of treatment in FMF, dosing of colchicine, colchicine toxicity, addressing liver function test abnormalities in FMF patients, additional disease-modifying antirheumatic drugs (DMARDs), and use of biologics in FMF. Primary care physicians need to be aware of these aspects of treatment because they can affect multiple organ systems and require close monitoring by all the patient's health care providers.

**A. Sammut, MD**

---

**Chikungunya Viral Arthritis in the United States: A Mimic of Seronegative Rheumatoid Arthritis**

Miner JJ, Aw Yeang HX, Fox JM, et al (Washington Univ School of Medicine, St Louis, MO)

*Arthritis Rheumatol* 67:1214-1220, 2015

---

*Objective.*—Chikungunya virus (CHIKV) is an arthritogenic mosquito-transmitted alphavirus that spread to the Caribbean in 2013 and to the US in 2014. CHIKV-infected patients develop inflammatory arthritis that can persist for months or years, but little is known about the rheumatologic and immunologic features of CHIKV-related arthritis in humans, particularly as compared to rheumatoid arthritis (RA). The purpose of this study was to describe these features in a group of 10 American travelers who were nearly simultaneously infected while visiting Haiti in June 2014.

*Methods.*—Patient history was obtained and physical examination and laboratory tests were performed. All patients with CHIKV-related arthritis had detectable levels of anti-CHIKV IgG. Using cytometry by time-of-flight (CyTOF), we analyzed peripheral blood mononuclear cells in CHIKV-infected patients, healthy controls, and patients with untreated, active RA.

*Results.*—Among 10 CHIKV-infected individuals, 8 developed persistent symmetric polyarthritis that met the American College of Rheumatology/

European League Against Rheumatism 2010 criteria for (seronegative) RA. CyTOF analysis revealed that RA and CHIKV-infected patients had greater percentages of activated and effector CD4+ and CD8+ T cells than healthy controls.

*Conclusion.*—In addition to similar clinical features, patients with CHIKV infection and patients with RA develop very similar peripheral T cell phenotypes. These overlapping clinical and immunologic features highlight a need for rheumatologists to consider CHIKV infection when evaluating patients with new, symmetric polyarthritis.

► Chikungunya virus (CHIKV) is a mosquito-transmitted virus that was first reported in Africa in the 1950s. Outbreaks have subsequently occurred in Africa, Asia, Europe, and the regions of the Indian and Pacific Oceans. In 2013, it was reported in the Caribbean and subsequently in Florida. There is great potential for CHIKV to spread throughout the United States. The most common symptoms of CHIKV are fever, joint pain, and rash.

The authors of this article reported on 10 travelers to Haiti who developed CHIKV at the same time. They found that 8 of the 10 travelers developed chronic arthritis that was similar to seronegative rheumatoid arthritis (RA). Not only did the clinical features meet the criteria for the diagnosis of RA, but the immunophenotypes of the cells tested in the synovium were similar to those seen in patients with early, untreated RA. A limitation of this study is the small number of patients; however, that being said, all of the patients developed CHIKV around the same time and were monitored and proven to have CHIKV. The findings suggest that CHIKV be considered in the differential diagnosis of patients who develop chronic arthritis and have a relevant travel history. Unfortunately, the chronic arthritis associated with CHIKV typically does not respond to immunosuppression, making it a form of chronic arthritis that is more difficult to manage.

This summer, many of my patients were traveling to the Caribbean and to Florida, and I made it a point to counsel them on preventing mosquito bites. Travelers can protect themselves from mosquito bites with insect repellent, staying in places with air conditioning, with the use of window screens, and by wearing long sleeves and pants.

**A. Sammut, MD**

**PART TWO**

# INFECTIOUS DISEASE

NANCY M. KHARDORI, MD, PhD

# Introduction

This year, the "news" has been about the Zika virus following in quick succession to Ebola virus last year. Since 1947, it caused sporadic cases of infection in Africa and Southeast Asia. Large outbreaks were reported from Micronesia in 2007 and from French Polynesia in 2013. The first local transmission in the Americas occurred in May 2015. Active transmission of the virus has been reported from 48 countries in a short period of time. The unique association of congenital infection by this virus with devastating neurological consequences has become a grave public health concern. The infection in adults is mostly asymptomatic, making diagnosis difficult and currently there is no treatment or vaccine. A number of vaccine candidates are under study.

The ongoing resistance and dwindling number of antibiotics available for treatment of common infections is being addressed through a number of ways including the study of newer classes of antibiotics and novel treatment strategies. A new antibiotic Solithromycin (an oral fluroketolide) was reported as being 100% effective for treatment of culture-proven gonorrhea at genital and extra-genital sites. For other gram negative bacteria, particularly multi-resistant ones, not much has been found or added. On the other hand, a long list of antibiotics has become available for treatment of gram positive pathogens including MRSA and VRE. Using a combination of Vancomycin and Beta lactams for MRSA has been shown to shorten the duration of therapy in a multicenter randomized controlled trial. An antibody antibiotic conjugate targets S. aureus inside the host cells in an experimental mouse model. If this concept works in human infections, complications from persistence of viable S. aureus inside host cells in spite of antimicrobial therapy will decrease significantly. Using whole genome sequencing, the demonstration that alternating antibiotic treatments constrain evolutionary paths to multidrug resistance brings back for consideration the concept of antibiotic cycling or rotation for groups of patients in the interest of retaining their efficacy. The search for "ideal" killer phages to treat resistant bacterial infections has recently picked up and phage therapy may become a reality. Echinocandin resistance in candida species, in particular C. glabrata, points to the problem of emerging resistance to antifungals on the horizon.

Clostridium difficile continues to cause significant morbidity and mortality in the hospitalized patient population. Some of the more recent increase in the rate seems to be related to "overcall" caused by the use of PCR only for testing. An algorithm of screening tests, GDH or PCR followed by or with toxin testing, seems to be more appropriate. The controversy over the use of contact precaution for MRSA has finally settled in favor of focusing on the adherence to good hand hygiene practices and standard precautions except for patients with uncontrolled wound drainage or respiratory secretions.

The use of Matrix-Assisted Laser Desorption Ionization-Time of Flight Mass Spectrometry (MALDI-TOF MS) for identification of bacteria and yeast is becoming more available. Its use for identification of mycobacteria and norcardia species has now been shown to be feasible in spite of involving more complex technology.

The demonstration that asymptomatic humans transmit dengue virus to mosquitoes brings a fundamental change in the current paradigm for epidemiology and control of dengue virus disease. The genotype spectrum of Hepatitis C virus has now been extended to genotype 7 which may have an impact on management strategies. This year, the report of a stable trimeric influenza hemagglutinin stem as a broadly protective immunogen adds to the list of potential universal as opposed to seasonal vaccines for influenza. VirScan, a comprehensive method for serological profiling, paves the way for defining "human virome" and its role in health and disease. Speaking of viruses, not much has changed in the area of day to day HIV infection management. However, the quest for cure continues. Two publications discussed in this edition describe innovative molecular constructs designed to selectively kill the rare latently infected cells responsible for virologic and clinical relapse if antiretroviral treatment is interrupted. Most appropriately, the concept has been labeled "Cure by Killing".

Immunologic data discussed in one of the selections for this issue argues that the common view of vitamin D as an anti-inflammatory immune response modifier is an oversimplification. The data does not provide rationale for widespread self-medication with Vitamin D supplements for beneficial effect against bacteria or viruses.

Once again, I wish to gratefully acknowledge the excellent and timely assistance of Ms. Doris Murray in preparing my selected materials for submission to the 2016 Edition of Year Book of Medicine.

**Nancy M. Khardori, MD, PhD**

# 15 Bacterial Infections

**Impact of Policies on the Rise in Sepsis Incidence, 2000–2010**

Gohil SK, for the Centers for Disease Control and Prevention Epicenters Program (Univ of California, Irvine; et al)

*Clin Infect Dis* 62:695-703, 2015

*Background.*—Sepsis hospitalizations have increased dramatically in the last decade. It is unclear whether this represents an actual rise in sepsis illness or improved capture by coding. We evaluated the impact of Centers of Medicare and Medicaid Services (CMS) guidance after newly introduced sepsis codes and medical severity diagnosis-related group (MS-DRG) systems on sepsis trends.

*Methods.*—In this retrospective cohort study of California hospitalizations from January 2000 to December 2010, sepsis was identified by *International Classification of Diseases, Ninth Revision* (ICD-9) coding (Dombrovskiy method). Sepsis-associated mortality rates were calculated. Logistic regression models evaluated variables associated with sepsis and mortality. Segmented regression time series analysis assessed changes in sepsis frequency for (1) baseline (January 2000 to September 2003); (2) post-CMS guidelines on sepsis coding (October 2003 to September 2007); and (3) after the introduction of MS-DRG (October 2007 to December 2010).

*Results.*—Annual hospitalizations with sepsis diagnoses tripled within a decade, from 21.1 to 59.9 cases per 1000 admissions, with a 2.8- and 2.0-fold increase in severe and nonsevere sepsis, respectively, whereas annual admissions remained unchanged and sepsis-associated mortality decreased. Greatest increases were seen for severe sepsis present on admission (3.8-fold increase). Increases in sepsis were temporally correlated with CMS coding guidance and MS-DRG introduction after adjustment for comorbidity and other factors.

*Conclusions.*—Sepsis rate increases were associated with introduction of CMS-issued guidance for new sepsis ICD-9 coding and MSDRGs. Coding artifact ("up-capture" of less severely ill septic patients) may be contributing to the apparent rise in sepsis incidence and decline in mortality. Epidemiologic trends based on administrative data should account for policy-related effects.

► In the United States, hospitalization for sepsis has steadily increased over the past 2 decades. Sepsis now ranks as the most expensive condition associated with hospitalization at 15.4 billion dollars annually.[1] Ongoing national and global efforts are being made to improve awareness, early recognition, diagnosis, and management of sepsis. In parallel, significant changes in sepsis coding criteria, definitions, and reimbursements have occurred. The introduction of *International Classification of Diseases, Ninth Revision* (ICD-9) codes in the 995.9x series in October 2002 allowed specific sepsis diagnosis within a single code. The Centers of Medicare and Medicaid Services (CMS)[2] updated the previous diagnosis-related group (DRG) reimbursement system into the current medical severity DRG (MS-DRG) system to tie reimbursements to medical severity. Whether the sepsis rate increases as measured by large-scale administrative data may at least in part represent "up-capture" of sepsis diagnosis in which patients not previously categorized as having sepsis might be more likely to be put into this category is the possibility explored in this study. If this is a possibility, such coding practices can have an important impact on the epidemiology of other parameters, including sepsis-associated mortality. This is a retrospective cohort study of hospitalizations in California from January 1, 2000, to December 31, 2010, using comprehensive statewide data from the California Mandatory Hospital Discharge Data Set with includes up to 25 sepsis administrative codes for medical and procedural diagnoses. The data show that a significant portion of increase in the reported incidence of sepsis is temporally related to CMS policy changes that affected sepsis coding and reimbursement. These changes seem to have led to the up-capture of sepsis-related codes. There has been a 3.6-fold increase in the primary diagnosis of sepsis with 1.4-fold decrease in pneumonia as the primary diagnosis and decrease in sepsis-associated mortality. The number of total admissions remained stable over the study period. The data strongly suggest preferential exchange of other infection diagnoses for sepsis diagnoses.

**N. M. Khardori, MD, PhD**

*References*

1. Hall MJ, Williams SN, DeFrances CJ, Golosinskiy A. Inpatient care for septicemia or sepsis: a challenge for patients and hospitals. *NCHS Data Brief*. 2011;(62):1-8.
2. Centers for Medicare and Medicaid Services. Medicare program: changes to the hospital inpatient prospective payment systems. 2007. https://www.cms.golv/Medicare/Medicare-Fee for Service-Payment/AcutelnpatientPPS/dowloads/cms.1533.fc.pdf. Accessed August 2014.

## Extensive Household Outbreak of Urinary Tract Infection and Intestinal Colonization due to Extended-Spectrum β-Lactamase–Producing *Escherichia coli* Sequence Type 131

Madigan T, Johnson JR, Clabots C, et al (Mayo Clinic, Rochester, MN; Univ of Minnesota, Minneapolis)
*Clin Infect Dis* 61:e5-e12, 2015

*Background.*—Reasons for the successful global dissemination of multidrug-resistant *Escherichia coli* sequence type 131 (ST131) are undefined, but may include enhanced transmissibility or ability to colonize the intestine compared with other strains.

*Methods.*—We identified a household in which 2 young children had urinary tract infection (UTI) caused by an extended-spectrum β-lactamase (ESBL)–producing, multidrug-resistant ST131 *E. coli* strain. We assessed the prevalence of ST131 intestinal colonization among the 7 household members (6 humans, 1 dog). Fecal samples, collected 3 times over a 19-week period, were cultured selectively for *E. coli*. Isolates were characterized using clone-specific polymerase chain reaction to detect ST131 and its ESBL-associated *H*30Rx subclone, pulsed-field gel electrophoresis, extended virulence genotyping, and antimicrobial susceptibility testing.

*Results.*—In total, 8 different *E. coli* pulsotypes (strains) were identified. The index patient's urine isolate represented ST131-*H*30Rx strain 903. This was the most widely shared and persistent strain in the household, colonizing 5 individuals at each sampling. In contrast, the 7 non-ST131 strains were each found in only 1 or 2 household members at a time, with variable persistence. The ST131 strain was the only strain with both extensive virulence and antimicrobial resistance profiles.

*Conclusions.*—An ESBL-producing ST131-*H*30Rx strain caused UTI in 2 siblings, plus asymptomatic intestinal colonization in multiple other household members, and was the household's most extensively detected and persistent fecal *E. coli* strain. Efficient transmission and intestinal colonization may contribute to the epidemiologic success of the H30Rx subclone of *E. coli* ST131.

▶ *Escherichia coli* strains causing extraintestinal infections (ExPEC) including urinary tract infections (UTIs) colonize the human intestinal tract but have enhanced capacity to cause extraintestinal infections.[1] There has been a rapid global emergence and spread of antimicrobial-resistant ExPEC strains largely due to the colonial expansion of a single sequence type, ST131. Few studies have assessed uninfected household contacts of patients with ST131 infection.

The authors of this study identified a household with UTI in 2 young children caused by an ESBL-producing multidrug-resistant ST131 *E coli* strain. The children lacked the traditional risk factors for antimicrobial resistance. All household members were evaluated for intestinal colonization with antibiotic resistant *E coli* over a 19-week period. A total of 18 stool samples were provided by 6 human household members (3 each at 0, 10, and 19 weeks). No *E coli* was found in the single fecal specimen from the pet dog. Clone specific polymerase chain reaction, pulsed-field electrophoresis, extended virulence genotyping, and antimicrobial susceptibility were performed on all isolates. *E coli* ST131 was highly prevalent and persistent over the 19-week study period as an intestinal colonizer among all human household members. The mother shared more strains than the father with the children. The data provide evidence that *E coli* ST131 is a persistent intestinal colonizer that is efficiently transmitted among household members. The health care employment history of parents suggests possible acquisition of the strain from a health care associated reservoir and importation into the household. This colony includes highly resistant and virulent strains with a superior ability to colonize the human intestinal tract and to spread among household contacts, putting children without traditional risk factors for antibiotic resistance at risk of severe and potentially life-threatening infection.

**N. M. Khardori, MD, PhD**

*Reference*

1. Johnson JR, Russo TA. Extraintestinal pathogenic *Escherichia coli*: "The other bad *E. coli*". *J Lab Clin Med.* 2002;139:155-162.

---

**Combination of Vancomycin and β-Lactam Therapy for Methicillin-Resistant *Staphylococcus aureus* Bacteremia: A Pilot Multicenter Randomized Controlled Trial**

Davis JS, for the Combination Antibiotics for MEthicillin Resistant *Staphylococcus aureus* (CAMERA) study group and for the Australasian Society for Infectious Diseases Clinical Research Network (Menzies School of Health Res, Casuarina Northern Territory, Australia; et al)

*Clin Infect Dis* 62:173-180, 2016

---

*Background.*—In vitro laboratory and animal studies demonstrate a synergistic role for the combination of vancomycin and antistaphylococcal β-lactams for methicillin-resistant *Staphylococcus aureus* (MRSA) bacteremia. Prospective clinical data are lacking.

*Methods.*—In this open-label, multicenter, clinical trial, adults with MRSA bacteremia received vancomycin 1.5 g intravenously twice daily and were randomly assigned (1:1) to receive intravenous flucloxacillin 2 g every 6 hours for 7 days (combination group) or no additional therapy (standard therapy group). Participants were stratified by hospital and randomized in permuted blocks of variable size. Randomization codes were kept in sealed, sequentially numbered, opaque envelopes. The primary outcome was the duration of MRSA bacteremia in days.

*Results.*—We randomly assigned 60 patients to receive vancomycin (n = 29), or vancomycin plus flucloxacillin (n = 31). The mean duration of bacteremia was 3.00 days in the standard therapy group and 1.94 days in the combination group. According to a negative binomial model, the mean time to resolution of bacteremia in the combination group was 65% (95% confidence interval, 41%–102%; *P* = .06) that in the standard therapy group. There was no difference in the secondary end points of 28- and 90-day mortality, metastatic infection, nephrotoxicity, or hepatotoxicity.

*Conclusions.*—Combining an antistaphylococcal β-lactam with vancomycin may shorten the duration of MRSA bacteremia. Further trials with a larger sample size and objective clinically relevant end points are warranted.

Australian New Zealand Clinical Trials Registry: ACTRN 12610000940077 (www.anzctr.org.au) (Table 3).

▶ The all cause 30-day mortality was recently shown to be 30% for methicillin-resistant *Staphylococcus aureus* (MRSA) bacteremia compared to 17.7% for

TABLE 3.—Primary Outcome Measure

| Population[a] | Duration of Bacteremia, d[b] | | Ratio of Means (95% CI) | P Value |
|---|---|---|---|---|
| | Standard Therapy | Combination Therapy | | |
| ITT population | | | | |
| Mean (SD) | 3.00 (3.35) | 1.94 (1.79) | 0.65 (0.41–1.02) | .06 |
| Median (IQR) | 1 (1–2) | 1 (1–4) | ... | ... |
| Per-protocol population | | | | |
| Mean (SD) | 2.92 (3.37) | 1.82 (1.59) | 0.62 (0.38–1.01) | .055 |
| Median (IQR) | 1 (1–2) | 1 (1–4) | ... | ... |

Abbreviations: CI, confidence interval; IQR, interquartile range; ITT, intention-to-treat; SD, standard deviation.
[a]The ITT population included 29 patients in the standard therapy and 31 in the combination therapy group; the per-protocol population, 26 and 28 patients, respectively.
[b]Duration of bacteremia in days follows a negative binomial distribution.
Reprinted from Davis JS, for the Combination Antibiotics for MEthicillin Resistant *Staphylococcus aureus* (CAMERA) Study Group and for the Australasian Society for Infectious Diseases Clinical Research Network. Combination of vancomycin and β-lactam therapy for methicillin-resistant *Staphylococcus aureus* bacteremia: a pilot multicenter randomized controlled trial. *Clin Infect Dis*. 2016;62:173-180, with permission from The Author.

bacteremia due to methicillin-susceptible *S aureus* (MSSA). The higher mortality associated with MRSA has been attributed to differences in underlying host factors and/or limitations of vancomycin, the most commonly used antistaphylococcal agent.[1] Vancomycin is known to demonstrate slow bacterial killing, poorer tissue penetration, and slower clearance of bacteremia, all of which lead to higher mortality.[2] The more recent anti-MRSA agents like linezolid, daptomycin, and ceftaroline have all been found to be noninferior to vancomycin for MRSA bacteremia. They are all associated with high cost and higher risk of adverse effects.

This is a pilot multicenter randomized controlled trial of a combination of vancomycin and betalactam therapy for MRSA bacteremia. Patients were recruited in a 1:1 randomization fashion at 7 Australian hospitals between January 2011 and May 2014. Using other standard management for MRSA bacteremia, patients were randomized to receive either vancomycin alone or a combination of vancomycin plus intravenous flucloxacillin. The primary end point of duration of MRSA bacteremia in days and secondary end points of nephrotoxicity, hepatotoxicity, all cause 90-day mortality, recurrence of bacteremia, metastatic complications during the first 10 days and requirement for intensive care unit admission or development of septic shock after randomization were assessed. As shown in Table 3, there is a difference in primary outcome in both intent to treat and per-protocol population with *P* values of .06 and .055, respectively. The addition of nafcillin or oxacillin to daptomycin has previously shown to clear persistent MRSA bacteremia. In vitro, 17 studies have demonstrated synergy between vancomycin and betalactams against MRSA and VISA. The proposed mechanisms include potentiation of host defense peptide activity against *S aureus* and reduced transcription of mecA with increased susceptibility to betalactams.[3,4]

**N. M. Khardori, MD, PhD**

*References*

1. Deresinski S. Vancomycin: does it still have a role as an antistaphylococcal agent? *Expert Rev Anti Infec Ther.* 2007;5:393-401.
2. Lodise TP Jr, McKinnon PS, Levine DP, Rybak MJ. Impact of empirical-therapy selection on outcomes of intravenous drug users with infective endocarditis caused by methicillin-susceptible *Staphylococcus aureus. Antimicrob Agents Chemother.* 2007;51:3731-3733.
3. Sakoulas G, Okumura CY, Thienphrapa W, et al. Nafcillin enhances innate immune-mediated killing of methicillin-resistant *Staphylococcus aureus. J Mol Med (Berl).* 2014;92:139-149.
4. Ortwine JK, Werth BJ, Sakoulas G, Rybak MJ. Reduced glycopeptide and lipopeptide susceptibility in *Staphylococcus aureus* and the "seesaw effect": taking advantage of the back door left open? *Drug Resist Update.* 2013;16:73-79.

## Increased Risk of Pyogenic Liver Abscess Among Patients With Colonic Diverticular Diseases: A Nationwide Cohort Study

Tsai M-S, Lee H-M, Hsin M-C, et al (E-Da Hosp and I-Shou Univ, Kaohsiung, Taiwan; et al)
*Medicine* 94:e2210, 2015

Whether patients with diverticular diseases exhibit a higher risk of developing pyogenic liver abscess (PLA) remains inconclusive.

From the inpatient claims in Taiwan's National Health Insurance Research Database, we identified 54,147 patients diagnosed with diverticulosis in the 1998 to 2010 period and 216,588 controls without the disorder. The 2 cohorts were matched by age, sex, and admission year, and were followed up until the end of 2010 to estimate the risk of PLA.

Overall, the incidence of PLA was 2.44-fold higher in the diverticular-disease group than in the controls (11.5 vs 4.65 per 10,000 person-year). The adjusted hazard ratio (aHR) of PLA was 2.11 (95% confidence interval [CI], 1.81–2.44) for the diverticular-disease group, according to a multivariate Cox proportional hazards regression model. The age specific data showed that the aHR for the diverticular-disease group, compared with the controls, was the highest inpatients younger than 50 years old (aHR, 4.03; 95% CI, 2.77–5.85). Further analysis showed that the diverticular-disease group exhibited an elevated risk of PLA regardless of whether patients had diverticulitis.

The patients with diverticular diseases exhibited a higher risk of PLA (Table 1).

▶ Liver abscesses caused by bacteria (pyogenic liver abscess [PLA]) is a serious infection that can be fatal without prompt recognition and treatment.[1] The underlying risk factors and the microbiology of PLA differs in various parts of the world. Diverticular diseases of the colon are a common health problem worldwide and most frequently observed pathology on routine colonoscopy. In those older than 45 years, the prevalence of diverticular disease is around 33%. The breakdown of colonic mucosal barrier is a risk factor for multiple complications including PLA. The colonic mucosal defects serve as a source of

**TABLE 1.**—Characteristics of Patients Between Patients With Diverticular and Patients Without Diverticular

| | Diverticular | | | | |
|---|---|---|---|---|---|
| | Yes (N = 54,147) | | No (N = 216,588) | | |
| | n | % | n | % | *P*-Value |
| Age, year | | | | | 0.99 |
| ≦49 | 20,089 | (37.1) | 80,356 | (37.1) | |
| 50–64 | 12,634 | (23.3) | 50,536 | (23.3) | |
| ≥65 | 21,424 | (39.6) | 85,696 | (39.6) | |
| Mean (SD)* | 57.7 | (18.1) | 57.2 | (18.1) | 0.001 |
| Gender | | | | | 0.99 |
| Female | 23,953 | (44.2) | 95,812 | (44.2) | |
| Male | 30,194 | (55.8) | 120,776 | (55.8) | |
| Comorbidity | | | | | |
| Diabetes mellitus | | | | | <0.001 |
| Hypertension | 16,871 | (31.2) | 35,861 | (16.6) | <0.001 |
| Hyperlipidemia | 4564 | (8.43) | 9394 | (4.34) | <0.001 |
| Cancer | 2397 | (4.43) | 7804 | (4.43) | <0.001 |
| COPD | 4267 | (7.88) | 7904 | (3.65) | <0.001 |
| Heart failure | 3002 | (5.54) | 5911 | (2.73) | <0.001 |
| Choledocholithiasis | 4759 | (8.79) | 6413 | (2.96) | <0.001 |
| Alcoholic liver disease | 1167 | (2.16) | 1074 | (0.50) | <0.001 |
| Liver cirrhosis | 1917 | (3.54) | 2439 | (1.13) | <0.001 |
| Cholangitis | 836 | (1.54) | 1113 | (0.51) | <0.001 |
| Cholecystitis | 1614 | (2.98) | 1718 | (0.79) | <0.001 |
| Pancreatic diseases | 1893 | (3.50) | 2120 | (0.98) | <0.001 |

Chi-square test. COPD = chronic obstructive pulmonary disease, SD = standard deviation.
**t*-test.
Reprinted from Tsai M-S, Lee H-M, Hsin M-C, et al. Increased risk of pyogenic liver abscess among patients with colonic diverticular diseases: a nationwide cohort study. *Medicine*. 2015;94:e2210, with permission from Wolters Kluwer Health, Inc.

hematogenous pathogens to the liver by invasion into the portal system.[2] In Asia PLA has been shown to be associated with diabetes mellitus or a cryptogenic etiology.[3]

This study analyzes Taiwan's National Health Insurance Research Database (NHIRD) composed of de-identified medical claims from 99% of the 23 million residents. *International Classification of Disease* (9th revision) codes for newly diagnosed diverticular diseases including diverticulosis and diverticulitis between 2000 and 2011 were used for the study. As shown in Table 1, the principal diseases, including hypertension, hyperlipidemia, chronic obstructive pulmonary disease, cancer, heart failure, choledocholithiasis, cirrhosis, cholangitis, cholecystitis, pancreatic diseases, and percutaneous aspiration of the gallbladder and biliary tract, were higher in the diverticular disease cohort. Comparing the incidence of PLA in the 2 groups, diverticular diseases were associated with a significantly higher risk of PLA (2.44-fold). The adjusted hazards ratio for developing PLA during follow-up was 2.10 for the diverticular disease cohort compared to nondiverticular disease cohort. The incidence and relative risk of PLA was significantly higher in patients with diverticulosis (2.26) followed by patients with diverticulitis (1.98). Recent studies have reported a lower but still significant in-hospital mortality (2.5%–10%) for PLA mostly related to delayed diagnosis.[4] The data in this study point to the possibility of direct bacterial translocation through intact intestinal mucosa.

**N. M. Khardori, MD, PhD**

*References*

1. Cerwenka H, Bacher H, Werkgartner G, et al. Treatment of patients with pyogenic liver abscess. *Chemotherapy.* 2005;51:366-369.
2. Jeong SW, Jang JY, Lee TH, et al. Cryptogenic pyogenic liver abscess as the herald of colon cancer. *J Gastroenterol Hepatol.* 2012;27:248-255.
3. Wang J, Yan Y, Xue X, et al. Comparison of pyogenic liver abscesses caused by hypermucoviscous *Klebsiella pneumoniae* and non-*Klebsiella pneumoniae* pathogens in Beijing: a retrospective analysis. *J Int Med Res.* 2013;41:1088-1097.
4. Rahimian J, Wilson T, Oram V, et al. Pyogenic liver abscess: recent trends in etiology and mortality. *Clin Infect Dis.* 2004;39:1654-1659.

## Asymptomatic Bacteriuria Treatment Is Associated With a Higher Prevalence of Antibiotic Resistant Strains in Women With Urinary Tract Infections

Cai T, Nesi G, Mazzoli S, et al (Santa Chiara Regional Hosp, Trento, Italy, Univ of Florence, Italy; Univ of Pisa, Italy)
*Clin Infect Dis* 61:1655-1661, 2015

*Background.*—Women suffering from recurrent urinary tract infections (rUTIs) are routinely treated for asymptomatic bacteriuria (AB), but the consequences of this procedure on antibiotic resistance are not fully known. The aim of this study was to evaluate the impact of AB treatment on antibiotic resistance among women with rUTIs.

*Methods.*—The study population consisted of 2 groups of women who had previously been enrolled in a randomized clinical trial: group A was not treated, and group B was treated. All women were scheduled for follow-up visits every 6 months, or more frequently if symptoms arose. Microbiological evaluation was performed only in symptomatic women. All women were followed up for a mean of 38.8 months to analyze data from urine cultures and antibiograms.

*Results.*—The previous study population consisted of 673 women, but 123 did not attend the entire follow-up period. For the final analysis, 257 of the remaining 550 patients were assigned to group A, and 293 to group B. At the end of follow-up, the difference in recurrence rates was statistically significant ($P < .001$): 97 (37.7%) in group A versus 204 (69.6%) in group B. Isolated *Escherichia coli* from group B showed higher resistance to amoxicillin–clavulanic acid ($P = .03$), trimethoprim-sulfamethoxazole ($P = .01$), and ciprofloxacin ($P = .03$) than that from group A.

*Conclusions.*—This study shows that AB treatment is associated with a higher occurrence of antibiotic-resistant bacteria, indicating that AB treatment in women with rUTIs is potentially dangerous.

► Asymptomatic bacteriuria (AB) is defined as the presence of bacteria in urine without signs and symptoms of urinary tract infection (UTI). Treatment for AB is generally recommended only during pregnancy and before urologic surgery in men.[1] However, the overuse and inappropriate use of antibiotics in this setting has been recognized to lead to increased antimicrobial resistance as well as higher health care costs. AB is treated in women without any clear indication for treatment and with a high risk of selecting multidrug-resistant bacteria. Cai et al in a randomized controlled clinical study demonstrated that during a 1-year period, treating AB in patients with "recurrent" UTI was associated with a higher rate of symptomatic UTIs.[2] These findings suggest that AB may play a protective role in preventing symptomatic recurrence of UTI. This study investigated the impact of AB treatment in women with a history of UTIs on the development of antibiotic-resistant bacteria.

The study population is 550 women of 673 women used in the recurrence rate study by the same group of investigators. All patients had scheduled follow-ups every 6 months, or more often in the case of recurring symptoms. All episodes of symptomatic UTIs were recorded and treated with antibiotics based on antimicrobial susceptibility testing. Microbiological evaluation was performed only in symptomatic patients. Of the 550 enrolled patients, 257 were assigned to the no treatment group (Group A) and 293 to the treatment group (Group B). A statistically significant difference was noted in recurrence rates between the 2 groups (37.7% in Group A vs 69.6% in Group B). The bacteria (*Escherichia* coli) isolated from Group B showed higher resistance to amoxicillin-clavulanic acid, trimethoprim-sulfamethoxazole, and ciprofloxacin. These data provide evidence for double jeopardy in treating AB with antibiotics.

**N. M. Khardori, MD, PhD**

*References*

1. Hooton TM, Scholes D, Stapleton AE, et al. A prospective study of asymptomatic bacteriuria in sexually active young women. *N Engl J Med.* 2000;343:992-997.
2. Cai T, Mazzoli S, Mondaini N, et al. The role of asymptomatic bacteriuria in young women with recurrent urinary tract infections: to treat or not to treat? *Clin Infect Dis.* 2012;55:771-777.

## Capsule Switching and Antimicrobial Resistance Acquired during Repeated *Streptococcus pneumoniae* Pneumonia Episodes

Chang B, Nariai A, Sekizuka T, et al (Natl Inst of Infectious Diseases, Tokyo, Japan; Yokohama Minami Kyosai Hosp, Kanagawa, Japan; et al)
*J Clin Microbiol* 53:3318-3324, 2015

*Streptococcus pneumoniae* colonizes the nasopharyngeal mucus in healthy people and causes otitis media, pneumonia, bacteremia, and meningitis. In this study, we analyzed an *S. pneumoniae* strain that caused 7 repeated pneumonia episodes in an 80-month-old patient with cerebral palsy during a period of 25 months. A total of 10 *S. pneumoniae* strains were obtained from sputum samples, and serotype 6B was isolated from samples from the first 5 episodes, whereas serotype 6A was isolated from samples from the last 2. Whole-genome sequencing showed clonality of the 10 isolates with 10 single nucleotide polymorphisms (SNPs) in the genomes. Among these SNPs, one single point mutation in the *wciP* gene was presumed to relate to the serotype switching from 6B to 6A, and the other mutations in *parC* and *gyrA* were related to fluoroquinolone resistance. These results suggested that an *S. pneumoniae* strain, which asymptomatically colonized the patient's nasopharynx or was horizontally transmitted from an asymptomatic carrier, caused the repeated pneumonia events. Phenotypic variations in the capsule type and antimicrobial susceptibility occurred during the carrier state. Hyporesponsiveness to serotypes 6B and 6A of *S. pneumoniae* was found even after vaccination with the 7-valent pneumococcal conjugate vaccine and the 23-valent pneumococcal polysaccharide vaccine. After an additional vaccination with the 13-valent pneumococcal conjugate vaccine, opsonic activities for both serotypes 6A and 6B significantly increased and are expected to prevent relapse by the same strain.

▶ Invasive disease caused by *Streptococcus pneumoniae* is preceded by colonization, which is also responsible for transmission.[1] The widespread use of 7- and now 13-valent pneumococcal conjugate vaccines has reduced the incidence of pneumococcal infections and the colonization rate by vaccine serotypes but has not affected overall colonization.[2,3] Also, breakthrough infections and some unusual vaccine failures have been reported.[4]

The authors of this article have observed repeated pneumococcal pneumonia episodes in a child with congenital cerebral palsy and multiple severe handicaps since 2011. An additional 6 pneumococcal pneumonia episodes occured in the 24 months following PCV7 vaccination and earlier PPSV23. This study analyzes 10 *S pneumoniae* isolated from the 7 pneumonia episodes using serotyping, antimicrobial susceptibility testing, molecular typing (MLST), whole genome sequencing (WGS), and host immune response against *S pneumoniae*. The same *S pneumoniae* strain ST 4250 (Serotype 6B) or a closely related genetic strain was identified as the cause of infection during all episodes. This serotype is present in both PCV7 and PPSV23. Hyporesponsiveness to 6B in PCV7 in children has been reported. Only 1 more strain, ST4240, belonging to serotype 6B was isolated in Japanese children between 2007 and 2014. Sustained colonization by the ST4250 strain in the patient's nasopharyngeal mucosa was suspected. However, only normal flora and no *S pneumoniae* was recovered between episodes of infection. Pneumonia was acute each time, completely cured, and did not cause a biofilm. Only 10 single nucleotide polymorphisms were detected in this strain pointing to low frequency of recombination.

The cause of hyporesponsiveness to 6B serotype in PPSV23 in this patient is not clear. However, results suggest that insufficient opsonization activity against serotype B or horizontal transmission may be the reason for repeated infections. The switch from 6B to 6A serotype after the 5th episode along with development of fluoroquinolone resistance favors that conclusion. Further vaccination with PCV13 led to effective 6B and 6A specific antibody production. The likelihood of horizontal transmission in this patient emphasizes the significance of routine precautions to prevent transmission.

**N. M. Khardori, MD, PhD**

*References*

1. Simell B, Auranen K, Kayhty H, Goldblatt D, Dagan R, O'Brien KL. Pneumococcal Carriage Group. The fundamental link between pneumococcal carriage and disease. *Expert Rev Vaccines*. 2012;11:841-855.
2. Simonsen L, Taylor RJ, Schuck-Paim C, Lustig R, Haber M, Klugman KP. Effect of 13-valent pneumococcal conjugate vaccine on admissions to hospital 2 years after its introduction in the USA: a time series analysis. *Lancet Respir Med*. 2014;2:387-394.
3. Lee GM, Kleinman K, Pelton SI, et al. Impact of 13-valent pneumococcal conjugate vaccination on Streptococcus pneumoniae carriage in young children in Massachusetts. *J Pediatric Infect Dis Soc*. 2014;3:23-32.
4. Oishi T, Ishiwada N, Matsubara K, et al. Japanese IPD Study Group. Low opsonic activity to the infecting serotype in pediatric patients with invasive pneumococcal disease. *Vaccine*. 2013;31:845-849.

# 16 Viral Infections

**Zika Virus and Pregnancy: What Obstetric Health Care Providers Need to Know**

Meaney-Delman D, Rasmussen SA, Staples JE, et al (Ctrs for Disease Control and Prevention, Atlanta, GA)

*Obstet Gynecol* 127:642-648, 2016

Zika virus is a flavivirus transmitted by *Aedes (Stegomyia)* species of mosquitoes. In May 2015, the World Health Organization confirmed the first local transmission of Zika virus in the Americas in Brazil. The virus has spread rapidly to other countries in the Americas; as of January 29, 2016, local transmission has been detected in at least 22 countries or territories, including the Commonwealth of Puerto Rico and the U.S. Virgin Islands. Zika virus can infect pregnant women in all three trimesters. Although pregnant women do not appear to be more susceptible to or more severely affected by Zika virus infection, maternal–fetal transmission has been documented. Several pieces of evidence suggest that maternal Zika virus infection is associated with adverse neonatal outcomes, most notably microcephaly. Because of the number of countries and territories with local Zika virus transmission, it is likely that obstetric health care providers will care for pregnant women who live in or have traveled to an area of local Zika virus transmission. We review information on Zika virus, its clinical presentation, modes of transmission, laboratory testing, effects during pregnancy, and methods of prevention to assist obstetric health care providers in caring for pregnant women considering travel or with a history of travel to areas with ongoing Zika virus transmission and pregnant women residing in areas with ongoing Zika virus transmission.

▶ The first local mosquito-to-human transmission of Zika virus in the Americas (Brazil) was confirmed by the World Health Organization in May 2015. Based on the rapid spread of the virus through the country, Brazilian Ministry of Health estimated that 440 000 to 1 300 000 cases of Zika virus disease had occurred by the end of 2015.[1] The officials noted an unusual increase in the number of newborns with microcephaly in northeast Brazil in October 2015, and by the end of the year, more than 3500 newborns with microcephaly were reported nationally.[2] Zika virus, first identified in 1947 in Uganda in a monkey, is a mosquito-borne flavivirus. In contrast to malaria parasite transmitted by Anophetes type of mosquito, Zika virus is transmitted by the *Aedes* species, most commonly *Aedes aegypti*, which also transmits yellow fever, dengue, and chikungunya viruses. *Aedes albopictus* is the other mosquito species known to transmit Zika virus.

This article is the current commentary on Zika virus and pregnancy with particular attention to prevention recommendations for pregnant American women. In the United States, *A aegypti* has a limited presence in the South, but *A albopictus* has a wider distribution across the Southeastern United States and into the Midwest.[3] Genetic analysis of the currently spreading virus suggests that the Zika virus in Brazil originated from viral strains circulating in French Polynesia and nearby islands during the outbreak of 2013–2014. After the incubation period of 2 days to 2 weeks, the disease is asymptomatic in about 80% of infected humans. In the other 20% symptoms are mild, nonspecific, and indistinguishable from a number of other infections. Guillian-Barre syndrome has been reported as a complication, but severe illness is uncommon and deaths rare. Maternal-fetal transmission occurs throughout pregnancy. Although the full spectrum of congenital Zika virus infection is unknown, microcephaly, brain atrophy, ventricular enlargement, intracranial calcification, ocular defects, scalp rugae, and joint contractures have been reported. The latest information on all aspects, including prevention on Zika virus and pregnancy, is available on the Centers for Disease Control and Prevention website.

**N. M. Khardori, MD, PhD**

*References*


1. Hennessey M, Fischer M, Staples JE. Zika virus spreads to new areas—Region of the Americas, May 2015–January 2016. *MMWR Morb Mortal Wkly Rep*. 2016; 65:55-58.
2. Pan American Health Organization, World Health Organization. Epidemiological update: neurological syndrome, congenital anomalies, and Zika virus infection. 2016. http://www.paho.org/hq/indes-php?option=com_docman&task=doc_download&Itemid=&gid=32879/&lang=en. Accessed January 17, 2016.
3. Kraemer MU, Sinka ME, Duda KA, et al. The global distribution of the arbovirus vectors Aedes aegypti and Ae. albopicuts. *Elife*. 2015;4:e08347.


## HIV: Cure by killing

Richman DD (Univ of California San Diego)
*Nature* 528:198-199, 2015

*Background.*—Combination antiretroviral drug therapy to suppress HIV infection and its complications does not eradicate the virus, but rather allows the formation of a latent reservoir of cells that have HIV DNA integrated into the host cell chromosomes. If therapy is interrupted, the patient can experience a raging infection. Cure will only be achieved if the reservoir is eradicated, and only then can the patient discontinue the costly, inconvenient, and often disabling treatment. A couple of innovative molecular constructs have been proposed to selectively kill these rare, latently infected cells and achieve a cure.

*Methods.*—For latently infected cells to be targeted, the virus must be activated to recommence its replication cycle. Few of the infected cells have responded to currently used agents. Additionally, destroying these cells may rely on the patient's immune response, which is already compromised and may be linked to the initial viral agent, not a mutated version. These problems are being addressed by using protein constructs that combine the binding specificities of two different antibodies, with one binding to a broad spectrum of HIV envelope proteins found on the surface of actively infected cells and the other to the molecule CD3, which is found on the surface of all T cells. This approach is designed to direct the $CD8^+$ subset of T cells, with their cell-killing ability, to kill latently infected cells that are expressing envelope proteins. Binding to CD3 allows any $CD8^+$ T cells to be targeted to the infected cells. This eliminates the need to have the T cells specifically bind to the HIV surface glycoproteins.

*Results.*—In vitro results indicate that these approaches directly kill the cells as desired. One construct achieved ex vivo efficacy as well. With the other construct, the CD3-binding arm not only activates cytotoxic $CD8^+$ T cells but also activates the latently infected CD4 T cells to express envelope proteins, allowing these cells to be killed. More studies are needed to provide the evidence that there is substantial killing ability with this construct ex vivo.

*Barriers to Success and Conclusions.*—Several biological features must be overcome. First, only one in a million $CD4^+$ T cells in HIV-infected persons is latently infected, so these cells are difficult to detect and measure. Second, none of the agents that induce HIV antigen expression in most latently infected cells do so without affecting non-infected cells. Third, the latent reservoir may include cells in anatomical compartments that large protein constructs cannot penetrate.

Several developmental hurdles also must be addressed. First, in vitro efficacy may not be seen in vivo. Second, target cells and cytotoxic cells may not be as dense or uniformly distributed in actual tissues as in cell cultures. Third, no envelope-binding antigen binds to all HIV envelopes. Fourth, researchers must address the possibility that the virus will mutate and escape recognition. Off-target effects can also be a concern, and protein constructs can induce immune responses, which complicate results.

Constructs that can generate bifunctional capabilities offer an innovative approach to the problem of curing HIV. More work is needed (Fig 1).

▶ The current antiretroviral therapy suppresses HIV replication cycle, resulting in preservation of host immunity and prevention of complications. The replication cycle involves the integration of HIV DNA into the genome of host cells and the generation of new viral particles. The new viral particles are released by budding from the cell. The small proportion of cells that survive the lytic effect of infection go on to form a latent reservoir with HIV DNA integrated into host cell chromosomes. Interruption or resistance to antiretroviral drugs initiates the replication cycle again. For a full cure to occur in the absence of continued antiviral treatment, the reservoir must be eradicated. Drugs such as histone deacetylase inhibitors are designed to induce the transcription of viral RNA and restart of the replication cycle. However, only a small number of

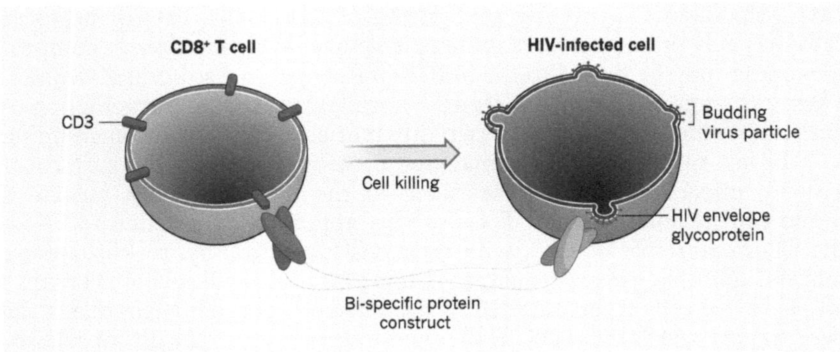


FIGURE 1.—Bi-specific constructs. Sung *et al.*[1] and Pegu *et al.*[2] present two different protein constructs that combine sections of two monoclonal antibodies: one antibody binds to the CD3 molecule expressed on the surface of all T cells of the immune system, and the other binds to envelope proteins of the HIV virus, which are expressed on the surface of infected cells. These constructs direct $CD8^+$ (cytotoxic) T cells to kill HIV-infected cells, regardless of whether receptors on the $CD8^+$ T cell have specificity for the virus. This targeting is designed to increase the efficiency of the anti-HIV immune response and to help clear rare, latently infected cells. *Editor's Note*: Please refer to original journal article for full references. (Reprinted from Richman DD. HIV: cure by killing. *Nature*. 2015;528:198-199, with permission from Macmillan Publishers Limited.)

latently infected cells respond to them. More importantly, this approach is dependent on subsequent destruction of the activated cells by patients' immune response, which may be impaired or targeted against the initially infecting virus that may have escaped immune recognition by mutating. Two recent publications describe innovative molecular constructs designed to selectively kill these rare and latently infected cells.[1,2] Two protein constructs (conceptually similar) combine the binding specificities of 2 antibodies (Fig 1). One antibody binds to the CD3 molecule displayed on the surface of all T cells, and the other binds to a broad spectrum of HIV envelope proteins on the surface of actively infected cells typically CD4. The use of CD3 present on all T cells directs the CD8 (cytotoxic cells) to target the infected cells circumventing the need for these cells to specifically bind to HIV surface glycoproteins. In vitro data presented by both groups show direct killing of cells that express HIV envelope proteins by CD8 cells independent of their antigen specificity. The CD3 binding arm of the construct not only activated cytotoxic CD8 T cells, but also induced infected CD4 cells to express HIV envelope proteins and their killing by the CD8 cells.[2] The Dual-Affinity Re-Targeting (DART) construct killed cells taken from patients with viral suppression from antiretroviral therapy after they had been induced to express envelope proteins by phytohaemagglutinin or histone deacetylase inhibitor. The findings are an early step in the direction of curing HIV infection by killing the virus in latently infected cells.

**N. M. Khardori, MD, PhD**

*References*

1. Sung JAM, Pickeral J, Liu L, et al. Dual-affinity re-targeting proteins direct T cell-mediated cytolysis of latently HIV-infected cells. *J Clin Invest.* 2015;125: 4077-4090.
2. Pegu A, Asokan M, Wu L, et al. Activation and lysis of human CD4 cells latently infected with HIV-1. *Nature Commun.* 2015;6:8447.

**Asymptomatic humans transmit dengue virus to mosquitoes**

Duong V, Lambrechts L, Paul RE, et al (Institut Pasteur in Cambodia, Phnom Penh; Institut Pasteur, Paris, France; Centre National de la Recherche Scientifique, Paris, France; et al)

*Proc Natl Acad Sci U S A* 112:14688-14693, 2015

Three-quarters of the estimated 390 million dengue virus (DENV) infections each year are clinically inapparent. People with inapparent dengue virus infections are generally considered dead-end hosts for transmission because they do not reach sufficiently high viremia levels to infect mosquitoes. Here, we show that, despite their lower average level of viremia, asymptomatic people can be infectious to mosquitoes. Moreover, at a given level of viremia, DENV-infected people with no detectable symptoms or before the onset of symptoms are significantly more infectious to mosquitoes than people with symptomatic infections. Because DENV viremic people without clinical symptoms may be exposed to more mosquitoes through their undisrupted daily routines than sick people and represent the bulk of DENV infections, our data indicate that they have the potential to contribute significantly more to virus transmission to mosquitoes than previously recognized.

▶ Virus transmission to mosquitoes from infected humans leading to ongoing transmission is considered a critical step in the epidemiology of diseases caused by dengue viruses (DENV-1—DENV-4). Infected humans are able to transmit this virus to mosquitoes from 2 days before to 2 days after the onset of symptoms. Of the 390 million dengue virus infections each year, about 300 million (75%) are clinically inapparent. Because of the low-level viremia in patients with clinically inapparent infection, they are generally considered dead-end hosts for transmission. In the only study that reported viral RNA quantification in a limited number of asymptomatic patient did not detect a significantly lower viremia and infectiousness to mosquitoes was not evaluated.[1]

In this study researchers have focused on patients who are asymptomatic or have insufficient symptoms to be detected by existing clinical definition and surveillance symptoms. Based on an earlier publication, they defined "inapparent" or "subclinical" interchangeably to denote infections confirmed by virus detection or seroconversion in patients with insufficient symptoms and not detected by current clinical definitions or epidemiologic methods.[2] "Asymptomatic" was defined as a confirmed DENV infection in the complete absence of reported or detected clinical features. The study design allowed identification of viremia in people before the onset of fever and associated symptoms. The study groups (all over age 4 years) were exposed to mosquitoes from 3 days before to 8 days after the onset of symptoms. The significant and surprising finding in this study is that DENV-infected patients with no detectable symptoms or before the onset of symptoms are significantly more infectious to mosquitoes than symptomatic patients. Such patients may actually be exposed to more mosquitoes through their undisrupted daily routine. At given levels of viremia, asymptomatic subjects were markedly more infectious to mosquitoes than sick symptomatic patients. These results make a fundamental change in the current paradigm for epidemiology and control of DENV based on the focus on patient with apparent illness.

**N. M. Khardori, MD, PhD**

*References*

1. Duong V, Ly S, Lorn Try P, et al. Clinical and virological factors influencing the performance of a NS1 antigen-capture assay and potential use as a marker of dengue disease severity. *PLoS Negl Trop Dis.* 2011;5:e1244.
2. Grange L, Simon-Loriere E, Sakuntabhai A, Gresh L, Paul R, Harris E. Epidemiological risk factors associated with high global frequency of inapparent dengue virus infections. *Front Immunol.* 2014;5:280.

## Analysis of Varicella-Zoster Virus in Temporal Arteries Biopsy Positive and Negative for Giant Cell Arteritis

Nagel MA, White T, Khmeleva N, et al (Univ of Colorado School of Medicine, Aurora; et al)
*JAMA Neurol* 72:1281-1287, 2015

*Importance.*—Giant cell arteritis (GCA) is the most common systemic vasculitis in elderly individuals. Diagnosis is confirmed by temporal artery (TA) biopsy, although biopsy results are often negative. Despite the use of corticosteroids, disease may progress. Identification of causal agents will improve outcomes. Biopsy-positive GCA is associated with TA infection by varicella-zoster virus (VZV).

*Objective.*—To analyze VZV infection in TAs of patients with clinically suspected GCA whose TAs were histopathologically negative and in normal TAs removed post mortem from age-matched individuals.

*Design, Setting, and Participants.*—A cross-sectional study for VZV antigen was performed from January 2013 to March 2015 using archived, deidentified, formalin-fixed, paraffin-embedded GCA-negative, GCA-positive, and normal TAs (50 sections/TA) collected during the past 30 years. Regions adjacent to those containing VZV were examined by hematoxylin-eosin staining. Immunohistochemistry identified inflammatory cells and cell types around nerve bundles containing VZV. A combination of 17 tertiary referral centers and private practices worldwide contributed archived TAs from individuals older than 50 years.

*Main Outcomes and Measures.*—Presence and distribution of VZV antigen in TAs and histopathological changes in sections adjacent to those containing VZV were confirmed by 2 independent readers.

*Results.*—Varicella-zoster virus antigen was found in 45 of 70 GCA-negative TAs (64%), compared with 11 of 49 normal TAs (22%) (relative risk [RR] = 2.86; 95%CI, 1.75-5.31; $P < .001$). Extension of our earlier study revealed VZV antigen in 68 of 93 GCA-positive TAs (73%), compared with 11 of 49 normal TAs (22%) (RR = 3.26; 95%CI, 2.03-5.98; $P < .001$). Compared with normal TAs, VZV antigen was more likely to be present in the adventitia of both GCA-negative TAs (RR = 2.43; 95% CI, 1.82-3.41; $P < .001$) and GCA-positive TAs (RR = 2.03; 95% CI, 1.52-2.86; $P < .001$). Varicella-zoster virus antigen was frequently found in perineurial cells expressing claudin-1 around nerve bundles. Of 45 GCA-negative participants whose TAs contained VZV antigen, 1 had histopathological features characteristic of GCA, and 16 (36%) showed adventitial inflammation adjacent to viral antigen; no inflammation was seen in normal TAs.

*Conclusions and Relevance.*—In patients with clinically suspected GCA, prevalence of VZV in their TAs is similar independent of whether biopsy results are negative or positive pathologically. Antiviral treatment may confer additional benefit to patients with biopsy-negative GCA treated with corticosteroids, although the optimal antiviral regimen remains to be determined.

▶ The hallmark of pathological diagnosis of Giant Cell arteritis (GCA) is inflammation and necrosis in the arterial media, multinucleated giant cells and/or epithelioid macrophages on temporal artery biopsy. Due to skip lesions, pathological results on temporal artery biopsy are negative in many clinically suspected cases. In a recent study, varicella-zoster virus (VZV) was found in 74% (61 of 82) GCA-positive temporal artery biopsies.[1] Furthermore, VZV was demonstrated in temporal arteries from patients with clinically suspected but pathologically negative GCA.[2] Histopathological reexamination of sections adjacent to those containing VZV antigen in a GCA-negative temporal artery revealed classic findings of GCA resulting in a change of pathologic diagnosis.[3]

This report is based on the search for VZV antigen in archived temporal arteries from patients with clinically suspected GCA and negative biopsy results. VZV antigen was found in 27% of normal, 64% of GCA negative and 73% of GCA positive temporal arteries (TAs). The study was performed on archived de-identified formalin-fixed paraffin embedded TAs more than 30 years. There were 49 normal, 70 GCA-negative, and 93 GCA-positive TAs in the study conducted between 2013 and 2015. Fifty sections per TA were studied. These findings point to a strong association between VZV and GCA with VZV antigen present in most clinically suspected GCA with or without pathological hallmarks. The findings make a case for the additional benefit provided by antiviral treatment to patients treated with corticosteroids for clinical diagnosis of GCA.

**N. M. Khardori, MD, PhD**

*References*


1. Gilden D, White T, Khmeleva N, et al. Prevalence and distribution of VZV in temporal arteries of patients with giant cell arteritis. *Neurology.* 2015;84:1948-1955.
2. Mathias M, Nagel MA, Khlevela N, et al. VZV multifocal vasculopathy with ischemic optic neuropathy, acute retinal necrosis and temporal artery infection in the absence of zoster rash. *J Neurol Sci.* 2013;325:180-182.
3. Gildren D, White TM, Nagae L, Gurdin WH, Boyer PJ, Nagel MA. Successful antiviral treatment of giant cell arteritis and Takayasu arteritis. *JAMA Neurol.* 2015;72:943-946.


**Hepatitis E virus and the safety of plasma products: investigations into the reduction capacity of manufacturing processes**

Farcet MR, Lackner C, Antoine G, et al (Global Pathogen Safety, Vienna, Austria)

*Transfusion* 56:383-391, 2016

*Background.*—Hepatitis E virus (HEV) has been transmitted by transfusion of labile blood products and the occasional detection of HEV RNA in plasma pools indicates that HEV viremic donations might enter the manufacturing process of plasma products. To verify the safety margins of plasma products with respect to HEV, virus reduction steps commonly used in their manufacturing processes were investigated for their effectiveness to reduce HEV.

*Study Design and Methods.*—Detection methods for HEV removal (by reverse transcription quantitative polymerase chain reaction) and inactivation (using an infectivity assay) were established. Immunoaffinity chromatography and 20-nm virus filtration for Factor (F)VIII, cold ethanol fractionation, and low-pH treatment for immunoglobulin, heat treatment for human albumin, and 35-nm nanofiltration for FVIII inhibitor-bypassing activity (FEIBA) were investigated for their capacity to reduce HEV or the physicochemically similar viruses feline calicivirus (FCV) and hepatitis A virus (HAV).

*Results.*—For FVIII, HEV reduction of 3.9 and more than 3.9 log was demonstrated for immunoaffinity chromatography and 20-nm nanofiltration, respectively, and the cold ethanol fractionation for immunoglobulin removed more than 3.5 log of HEV, to below the limit of detection (LOD). Heat treatment of human albumin inactivated more than 3.1 log of HEV to below the LOD and 35-nm nanofiltration removed 4.0 log of HEV from the FEIBA intermediate. The results indicated HAV rather than FCV as the more relevant model virus for HEV.

*Conclusion.*—Substantial HEV reduction during processes commonly used in the manufacturing of plasma products was demonstrated, similar to that previously demonstrated for HAV.

▶ Hepatitis E virus (HEV), genotypes 1 and 2, cause large epidemics of acute viral hepatitis in many tropical and subtropical countries through fecal-oral route transmission. The genotypes 3 and 4 have been recognized as zoonotic, primarily foodborne (mainly after consumption of raw or undercooked pork products) pathogens in industrialized countries. Seroprevalence rates of 10% to 53% has been reported in blood donors in a number of European countries and in the US general population pointing to a significant proportion of typically asymptomatic HEV infection.[1,2] HEV has been transmitted by blood transfusion.[3] Low-level concentration of HEV RNA was detected in 10% of plasma pools for fractionation, although a screening of coagulation factor concentrates at the end of the process were free of HEV RNA. This disparity is consistent with higher test sensitivity at the plasmic pool level and virus reduction during the manufacturing process. Because of the difficulty of growing HEV, it has not been possible to establish infectivity protocols. Hepatitis A virus (HAV) and feline calcivirus (FCV) are taxonomically closely related and are similar to HEV in physicochemical properties.

In this study, HAV and FCV were used as surrogate viruses in clearance studies and evaluated as potential model viruses for HEV. Using HAV and FCV infectivity assays for virus clearance studies in parallel with HEV RNA achieved substantial HEV reduction during processes that are commonly used in the manufacturing of plasma products. HAV rather than FCV inactivation during heat treatment was similar to the inactivation achieved for HEV. The findings are consistent with HAV rather than FCV being a more relevant model virus for HEV.

**N. M. Khardori, MD, PhD**

*References*

1. Slot E, Hogema B, Riezebos-Brilman A, et al. Silent hepatitis E virus infection in Dutch blood donors, 2011 to 2012. *Euro Surveill.* 2013;18. pii:20550.
2. Xu C, Wang RY, Schechterly CA, et al. An assessment of hepatitis E virus (HEV) in US blood donors and recipients: no detectable HEV RNA in 1939 donors tested and no evidence for HEV transmission to 362 prospectively followed recipients. *Transfusion.* 2013;53:2505-2511.
3. Matsubayashi K, Kang JH, Sakata H, et al. A case of transfusion-transmitted hepatitis E caused by blood from a donor infected with hepatitis E virus via zoonotic flood-borne route. *Transfusion.* 2008;48:1368-1375.

## Hepatitis C Virus Genotype 7, a New Genotype Originating from Central Africa

Murphy DG, Sablon E, Chamberland J, et al (Institut National de Santé Publique du Québec, Sainte-Anne-de-Bellevue, Canada; Innogenetics NV, Ghent, Belgium; et al)
*J Clin Microbiol* 53:967-972, 2015

We report a new hepatitis C virus (HCV) genotype identified in patients originating from the Democratic Republic of Congo. The prototype QC69 virus is shown to be a new lineage distinct from genotypes 1 to 6. Three additional patients were also found to be infected by a virus from this lineage, confirming its circulation in humans. We propose that these viruses be classified into HCV genotype 7.

▶ Hepatitis C virus (HCV) is estimated to infect 3% of the world's population. The availability of antibody and nucleic acid testing has essentially eliminated the transmission through blood components. The predominant mode of transmission in industrialized countries now is through intravenous drug use. The persistent presence of HCV in areas of Africa and Asia suggests alternative modes of transmission most likely through exposure to blood. Since its identification in the late 1980s, 6 major genotypes of HCV have been recognized. Genotypes 1, 2, 3, 4, and 6 have been divided further into a series of subtypes based on their high genetic diversity. The genotypes differ from each other by 30% and subtypes by 15% to 25% at the nucleotide level.

In this article, a new genotype of HCV is reported in 4 subjects originating from the Democratic Republic of Congo (DRC). The complete genome sequence of 1 isolate (QC69) and the partial genome sequences of 3 other isolates were studied. The findings show that these 4 isolates are genetically distinct from genotypes 1 to 6 and cluster together. This is the first addition to the HCV genotypes in 20 years.[1,2] The considerable level of genetic diversity in genotype 7 suggests that it has propagated and maintained for a long time in the DRC. However, it is not highly prevalent in DRC or may be limited to certain regions. In Quebec, Canada, NS5B analysis has been done to determine HCV genotype in more than 17 000 subjects. All 7 genotypes, many subtypes, and various unclassified variants have been found in local and/or immigrant populations. In addition to understanding epidemiology and evolution of HCV, genotypes are clinically relevant because current treatment regimens are tailored to efficacy for the infecting genotype.[3]

**N. M. Khardori, MD, PhD**

*References*

1. Simmonds P, Bukh J, Combet C, et al. Consensus proposals for a unified system of nomenclature of hepatitis C virus genotypes. *Hepatology.* 2005;42:962-973.
2. Smith DB, Bikh J, Kuiken C, et al. Expanded classification of hepatitis C virus into 7 genotypes and 67 subtypes: updated criteria and genotype assignment web resource. *Hepatology.* 2014;59:318-327.
3. American Association for the Study of Liver Diseases, Infectious Diseases Society of America. Recommendations for testing, managing and treating hepatitis C. 2014. http://www.hcvguidelines.org.

# 17 Fungal Infections

**Echinocandin Resistance in *Candida***

Perlin DS (New Jersey Med School—Rutgers Biomedical and Health Sciences, Newark)

*Clin Infect Dis* 61:S612-S617, 2015

Invasive fungal infections are an important infection concern for patients with underlying immunosuppression. Antifungal therapy is a critical component of patient care, but therapeutic choices are limited due to few drug classes. Antifungal resistance, especially among *Candida* species, aggravates the problem. The echinocandin drugs (micafungin, anidulafungin, and caspofungin) are the preferred choice to treat a range of candidiasis. They target the fungal-specific enzyme glucan synthase, which is responsible for the biosynthesis of a major cell wall polymer. Therapeutic failure involves acquisition of resistance, although it is a rare event among most *Candida* species. However, in some settings, higher-level resistance has been reported among *Candida glabrata*, which is also frequently resistant to azole drugs, resulting in difficult-to-treat multidrug-resistant strains. The mechanism of echinocandin resistance involves amino acid changes in "hot spot" regions of *FKS* encoded subunits of glucan synthase, which decreases the sensitivity of enzyme to drug, resulting in higher minimum inhibitory concentration values. The cellular processes promoting the formation of resistant *FKS* strains involve complex stress response pathways that yield a variety of adaptive compensatory genetic responses. Standardized broth microdilution techniques can be used to distinguish *FKS* mutant strains from wild type, but testing *C. glabrata* with caspofungin should be approached cautiously. Finally, clinical factors that promote echinocandin resistance include prophylaxis, host reservoirs including biofilms in the gastrointestinal tract, and intra-abdominal infections. An understanding of clinical and molecular factors that promote echinocandin resistance is critical to develop better diagnostic tools and therapeutic strategies to overcome resistance.

▶ Echinocandins have become front-line agents for presumptive antifungal use due to their broad spectrum of activity, development of resistance to azoles, and adverse events associated with amphotericin B. Resistance of *Candida* species to echinocandins was first reported in 2005 and has remained relatively low (3%) for *Candida albicans* and most other *Candida* species. However, echinocandin resistance is increasing in *Candida glabrata* (8%–9.3%), made worse by the fact that cross-resistance to azole antifungal agents is seen in as many isolates.[1] The echinocandin resistance in *C glabrata* rose from 2%–3% to 13% at Duke Hospital over a period of 10 years. A recent study has shown regional difference in echinocandin resistance in *C glabrata*. The widespread use of echinocandin and azole prophylaxis in many hospitals has lead to an epidemiologic shift with *C glabrata* becoming the dominant fungal blood stream pathogen.[2] Echinocandin resistance is acquired during therapy and is associated with amino acid changes in hot-spot regions of the *FKS* subunits of glucan synthase, yielding cells with thickened cell walls. There is no documented horizontal transmission probably because the development of *FKS*-mediated echinocandin resistance carries a fitness cost. This is a highly restricted mechanism in contrast to resistance to azole antifungals, which involves a wide array of mechanisms, including drug transporter, target site mutations, and target overexpression. The activity of echinocandins induces a variety of cellular stress response pathways creating drug-adapted persister states, which may ultimately break through and lead to *FKS*-resistant mutants. Direct molecular testing for the presence of *FKS* mutations may provide early and appropriate warning of echinocandin resistance. The reduction in host factors promoting resistance (ie, biofilm formation in the gastrointestinal tract, intra-abdominal candidiasis, and use of echinocandin prophylaxis) will lead to further reduction in morbidity and mortality.

**N. M. Khardori, MD, PhD**

*References*

1. Pfaller MA, Castanheira M, Lockhart SR, Ahlquist AM, Messer SA, Jones RN. Frequency of decreased susceptibility and resistance to echinocandins among fluconazole-resistant bloodstream isolates of Candida glabrata: results from the SENTRY Antimicrobial Surveillance Program (2006–2010) and the Centers for Disease Control and Prevention Population-Based Surveillance (2008–2010). *J Clin Microbiol*. 2012;50:1199-1203.
2. Lortholary O, Desnos-Ollivier M, Sitbon K, Fontanet A, Bretagne S, Dromer F. Recent exposure to capofungin or fluxonazole influences the epidemiology of candidemia: a prospective multicenter study involving 2,441 patients. *Antimicrob Agents Chemother*. 2011;55:532-538.

# 18 Tuberculosis

## Cathepsin G in Experimental Tuberculosis: Relevance for Antibacterial Protection and Potential for Immunotherapy

Walter K, Steinwede K, Aly S, et al (Res Ctr Borstel, Germany; Hannover Med School, Germany; Charité Univ Medicine Berlin, Germany; et al)
*J Immunol* 195:3325-3333, 2015

Neutrophil serine proteases, such as cathepsin G (CG) and neutrophil elastase (NE), have been implicated in the protective response against infections, including experimental mycobacterial infections. The goal of this study was to explore the role of CG in immunocompetent mice challenged aerogenically with *Mycobacterium tuberculosis*. We used genetically CG- or CG/NE-deficient mice to define the importance of these neutrophil serine proteases for antibacterial protection, granulomatous response, and survival. In addition, we explored the effect of intratracheally delivered liposomally encapsulated CG/NE as a therapeutic approach early during *M. tuberculosis* infection. Our data show that the presence of CG or CG/NE prolongs survival in *M. tuberculosis*–infected mice. However, CG is not directly involved in antibacterial defenses, and exogenous intratracheal administration of CG combined with NE does not reduce bacterial loads in the lungs of *M. tuberculosis*–infected mice.

▶ The relative contribution of macrophages, T cells, and cytokines in the inflammatory and protective antibacterial responses is unclear.[1] After inhalation, the initial permissive habitat for *Mycobacterium tuberculosis* is provided by alveolar macrophages. Subsequently, inflammatory T-cell and interferon-α activated macrophages acquire the capability to arrest the growth of *M tuberculosis* in the lung and limit the spread of bacteria to other organs and the environment.[2] Activated macrophages lead to growth arrest and killing of *M tuberculosis* by a number of bacteriostatic and bacteriocidal mechanisms, the most prominent being oxidative and nitrosative pathways. Macrophages have been shown to eliminate *M tuberculosis* more efficiently after phagocytosis of apoptotic neutrophils making it possible that neutrophil-derived bacteriocidal molecules play a role in early defenses against *M tuberculosis* infection.[3] Neutrophil serine proteases (eg, cathepsin [CG] and neutrophil elastase [NE]) have been implicated in defense against Gram-positive and Gram-negative bacteria and bacille Calmette–Guérin (BCG) infection in a mouse model. Deficiency in both CG and NE was associated with pronounced impairment in eliminating BCG than the deficiency of only CG. Administration of liposomal-CG and NE improved immunity against BCG.

In this research, the role of CG in immunocompetent mice infected by aerosolized *M tuberculosis* was studied using genetically CG- or CG/NE-deficient mice to define the role of neutrophil-derived serine proteases. Intratracheal use of liposomal CG/NE early during *M tuberculosis* infection was also studied. Premature death of CG- and CG/NE-deficient mice pointed to a modified chemokine and cytokine profile in their absence in mice infected with *M tuberculosis*. However, the cause for this was not a direct antibacterial effect by CG or CG/NE because intratracheal or orotracheal administration of liposomal CG and NE has no effect on the growth of *M tuberculosis* in the organs. The role of neutrophil serine proteases may be related to an unspecified dysregulation of inflammatory response.

**N. M. Khardori, MD, PhD**

*References*

1. Cooper AM, Torrado E. Protection versus pathology in tuberculosis: recent insights. *Curr Opin Immunol.*. 2012;24:431-437.
2. Kaufmann SH, Dorhoi A. Inflammation in tuberculosis: interactions, imbalances and interventions. *Curr Opin Immunol.*. 2013;25:441-449.
3. Tan BH, Meinken C, Bastain M, et al. Macrophages acquire neutrophil granules for antimicrobial activity against intracellular pathogens. *J Immunol.* 2006;177: 1864-1871.

# 19 Vaccines

**A stable trimeric influenza hemagglutinin stem as a broadly protective immunogen**

Impagliazzo A, Milder F, Kuipers H, et al (Crucell Vaccine Inst, Leiden, Netherlands; Crucell Vaccine Inst, San Diego, CA; et al)

*Science* 349:1301-1306, 2015

The identification of human broadly neutralizing antibodies (bnAbs) targeting the hemagglutinin (HA) stem revitalized hopes of developing a universal influenza vaccine. Using a rational design and library approach, we engineered stable HA stem antigens ("mini-HAs") based on an H1 subtype sequence. Our most advanced candidate exhibits structural and bnAb binding properties comparable to those of full-length HA, completely protects mice in lethal heterologous and heterosubtypic challenge models, and reduces fever after sublethal challenge in cynomolgus monkeys. Antibodies elicited by this mini-HA in mice and nonhuman primates bound a wide range of HAs, competed with human bnAbs for HA stem binding, neutralized H5N1 viruses, and mediated antibody-dependent effector activity.These results represent a proof of concept for the design of HA stem mimics that elicit bnAbs against influenza A group 1 viruses.

▶ The development of a universal vaccine against influenza offering protection against a wide range of strains and subtypes would eliminate the need for seasonal reformation of vaccines. In addition, it has the advantage of providing effective defense against viruses with pandemic potential. The recent discovery of broadly neutralizing human monoclonal antibodies (bnAbs) has paved the way for feasibility studies.[1] The majority of bnAbs are directed toward highly conformational epitopes in the hemagglutinin (HA) stem. If well exposed and properly presented, the HA stem has the potential to induce broad protective immunity against influenza. To generate a broadly protective soluble HA stem immunogen, it needs to be full length (FLHA) stable and without conformational changes, which have been shown to exhibit lower affinity with bnAbs related to FLHA.

The study describes the design and characterization of a series of soluble HA immunogens solely composed of the HA stem. Stabilized trimeric mini-HA #4900 as the final candidate demonstrated a unique ability to elicit broad and protective immune response in mice and nonhuman primates (*Macaca fascicularis*). In the primate studies, a single antigen dose was used with a potent adjuvant, which has been shown to have a favorable safety and immunogeniticity profile in a number of clinical trials.[2] The effect of this stabilized mini-HA stem immunogen was comparable to the improved immune response and protection demonstrated with stabilized respiratory syncytial virus F antigen. With the addressing of minimal doses of mini-HA and adjuvant for an optimal and broad protective response, this approach to human vaccination against influenza will become feasible.

**N. M. Khardori, MD, PhD**

*References*

1. Friesen RH, Lee PS, Stoop EJ, et al. A common solution to group 2 influenza virus neutralization. *Proc Natl Acad Sci U S A*. 2014;111:445-450.
2. Cox RJ, Pedersen G, Madhun AS, et al. Evaluation of a virosomal H5N1 vaccine formulated with Matrix M™ adjuvant in a phase I clinical trial. *Vaccine*. 2011;29: 8049-8059.

# 20 Clinical Diagnostics

**Evaluation of Matrix-Assisted Laser Desorption Ionization–Time of Flight Mass Spectrometry for Identification of *Mycobacterium* species, *Nocardia* species, and Other Aerobic Actinomycetes**

Buckwalter SP, Olson SL, Connelly BJ, et al (Mayo Clinic, Rochester, MN)

*J Clin Microbiol* 54:376-384, 2016

The value of matrix-assisted laser desorption ionization–time of flight mass spectrometry (MALDI-TOF MS) for the identification of bacteria and yeasts is well documented in the literature. Its utility for the identification of mycobacteria and *Nocardia* spp. has also been reported in a limited scope. In this work, we report the specificity of MALDI-TOF MS for the identification of 162 *Mycobacterium* species and subspecies, 53 *Nocardia* species, and 13 genera (totaling 43 species) of other aerobic actinomycetes using both the MALDI-TOF MS manufacturer's supplied database(s) and a custom database generated in our laboratory. The performance of a simplified processing and extraction procedure was also evaluated, and, similar to the results in an earlier literature report, our viability studies confirmed the ability of this process to inactivate *Mycobacterium tuberculosis* prior to analysis. Following library construction and the specificity study, the performance of MALDI-TOF MS was directly compared with that of 16S rRNA gene sequencing for the evaluation of 297 mycobacteria isolates, 148 *Nocardia* species isolates, and 61 other aerobic actinomycetes isolates under routine clinical laboratory working conditions over a 6-month period. MALDI-TOF MS is a valuable tool for the identification of these groups of organisms. Limitations in the databases and in the ability of MALDI-TOF MS to rapidly identify slowly growing mycobacteria are discussed.

▶ Diagnostic microbiology is in the process of transitioning from conventional culture, biochemical identification and susceptibility testing to genomics- and proteomics-based methods. Matrix-assisted laser desorption ionization–time of flight mass spectrometry (MALDI-TOF MS) has been studied extensively and being used for identification of bacteria and yeast. MALDI-TOF MS is an efficient and effective method for the identification of microbes with significant reduction in time to reporting of microbiological results.[1]

There are more than 170 species of mycobacteria, more than 1200 *Nocardia* and hundreds of other aerobic actinomycete species among 16 genera.[2] Although a large number of these species are environmental organisms, some are clinically relevant and cause a spectrum of infections in human. The current standard method of identification of mycobacteria and aerobic actinomycetes is DNA sequencing using several recognized targets for species identification. Because it is technically complex and labor-intensive, many clinical laboratories do not routinely perform sequencing.

In this study the authors describe the development of a custom MALDI-TOF MS database for *Mycobacteria* spp (162), *Nocardia* spp (53), and other aerobic actinomycetes (43) and report its specificity for identification and head-to-head comparison with the manufacturer's database. Confirmation of an earlier described simplified processing and extraction method for *Mycobacteria* tuberculosis outside a BSL3 environment is also provided. The data provide a comprehensive description of the utility of MALDI-TOF MS for its use as an efficient and effective method for identification of *Mycobacteria*, *Nocardia*, and other aerobic actinomycetes. Analysis, however, is not as straightforward as for other groups of bacteria and yeasts. Additional upfront processing steps are needed for safety reasons and effective lysis of the organism to make proteins available for analysis.

**N. M. Khardori, MD, PhD**

*References*

1. Patel R. Matrix-assisted laser desorption ionization-time of flight mass spectrometry in clinical microbiology. *Clin Infect Dis*. 2013;57:564-572, http://dx.doi.org/10.1093/cid/cit247, 2013;.
2. Leibniz Institute DSMZ-German Collection of Microorganisms and Cell Cultures. Prokaryotic nomenclature up-to-date. 2015. http://www.dsmz.de/bacterial-diversity/prokaryotic-nomenclature-up-to-date.

# 21 Health Care Associated Infections

## Clinical Effectiveness of Mupirocin for Preventing *Staphylococcus aureus* Infections in Nonsurgical Settings: A Meta-analysis

Nair R, Perencevich EN, Blevins AE, et al (Univ of Iowa College of Public Health; Univ of Iowa; et al)
*Clin Infect Dis* 62:618-630, 2016

A systematic literature review and meta-analysis was performed to identify effectiveness of mupirocin decolonization in prevention of *Staphylococcus aureus* infections, among nonsurgical settings. Of the 15 662 unique studies identified up to August 2015, 13 randomized controlled trials, 22 quasi-experimental studies, and 1 retrospective cohort study met the inclusion criteria. Studies were excluded if mupirocin was not used for decolonization, there was no control group, or the study was conducted in an outbreak setting. The crude risk ratios were pooled (cpRR) using a random-effects model. We observed substantial heterogeneity among included studies ($I^2 = 80\%$). Mupirocin was observed to reduce the risk for *S. aureus* infections by 59% (cpRR, 0.41; 95% confidence interval [CI], .36–.48) and 40% (cpRR, 0.60; 95% CI, .46–.79) in both dialysis and nondialysis settings, respectively. Mupirocin decolonization was protective against S. aureus infections among both dialysis and adult intensive care patients. Future studies are needed in other settings such as long-term care and pediatrics.

▶ The risk of subsequent infection caused by *Staphylococcus aureus* in nasal carriers of the organism is 2 to 12 times higher than the noncarriers.[1] In nasal carriers, *S aureus* infections such as bloodstream and surgical site infections are caused predominately by endogenous strains.[2] Mupirocin is currently the topical antibacterial of choice for short-term eradication of *S aureus* carriage. Even though resistance development is rare after short-term use, sustained use of mupirocin-based decolonization regimens for general inpatients, particularly for prolonged periods, has resulted in emergence of resistance. It is possible the intervention would be useful for a select group of patients.

The authors of this study conducted a systematic literature review and meta-analysis on the effectiveness of mupirocin decolonization to prevent infections caused by *Staphylococcus aureus*. The data presented are on 15 662 nonduplicated abstracts and articles. Thirteen studies were randomized controlled trials.

Most common use of mupirocin was for nasal colonization, followed by application to dialysis catheter exit site, wounds, and umbilicus. Analysis of pooled data showed that decolonization reduced the risk for *S aureus* infection by 52%. In most studies, the proportion of *S aureus* infection was lower among colonized patients treated with mupirocin compared with colonized patients not treated with mupirocin. There was no difference in the magnitude of risk reduction for *S aureus* infection between universal and targeted decolonization and between single agent and combination with other agents. However, subgroup analysis demonstrated substantial heterogenicity among eligible studies.

The authors recommended mupirocin use in dialysis patients with risk of *S aureus* colonization with subsequent infection. Intensive care unit patients detected to be *S aureus* carriers on admission may also benefit. The potential for acquisition and transmission of mupirocin-resistant *S aureus* can be evaluated by testing for the mupR gene. Nonantimicrobial alternatives (eg, povidone-iodine, lysostaphin, tea tree oil, probiotics and antibody-directed photodynamic therapy) also need to be evaluated.

**N. M. Khardori, MD, PhD**

*References*

1. Wertheim HF, Melles DC, Vos MC, et al. The role of nasal carriage in *Staphylococcus aureus* infections. *Lancet Infect Dis.* 2005;5:751-762.
2. Verhoeven PO, Gagnaire J, Botelho-Nevers E, et al. Detection and clinical relevance of *Staphylococcus aureaus* nasal carriage: an update. *Expert Rev Anti Infect Ther.* 2014;12:75-89.

---

## Transfer efficiency of *Staphylococcus aureus* between nitrile exam gloves and nonporous fomites

Koenig DW, Korir-Morrison C, Hoffman DR (Kimberly-Clark Corporation, Neenah, WI; Kimberly-Clark Corporation, Roswell, GA)
*Am J Infect Control* 44:245-246, 2016

---

This report describes fomite transmission of *Staphylococcus aureus* amongst various surfaces. A contact transfer protocol was completed to evaluate the movement of *S aureus* between a person wearing nitrile gloves and either: handshaking with another person with gloved hands, touching a plastic cellular telephone back, or touching a stainless steel rod. The data in this preliminary study imply that the highest bacterial transfer is with metal surfaces followed by plastic. Interestingly, glove-to-glove transfer occurred but transfered less bacteria than a plastic or metal surface. The observations from this study point to the need to clearly define hygiene behaviors to reduce the potential of hand- and surface-mediated transmission (Table 2).

▶ Around 40% of health care–associated infections are attributed to cross-infection through the hands of health care personnel.[1] Transfer of bacteria can occur between gloved hands and a fomite.[2] Of particular concern are the formites or devices that do not undergo cleaning or decontamination between

**TABLE 2.**—Bacteria Recovered from Fomites After Contact Transfer Protocol

| Contact Transfer Order (First Fomite → Second Fomite → Third Fomite) | Bacteria Recovered from Second Fomite | Bacteria Recovered from Third Fomite |
|---|---|---|
| Glove → glove → glove | $5.5 \pm 4.4 \times 10^3$ | $3.0 \pm 3.3 \times 10^2$ |
| Telephone* → glove → telephone | $1.4 \pm 0.5 \times 10^6$ | $6.2 \pm 5.4 \times 10^4$ |
| SS → glove → SS | $2.7 \pm 0.8 \times 10^6$ | $9.0 \pm 3.4 \times 10^4$ |
| SS → glove → SS plus soil load† | $5.2 \pm 0.6 \times 10^6$ | $1.5 \pm 0.2 \times 10^5$ |

*NOTE.* Values are presented as colony forming units ± standard deviation.
*SS*, stainless steel rod.
*Plastic cellular telephone back.
†Bovine serum albumin (5% w/v) added to the inoculum.
Reprinted from Koenig DW, Korir-Morrison C, Hoffman DR. Transfer efficiency of *Staphylococcus aureus* between nitrile exam gloves and nonporous fomites. *Am J Infect Control.* 2016;44:245-246, with permission from Elsevier Inc.

patient visits. Noncritical medical devices are an important reservoir, and 25% to 79% have been shown to be contaminated by at least 1 organism. *Staphylococcus* species are the most commonly identified organism on these devices.

This study describes fomite transfer experiences of *S aureus* using 2 model surfaces and gloved hands. Movement of a well-characterized *S aureus* strain was studied between a person wearing nitrile gloves, handshaking with another person with gloved hands, or touching the back of a plastic cellular telephone or a 304 stainless steal rod. Table 2 summarizes the bacteria recovered from fomites after the contact transfer protocol was completed. The highest potential of transfer was shown to be with metal, followed by plastic, which was increased by the addition of a soil load. Glove-to-glove transfer occurred but is less likely to transfer bacteria than a plastic or metal surface. There is a need for infection-prevention strategies to be taken further than current protocols and to educate health care providers to refrain from touching surfaces or cellular phones during or after patient contacts. The other important observation from this study is that the presence of soil increases the transfer of *S aureus* to the second and third fomites in transfer events involving stainless steel and gloves.

**N. M. Khardori, MD, PhD**

*References*

1. Weber DJ, Rutala WA, Miller MB, Huslage K, Sickert-Bennett E. Role of hospital surfaces in the transmission of emerging health care-associated pathogens: norovirus, *Clostridium difficile*, and *Acinetobacter* species. *Am J Infect Control.* 2010; 38:S25-S33.
2. Ye D, Shan J, Huang Y, et al. A gloves-associated outbreak of imipenem-resistant Acinetobacter baumannii in an intensive care unit in Guangdong, China. *BMC Infect Dis.* 2015;15:179.

## Characteristics and Antibiotic Use Associated With Short-Term Risk of *Clostridium difficile* Infection Among Hospitalized Patients

Aldrete Sdel M, Magee MJ, Friedman-Moraco RJ, et al (Emory Univ School of Medicine, Atlanta, GA; Georgia State Univ School of Public Health, Atlanta; et al)

*Am J Clin Pathol* 143:895-900, 2015

*Objectives.*—Polymerase chain reaction (PCR) has been shown to have an excellent sensitivity and specificity for the detection of *Clostridium difficile* infection (CDI). Little is known about risk factors for CDI within 14 days of an initial negative test. We sought to determine the characteristics among hospitalized patients associated with risk of short-term acquisition of CDI.

*Methods.*—A case-control study was conducted. Cases were patients who converted from PCR negative to positive within 14 days. Each case was matched with three controls. Conditional logistic regression was used to estimate the association between patient characteristics and CDI.

*Results.*—Of the 30 patients in our study who had a positive PCR within 14 days of a first negative PCR (cases), 15 (50%) occurred within 7 days of the initial test. Cases had a higher proportion of intravenous vancomycin use in the previous 8 weeks (odds ratio [OR], 3.38; 95% confidence interval [CI], 1.34-8.49) and were less likely to have recent antiviral agent use (OR, 0.30; 95% CI, 0.11-0.83) compared with controls.

*Conclusions.*—In hospitalized patients, treatment with intravenous vancomycin within the prior 8 weeks of a first negative PCR test for *C difficile* is a risk factor for short-term risk for hospital-acquired CDI. Repeat testing guidelines for *C difficile* PCR should take into consideration patients who may be at high risk for short-term acquisition of CDI (Table 3).

▶ *Clostridium difficile*, identified as the bacterial agent responsible for antibiotic-associated diarrhea in the late 1970s, is now recognized as the leading cause of infectious hospital-acquired diarrhea. Patients become symptomatic typically in 2 to 3 days after colonization with toxigenic *C difficile* spores. Molecular testing (polymerase chain reaction [PCR]) is recognized as an important tool for *C difficile* infection (CDI) diagnosis with a sensitivity of 73% to 100% and specificity of 91% to 100%, respectively. Based on the high negative predictive value, it is recommended that PCR not be repeated within 7 days of a negative test.[1] The specific risk factors for short-term acquisition of CDI after a negative test are not known except for the fact that they are exclusively inpatients and are most likely to undergo expedited repeat testing.

This study was designed to determine the rate of short-term acquisition (within 14 days of a negative test) and antibiotic regimens associated with acquisition. In this case-control study, each case that converted from a negative to positive test within 14 days was matched with 3 controls. Starting from a large study number of 12 021 PCR tests, 1500 were repeat tested within 14 days. Of these 60 PCR tests, 30 patients were identified as short-term CDI

TABLE 3.—Conditional Logistic Regression Matched Odds Ratios for Patient Characteristics and Antibiotic Use Associated With Short-Term Acquisition of *Clostridium difficile*[a]

| Characteristic | OR (95% CI)[b] |
|---|---|
| Male sex | 1.87 (0.76-4.18) |
| Death (all causes) | 1.85 (0.54-6.28) |
| Intensive care unit stay[c] | 0.59 (0.24-1.45) |
| Diabetes mellitus[d] | 0.94 (0.35-2.47) |
| Coinfection[e] | 1.49 (0.58-3.82) |
| Proton pump inhibitor | 1.18 (0.37-3.73) |
| Recent GI procedure[f] | 2.41 (0.84-6.88) |
| End-stage renal disease | 1.72 (0.60-4.19) |
| Leukemia | 0.49 (0.17-1.38) |
| Solid tumor | 1.85 (0.54-6.28) |
| Chemotherapy[g] | 0.94 (0.37-2.40) |
| Stem cell transplant | 3.00 (0.19-47.96) |
| Solid organ transplant | 0.67 (0.14-3.09) |
| Antibiotic use 8 weeks prior to first PCR test[h] | |
| β-Lactam | 2.35 (0.91-6.07) |
| Quinolone | 1.10 (0.47-2.59) |
| Aminoglycoside | 0.50 (0.06-4.15) |
| Metronidazole | 0.67 (0.14-3.09) |
| Vancomycin IV | **3.38 (1.34-8.49)** |
| Acyclovir prophylaxis | **0.30 (0.11-0.83)** |
| Antibiotic use 14 days after first PCR test[h] | |
| β-Lactam | 0.81 (0.36-1.81) |
| Quinolone | 1.18 (0.47-2.98) |
| Aminoglycoside | 1.50 (0.38-6.00) |
| Metronidazole | 2.39 (0.95-6.06) |
| Vancomycin IV | 0.47 (0.19-1.16) |
| Vancomycin PO | **6.63 (1.27-34.74)** |
| Acyclovir prophylaxis | 0.51 (0.20-1.29) |

CI, confidence interval; GI, gastrointestinal; IV, intravenous; OR, odds ratio; PCR, polymerase chain reaction; PO, oral.
[a]OR matched on age and days to first PCR test.
[b]Bold signifies statistical significance.
[c]Intensive care unit stay within 7 days before or 48 hours after first PCR test.
[d]Defined as HbA1c of more than 6.5%.
[e]Infection of any type and any source at the time of PCR testing.
[f]GI procedure of any type within 8 weeks prior to first PCR test.
[g]Received chemotherapy for malignancy within the past 8 weeks.
[h]Other antibiotics analyzed but not shown were macrolides, trimethoprim-sulfamethoxazole, antifungals, linezolid, tetracyclines, clindamycin, aztreonam, daptomycin, and "others" (carbapenem, dapsone, meropenem, nitrofurantoin, and tigecycline). None was statistically significant.
Reprinted from Aldrete Sdel M, Magee MJ, Friedman-Moraco RJ, et al. Characteristics and antibiotic use associated with short-term risk of *clostridium difficile* infection among hospitalized patients. *Am J Clin Pathol*. 2015;143:895-900, with permission from American Society for Clinical Pathology.

acquisition within a 7-day window, during which time it is recommended that PCR not be repeated. The rate of short-term acquisition was 142 per 100 000 person years. Patient characteristics and antibiotic use associated with short-term acquisition of *C difficile* are shown in Table 3. The odds of previous intravenous (IV) vancomycin were more common among cases than controls before the initial postive PCR. Within the next 14 days, the odds of taking oral metronidazole or oral vancomycin (both established treatments for CDI) were more common among cases. Among antibiotic classes, IV vancomycin, vancomycin with betalactamase, and quinolones in the 8 weeks before first PCR increased the odds in cases. The percentage of negative to positive PCR within 14 days was 4.2%. The antibiotic history within the prior 8 weeks may be beneficial in predicting short-term acquisition of *C difficile*.

**N. M. Khardori, MD, PhD**

*Reference*

1. Luo RF, Banaei N. Is repeat PCR needed for diagnosis of *Clostridium difficile* infection? *J Clin Microbiol.* 2010;48:3738-3741.

---

## Degowning the controversies of contact precautions for methicillin-resistant *Staphylococcus aureus*: A review

Kullar R, Vassallo A, Turkel S, et al (Cubist Pharmaceuticals, Lexington, MA; Providence Saint John's Health Ctr, Santa Monica, CA; et al)
*Am J Infect Control* 44:97-103, 2016

---

*Background.*—Contact precautions (CPs) are recommended to prevent methicillin-resistant Staphylococcus aureus (MRSA) transmission in institutions. Rising doubts about CP effectiveness and recognition of unintended consequences for patients have raised questions about the benefit. The objective of this study was to evaluate the effectiveness and adverse outcomes associated with CPs for prevention of MRSA transmission.

*Methods.*—We searched PubMed, Embase, and the Cochrane Library for articles related to effectiveness and adverse outcomes of CPs in patients with MRSA. Criteria for inclusion included the following: articles conducted in the United States, articles performed in an acute care setting, articles that were not a case series or review, and those with standardized collection of data or inclusion of case and control groups. Results were summarized and examined for potential limitations. Recommendations were based on our findings.

*Results.*—CPs reduced MRSA transmission in epidemic settings and in instances with high compliance, but a decrease in infection rates was not shown. Unintended consequences of CPs include decreased health care provider (HCP) time spent with patients, low HCP compliance, decreased perceptions of comfort from patients, and greater likelihood of patient complaints and negative psychologic implications.

*Conclusion.*—In endemic settings, there are few data to support routine use of CPs to control the spread of MRSA. Education should be performed in hospitals to improve patients' perception of care and understanding of CPs when implemented and HCPs' adherence to good hand hygiene and standard precautions practices.

▶ In 2013, the Centers for Disease Control and Prevention (CDC) released its first ever report on antibiotic resistance threats in the United States. The report highlighted that every year more than 2 million individuals acquire infections caused by multidrug-resistant organisms (MDROs) resulting in at least 23 000 deaths. Contact precautions (CPs) that fall under the category of transmission-based precautions are recommended by the CDC to control the spread of MDROs including methicillin-resistant *Staphylococcus aureus* (MRSA). Contact precautions involve a private room for the patient and the use of gloves and gowns for every health care provider for every patient encounter.[1] At any given time, 15% of patients in hospitals are under CPs. Recent studies have raised questions about the benefits of CPs in preventing MRSA transmission in non-outbreak setting especially taking into account that there are unintended consequence.[2,3]

In this study, peer-reviewed articles from January 1996 to May 2015 were included to evaluate the effectiveness, quality of care, and adverse outcomes of CPs in patients with MRSA. The authors concluded that there remains a gap in the evidence supporting the direct benefit of CPs in preventing the spread of MRSA in non-outbreak endemic settings. They recommend that attention should be focused on adherence to good hand hygiene practices and the use of standard precautions for all patients with the use of gowns and gloves reserved for patients with uncontained wound drainage and/or uncontained respiratory secretions. In keeping with these recommendations, the results of the largest study on compliance with standard precautions was recently published on a French cohort of 1599 health care facilities, 14 968 patient wards and 203 840 health care workers. Except for minor irregularities, a high level of implementation of standard precautions was found.[4] Such studies along with efforts to bring SPs to the forefront of all infection prevention programs are needed in the United States.

**N. M. Khardori, MD, PhD**

*References*


1. Siegel JD, Rhinehart E, Jackson M, Chiarello L, Health Care Infection Control Practices Advisory Committee. 2007 guideline for isolation precautions; preventing transmission of infectious agents in health care settings. *Am J Infect Control.* 2007;35:S65-S164.
2. Harris AD, Pineles L, Belton B, et al. Universal glove and gown use and acquisition of antibiotic-resistant bacteria in the ICU: a randomized trial. *JAMA.* 2013;310: 1571-1580.
3. Edmond MB, Masroor N, Stevens MP, Ober J, Bearman G. The impact of discontinujing contact precautions for VRE and MRSA on device-associated infections. *Infect Control Hosp Epidemiol.* 2015;39:978-980.
4. Giard M, Laprungne-Garcia E, Caillat-Vallet E, et al. Compliance with standard precautions: results of a French national audit. *Am J Infect Control.* 2016;44:8-13.


---

## A Decade of Experience in Primary Prevention of *Clostridium difficile* Infection at a Community Hospital Using the Probiotic Combination *Lactobacillus acidophilus* CL1285, *Lactobacillus casei* LBC80R, and *Lactobacillus rhamnosus* CLR2 (Bio-K+)

Maziade P-J, Pereira P, Goldstein EJC (Pierre-Le Gardeur Hosp, Lachenaie, Quebec, Canada; David Geffen School of Medicine at UCLA)

*Clin Infect Dis* 60:S144-S147, 2015

---

In August 2003, the 284-bed community hospital Pierre-Le Gardeur (PLGH) in Quebec experienced a major outbreak associated with the

*Clostridium difficile* NAP1/027/BI strain. Augmented standard preventive measures (SPMs) were not able to control this outbreak. It was decided in February 2004 to give to every adult inpatient on antibiotics, without any exclusion, a probiotic (Bio-K+: *Lactobacillus acidophilus* CL1285, *Lactobacillus casei* LBC80R, and *Lactobacillus rhamnosus* CLR2) within 12 hours of the antibiotic prescription. Augmented SPMs were continued. The use of the probiotic in addition to SPMs was associated with a marked reduction of *C. difficile* infection (CDI). During the 10 years of observation, 44 835 inpatients received Bio- K+, and the CDI rate at PLGH declined from 18.0 cases per 10 000 patient-days and remained at low mean levels of 2.3 cases per 10 000 patient-days. Additionally, 10-year data collected by the Ministry of Health in Quebec comparing the CDI rate between Quebec hospitals showed that CDI rates at PLGH were consistently and continuously lower compared with those at similar hospitals. Blood cultures were monitored at PLGH for *Lactobacillus* bacteremia through the 10 years' experience, and no *Lactobacillus* bacteremias were detected. Despite the limitation of an observational study, we concluded that the probiotic Bio-K+ was safe and effective in decreasing our primary CDI rate (Table 1).

▶ The emergence of the fluoroquinolone-resistant epidemic *Clostridium difficile* strain NAP1/027 was first recognized through a marked increase in the incidence of *C difficile* infection (CDI) in Montreal and surrounding Quebec region in 2013.[1] Pierre-Le Gardeur Hospital (PLGH) in Lachenaie, Quebec, a

**TABLE 1.**—Augmented Standard Preventive Measures for the Prevention of *Clostridium difficile* Infection Used August 2003– February 2004 Without Response but Continued Throughout the Study

Isolation of CDI patients
- Clostridium difficile–infected patients were rapidly identified
- Isolation was in a dedicated area
- Dedicated hospital staff was assigned for CDI patients

Cleansing and disinfection
- Rigorous cleaning program was implemented, including disinfection of bathrooms, toilets, floors, and walls with PerCept (hydrogen peroxide)
- Special attention was paid to rooms previously occupied by patients with diarrhea
- Disinfection of medical equipment (cuffs, bedpans, etc) was performed after each use to reduce patient-to-patient contamination

Monitoring of antibiotic use
- Monitoring of antibiotic use, ie, second- and third-generation cephalosporins
- Moxifloxacin removed from the formulary

Hand washing and hand disinfection
- A team took care of washing hands of inpatients twice a day, 7 days a week, using a waterless antibacterial sanitizer
- This was done in addition to normal patient hand hygiene

Source: Adapted from Maziade et al [3] with permission.
*Editor's Note*: Please refer to original journal article for full references.
*Abbreviation*: CDI, *Clostridium difficile* infection.
Reprinted from Maziade P-J, Pereira P, Goldstein EJC. A decade of experience in primary prevention of *Clostridium difficile* infection at a community hospital using the probiotic combination *Lactobacillus acidophilus* CL1285, *Lactobacillus casei* LBC80R, and *Lactobacillus rhamnosus* CLR2 (Bio-K+). *Clin Infect Dis.* 2015;60:S144-S147, with permission from The Author.

284-bed community hospital without heart, thoracic, neurosurgery, or transplant units, has been using a policy of standard protective measures (SPMs) since 1998. In response to the outbreak in August 2003, the hospital instituted an augmented SPM (aSPMs) policy (Table 1). No impact on the outbreak was seen after implementation of aSPMs by February 2014. At that point, PLGH instituted a novel probiotic bundle used for every adult inpatient on antibiotics without any exclusion. The pharmacy was responsible for dispensing a daily oral dose of a probiotic formula containing 50 billion colony-forming units (CFU) of *Lactobacillus acidophilus* (CL1285), *Lactobacillus casei* (LBC80R) and *Lactobacillus rhamnosus* (CLR2) in all adult inpatients within 2 to 12 hours of initiation of any antibiotic prescription along with aSPMs. The regimen was continued for a minimum of 30 days or for 5 days after the last dose of antibiotic including patients discharged home on antibiotics. The published findings of 8-year follow-up had shown a reduction of 73% in CDI cases, 76.4% of severe cases, and 39% of relapses.[2]

This study summarizes the 10-year experience with this quasi-experimental prospective cohort using a combination of aSMPs and probiotic bundle. The reduction of CDI recurrences started in the first month of the combined program. Over the 10-year observation period involving 44 835 patients, the CDI rate at PLGH declined from 18 cases per 10 000 patient days and remained at a low mean of 2.3 cases per 10 000 patient days. The rates were consistently lower than the comparable hospitals in the region. No *Lactobacillus* bacteremias were detected. A mean per-patient savings of US $2769 were estimated.[3]

**N. M. Khardori, MD, PhD**

*References*

1. Warny M, Pepin J, Fang A, et al. Toxin production by an emerging strain of *Clostridium difficile* associated with outbreaks of severe disease in North America and Europe. *Lancet.* 2005;366:1079-1084.
2. Maziade PJ, Andriessen JA, Pereira P, Currie B, Goldstein EJ. Impact of adding prophylactic probiotics to a bundle of standard preventative measures for *Clostridium difficile* infections; enhanced and sustained decrease in the incidence and severity of infection at a community hospital. *Curr Med Res Opin.* 2013;29:1341-1347.
3. Kamdeu Fansi AA, Guertin JR, LeLorier J. Savings from the use of a probiotic formula in the prophylaxis of antibiotic-associated diarrhea. *J Med Econ.* 2012;15: 53-60.

## Overdiagnosis of *Clostridium difficile* Infection in the Molecular Test Era

Polage CR, Gyorke CE, Kennedy MA, et al (Univ of California Davis School of Medicine, Sacramento; et al)
*JAMA Intern Med* 175:1792-1801, 2015

*Importance.—Clostridium difficile* is a major cause of health care–associated infection, but disagreement between diagnostic tests is an ongoing barrier to clinical decision making and public health reporting. Molecular tests are increasingly used to diagnose *C difficile* infection

(CDI), but many molecular test-positive patients lack toxins that historically defined disease, making it unclear if they need treatment.

*Objective.*—To determine the natural history and need for treatment of patients who are toxin immunoassay negative and polymerase chain reaction (PCR) positive (Tox−/PCR+) for CDI.

*Design, Setting, and Participants.*—Prospective observational cohort study at a single academic medical center among 1416 hospitalized adults tested for *C difficile* toxins 72 hours or longer after admission between December 1, 2010, and October 20, 2012. The analysis was conducted in stages with revisions from April 27, 2013, to January 13, 2015.

*Main Outcomes and Measures.*—Patients undergoing *C difficile* testing-were grouped by US Food and Drug Administration–approved toxin and PCR tests as Tox+/PCR+, Tox−/PCR+, or Tox−/PCR−. Toxin results were reported clinically. Polymerase chain reaction results were not reported. The main study outcomes were duration of diarrhea during up to 14 days of treatment, rate of CDI-related complications (ie, colectomy, megacolon, or intensive care unit care) and CDI-related death within 30 days.

*Results.*—Twenty-one percent (293 of 1416) of hospitalized adults tested for *C difficile* were positive by PCR, but 44.7% (131 of 293) had toxins detected by the clinical toxin test. At baseline, Tox−/PCR+ patients had lower *C difficile* bacterial load and less antibiotic exposure, fecal inflammation, and diarrhea than Tox+/PCR+ patients ($P < .001$ for all). The median duration of diarrhea was shorter in Tox−/PCR+ patients (2 days; interquartile range, 1-4 days) than in Tox+/PCR+ patients (3 days; interquartile range, 1-6 days) ($P = .003$) and was similar to that in Tox−/PCR− patients (2 days; interquartile range, 1-3 days), despite minimal empirical treatment of Tox−/PCR+ patients. No CDI-related complications occurred in Tox−/PCR+ patients vs 10 complications in Tox+/PCR+ patients (0% vs 7.6%, $P < .001$). One Tox−/PCR+ patient had recurrent CDI as a contributing factor to death within 30 days vs 11 CDI-related deaths in Tox+/PCR+ patients (0.6% vs 8.4%, $P = .001$).

*Conclusions and Relevance.*—Among hospitalized adults with suspected CDI, virtually all CDI-related complications and deaths occurred in patients with positive toxin immunoassay test results. Patients with a positive molecular test result and a negative toxin immunoassay test result had outcomes that were comparable to patients without *C difficile* by either method. Exclusive reliance on molecular tests for CDI diagnosis without tests for toxins or host response is likely to result in overdiagnosis, overtreatment, and increased health care costs.

▶ The increases in the rate of *Clostridium difficile* infection (CDI) between 2000 and 2008 were attributed to the emergence of a novel, hypervirulent strain. At that point, more than 95% of laboratories were using toxin immunoassays for diagnosis. The introduction of molecular tests that are more sensitive and detect microbial DNA instead of toxin is now felt to be behind the more recent increase. Increases of 50% to 100% in rate of CDI have been reported after switching from toxin tests to molecular tests.[1,2] As the facilities adopted molecular tests, increases have been observed in the rate of publicly reported CDI. Because polymerase chain reaction (PCR) detects the presence of bacteria similarly to culture methods, the results are of uncertain clinical significance given that *C difficile* colonization is 5 to 10 times more common than CDI, and noninfectious causes of diarrhea are common.

This article addresses the question whether patients with negative toxin test results and positive molecular test results for CDI are simply colonized and the diarrhea is from an unrelated cause.

This study addresses 3 clinically relevant questions. First, the natural history of PCR-positive patients with negative toxin immunoassay results. Second, the outcomes in patients with PCR positive and toxin negative compared with those with positive PCR and toxin or those with both tests negative. Of the hospitalized adults evaluated for CDI 21% (293 of 1416) tested positive by PCR. However, only 44.7% (131 of 293) were toxin positive by the routinely used clinical toxin test. These patients did not experience adverse events without treatment for CDI. Virtually all CDI-related complications and deaths occurred in patients with detectable toxin by immunoassay. The data clearly show that molecular tests are not specific for CDI even in the presence of symptoms. The outcomes in patients with positive PCR and negative toxin tests were comparable to patients with both tests negative. As recommended by investigators in the United Kingdom, the US authors of this study recommend a 2-step screening test, such as PCR or glutamate dehydrogenase antigen detection, followed by a toxin test to confirm active infection.[3] In the future, quantitative PCR may be more reliable for clinical use.

**N. M. Khardori, MD, PhD**

*References*


1. Longtin Y, Trottier S, Brochu G, et al. Impact of the type of diagnostic assay on *Clostridium difficile* infection and complication rates in a mandatory reporting program. *Clin Infect Dis*. 2013;56:67-73.
2. Koo HL, Van JN, Zhao M, et al. Real-time polymerase chain reaction detection of asymptomatic *Clostridium difficile* colonization and rising *C. difficile*—associated disease rates. *Infect Control Hosp Epidemiol*. 2014;35:667-673.
3. Department of Health, United Kingdom. Updated guidance on the diagnosis and reporting of *Clostridium difficile*. https://www.gov.uk/government/publications/updated-guidance-on-the-diagnosis-and-reporting-of-clostridium-difficile. Accessed July 8, 2015.

# 22 Miscellaneous

---

**Vitamin D [1,25(OH)$_2$D$_3$] Differentially Regulates Human Innate Cytokine Responses to Bacterial versus Viral Pattern Recognition Receptor Stimuli**

Fitch N, Becker AB, HayGlass KT (Univ of Manitoba, Winnipeg, Canada)

*J Immunol* 196:2965-2972, 2016

---

Vitamin D plays multiple roles in regulation of protective and maladaptive immunity. Although epidemiologic studies link poor in vivo 25(OH)D status to increased viral respiratory infections, we poorly understand how vitamin D affects viral pattern recognition receptor (PRR)-driven cytokine production. In this study, we hypothesized that the biologically active metabolite of vitamin D, 1,25(OH)$_2$D$_3$, inhibits human proinflammatory and anti-inflammatory innate cytokine responses stimulated by representative bacterial or viral PRR ligands. Fresh PBMCs or CD14$^+$ monocytes were stimulated with TLR4, TLR7/8-selective ligands, or respiratory syncytial virus (RSV) ± 1,25(OH)$_2$D$_3$. Proinflammatory and anti-inflammatory responses resulting from TLR4 stimulation were inhibited ~50% in the presence of 1,25(OH)$_2$D$_3$. Conversely, its usage at physiologic through pharmacologic concentrations inhibited neither proinflammatory nor anti-inflammatory responses evoked by viral PRR ligands or infectious RSV. This differential responsiveness was attributed to the finding that TLR7/8, but not TLR4, stimulation markedly inhibited vitamin D receptor mRNA and protein expression, selectively reducing the sensitivity of viral PRR responses to modulation. 1,25(OH)$_2$D$_3$ also enhanced expression of IkBa, a potent negative regulator of NF-κB and cytokine production, in TLR4-stimulated monocytes while not doing so upon TLR7/8 stimulation. Thus, 1,25(OH)$_2$D$_3$ inhibits both proinflammatory and a broad panel of anti-inflammatory responses elicited by TLR4 stimulation, arguing that the common view of it as an antiinflammatory immune response modifier is an oversimplification. In viral responses, it consistently fails to modify TLR7/8- or RSV stimulated innate cytokine production, even at supraphysiologic concentrations. Collectively, the data call into question the rationale for increasingly widespread self-medication with vitamin D supplements.

► Vitamin D deficiency has been linked to a large number of human diseases, including infection. This has led to change of self-medication with vitamin C in the 1970s and 1980s to self-medication with vitamin D in many countries. The biologically active metabolite 1,25(OH)$_2$D$_3$ acts on the immune system at multiple levels. Its effect on antimicrobial peptide production is well studied.[1]

However, the effect of vitamin D on immune regulation, specifically cytokine production by the innate immune response that programs subsequent adoptive immune response, is not well characterized.

This study was started to test the hypothesis that 1,25$(OH)_2D_3$ acts on innate immune cells of healthy humans to decrease proinflammatory and to enhance protective anti-inflammatory cytokine and chemokine responses after stimulation with both well-defined synthetic and infectious viral stimuli. The authors conclude that active metabolite of vitamin D exerts a qualitatively different impact on TLR4 versus TLR7/8-stimulated innate immunity in humans. TLR4-dependent proinflammatory and anti-inflammatory cytokine and chemokine responses were strongly inhibited in the presence of vitamin D. In contrast, TLR7/8-dependent responses were unaffected throughout the dose range from physiologic to pharmacologic. These findings translate into a differential susceptibility of bacterial versus viral purified pattern recognition (PRR) ligands to vitamin D modulation. This is the first report of differential susceptibility of bacterial versus viral PRR responses to Vitamin D modulation. The data clearly argue for more critical assessment of linking the presumed protective benefits of vitamin D to prevention and/or resolution of viral infections in healthy populations. They also point to the fact that the common view of vitamin D as an anti-inflammatory immune response modifier is an oversimplification because both proinflammatory and anti-inflammatory responses elicited by TLR4 stimulation are inhibited. In conclusion, the data do not provide rationale for widespread self-medication with vitamin D supplements for beneficial effect against bacteria or viruses.

**N. M. Khardori, MD, PhD**

*Reference*

1. White JH. Vitamin D as an inducer of cathelicidin antimicrobial peptide expression: past, present and future. *J Steroid Biochem Mol Biol.* 2010;121:234-238.

---

### Your Viral Past: A Comprehensive Method for Serological Profiling to Explore the Human Virome

Burnham C-A, McAdam AJ (Washington Univ School of Medicine, St Louis, MO; Boston Children's Hosp, MA)
*Clin Chem* 62:426-427, 2016

---

*Background.*—Multiplexing of diagnostic tests allows the simultaneous assay for several different pathogens within a single test. Multiplex molecular assays are commonly used for pathogens and genetic markers of antibiotic resistance but are not as commonly employed for detecting antibodies specific to pathogens. The body's antibody responses to pathogens may take a week or longer to develop, but are often long-lived, so their detection could indicate present, recent, and long-past infections. The usefulness of the multiplexing approach becomes apparent when put in the context of the body's virome, or the collection of viruses in an individual. Although the microbiome can be studied for numbers of bacteria because they share the 16S rRNA gene, no conserved genetic signature exists for the broad detection and identification of viruses.

*Characterizing the Virome.*—The VirScan test uses a novel array approach that can provide comprehensive serological profiles of viruses using a synthetic human virome. Immunoprecipitation is combined with next-generation sequencing of a bacteriophage library containing peptides that represent viruses that infect humans. The DNA microarray and bacteriophage display is combined to create a uniform picture of viral peptides, then next-generation sequencing is used to determine the sequence of the DNA encoding the peptides recognized by the antibodies in blood samples of subjects. As a result, researchers can look into the interactions between the human immune system and the virome. VirScan detects not just recent or current viral infection but also potentially the cumulative history of viral infections over the lifetime of the individual.

*Application.*—The VirScan assay was used to profile 569 persons from various continents of varying ages and with varying HIV status. Viral antibody detection varied with age, geographic area, and HIV status. In persons less than age 10 years, antibodies to fewer viruses were detected compared to older, geographically matched controls, but antibodies to some viruses associated with childhood were often detected in the children. An average serologic evidence of infection with 10 viral species was found per person, but the results ranged up to 62 viruses in five persons and up to 84 viruses in two persons.

*Limitations.*—Medications such as IVIg and immunosuppressive agents interfere with the results. Further tests are needed to validate the VirScan assay results. The assay may be limited in its ability to analyze antibiotic sensitivity for some viruses. In addition, the test antigens were limited to those viruses known to infect humans, so the assay will not detect antibodies against emerging or new viruses.

*Conclusions.*—VirScan is one tool that will help to expand our understanding of human virome status. As costs decrease and more advances are made in sample preparation and bioinformatics, more clinical laboratories will be able to perform these assays and possibly obtain information about the role of viruses in chronic disease and cancer as well as immune system function.

▶ Infectious disease diagnostics are in a phase of rapid advancement and change from culture-based traditional methods to genome and proteome-based methods. A major advantage of newer methods is multiplexing to allow simultaneous testing for a number of different pathogens within a single assay. The multiplex molecular assays such as multiplex polymerase chain reaction are now approved by Food and Drug Administration for more than 20 pathogens and genetic markers of resistance from a single clinical specimen. Multiplex testing is much less available for detecting antibodies specific for pathogens. Although not helpful for early diagnosis, antibodies are often long lived and detect present, recent, or long-lasting infections. The ease with which bacteria can be studied has contributed vastly to the understanding of human Microbiome. The microorganism contained in our microbiome vary by body site and may contribute to individuals state of health and disease. It is now being recognized that we share our body with microorganisms other than bacteria including fungi and viruses. The so-called virome is a collection of viruses within an individual ranging from those viruses that cause acute infection (eg, influenza virus) to those that persist or cause latent infections (eg, cytomegalovirus). The knowledge regarding the impact of the virome on human health is in its early phase of study.[1] Large unbiased surveys have attempted to incriminate a viral etiology for diseases for which no specific virus has been implicated. The 16S rRNA gene is a common genetic element that bacteria share and is useful in investigating bacterial communities. On the other hand, a conserved genetic signature for viruses does not exist. A test called VirScan was recently described and uses a novel assay approach that can provide comprehensive serologic profiling for viruses using a synthetic human virome.[2] The method uses immunoprecipitation combined with next generation sequencing of a bacteriophage library containing peptides representing viruses known to infect humans. Serologic evidence of infection with 10 viral species was detected per person, antibodies to 62 viruses were noted in 5 individuals and to 84 viruses in 2 individuals. In addition to characterizing the virome, combination tests like VirScan can be used to detect viral nucleic acids in clinical samples containing peptides representing viruses known to infect humans for diagnostic purposes.

**N. M. Khardori, MD, PhD**

*References*

1. Wylie KM, Weinstock GM, Storch GA. Virome genomics: a tool for defining the human virome. *Curr Opin Microbiol.* 2013;16:479-484.
2. Xu GJ, Kula T, Xu Q, et al. Viral immunology. Conmprehensive serological profiling of human populations using a synthetic human virome. *Science.* 2015;348: aaa0698.

---

**Exposure to moxifloxacin and cytomegalovirus replication is associated with skin squamous cell carcinoma development in lung transplant recipients**

Gerber SR, Seifert B, Inci I, et al (Univ Hosp Zurich, Switzerland; Univ of Zurich, Switzerland)

*J Eur Acad Dermatol Venereol* 29:2451-2457, 2015

---

*Background.*—Lung transplant recipients (LTR) are at increased risk for squamous cell carcinoma of the skin (SCC), but risk factors (RF) are incompletely understood.

*Objective.*—To assess associations between exposure to certain medications and viral infections, and subsequent SCC development.

*Methods.*—Retrospective study examining incidence and potential RF for SCC in LTR transplanted from 1992 to 2010 followed up at one centre. Cumulative incidence and Cox proportional hazards regression models were used to evaluate RF in the first year post-transplant for SCC formation during the follow-up.

*Results.*—In 205 analysed LTR, 46 patients were diagnosed with SCC during a median follow-up of 4.9 years. The cumulative incidences of first SCC were 16.7% and 34.1%, for 5 and 10 years post-transplantation respectively. Multivariable analysis identified CMV replication (HR 7.69, 95% CI 2.93–20.2, $P < 0.001$) and moxifloxacin exposure (HR 2.35, 95% CI 1.15–4.81, $P = 0.020$) during the first year post-transplantation as independent RF for SCC development during follow-up.

*Conclusion.*—In our cohort, moxifloxacin use and CMV replication during the first year post-transplantation were associated with increased risk for SCC. These two factors could be indicators of over-immunosuppression. Their role in SCC development requires investigations in larger cohorts and prospective studies.

► As the number of solid organ transplant recipients (SOTRs) and survivors are increasing, the risk for subsequent development of malignancies is likewise increasing.[1] Keratinocyte skin cancers, squamous cell carcinoma (SCC) and basal cell carcinoma are the most common posttransplant malignancies in populations of European descent. The incidence of SCC in this population depends on the ultraviolet radiation (UVR) exposure and prevalence of the cancer in the general population with a marked geographic variation. In general, the incidence rates of SCC in SOTRs are 20- to 250-fold higher than the general population.

This retrospective study from 1992 to 2010 reports on the association between exposure medications and viral infection and development of SCC in 205 lung transplant recipients (LTRs). Male gender, sun exposure, UVR, skin type, duration, type and intensity of immunosuppression are known risk factors for development of SCC in SOTRs. The potential of voriconazole to cause photosensitization and enhance UVR-related skin cancer in SOTRs has been well reported.[2] Fluoroquinolones, also with photosensitizing potential, are among the antibiotics frequently used in SOTRs. In the present cohort of LTRs, the incidence of SCC was documented to be 22.4% during the median follow-up of 4.9 years. Some of the known risk factors for SCC were confirmed in this study. In addition, moxifloxacin exposure and duration of cytomegalovirus replication during the first year posttransplant were significantly and independently associated with development of SCC during follow-up. Exposure to other quinolones, including ciprofloxacin and levofloxacin, was not associated with increased incidence of SCC in this study. Interestingly, moxifloxacin has been reported to have milder photosensitization effect than other quinolones. The higher cumulative dose and/or other unidentified factors may be responsible for the association described with moxifloacin.

**N. M. Khardori, MD, PhD**

*Reference*

1. Williams K, Mansh M, Chin-Hong P, Singer J, Arron ST. Voriconazole-associated cutaneous malignancy: a literature review on photocarcinogenesis in organ transplant recipients. *Clin Infect Dis.* 2014;58:997-1002.

## Genome-Based Infection Tracking Reveals Dynamics of *Clostridium difficile* Transmission and Disease Recurrence

Kumar N, Miyajima F, He M, et al (Wellcome Trust Sanger Inst, Hinxton, UK; Univ of Liverpool, UK; et al)
*Clin Infect Dis* 62:746-752, 2016

*Background.*—Accurate tracking of *Clostridium difficile* transmission within healthcare settings is key to its containment but is hindered by the lack of discriminatory power of standard genotyping methods. We describe a whole-genome phylogenetic-based method to track the transmission of individual clones in infected hospital patients from the epidemic *C. difficile* 027/ST1 lineage, and to distinguish between the 2 causes of recurrent disease, relapse (same strain), or reinfection (different strain).

*Methods.*—We monitored patients with *C. difficile* infection in a UK hospital over a 2-year period. We performed whole-genome sequencing and phylogenetic analysis of 108 strains isolated from symptomatic patients. High-resolution phylogeny was integrated with in-hospital transfers and contact data to create an infection network linking individual patients and specific hospital wards.

*Results.*—Epidemic *C. difficile* 027/ST1 caused the majority of infections during our sampling period. Integration of whole-genome single nucleotide polymorphism (SNP) phylogenetic analysis, which accurately discriminated between 27 distinct SNP genotypes, with patient movement and contact data identified 32 plausible transmission events, including ward-based contamination (66%) or direct donor–recipient contact (34%). Highly contagious donors were identified who contributed to the persistence of clones within distinct hospital wards and the spread of clones between wards, especially in areas of intense turnover. Recurrent cases were identified between 4 and 26 weeks, highlighting the limitation of the standard <8-week cutoff used for patient diagnosis and management.

*Conclusions.*—Genome-based infection tracking to monitor the persistence and spread of *C. difficile* within healthcare facilities could inform infection control and patient management.

▶ Unlike most other health care–associated infection, *Clostridium difficile* infection (CDI) is transmitted by highly resistant spores that overcome standard infection prevention measures. Spores excreted by both asymptomatic carriers and symptomatic patients excrete *C difficile* spores, leading to spread by direct (person-to-person) or indirect (environmental) modes of transmission. The key to the containment of *C difficile* is accurate tracking, which has been difficult to accomplish because of the lack of discriminatory power of standard genotyping methods. As for other bacterial pathogens, high-throughput, whole-genome sequencing (WGS) has been successful in investigating *C difficile* at the global, national, and local levels.[1]

This study combines WGS with detailed epidemiological data to monitor *C difficile* 027/ST1, its persistence, and its transmission over a 2-year period within a large university hospital in Liverpool, United Kingdom. The investigators adopted an epidemiological model that identifies the most plausible *C difficile* transmission events based on shared time and location of patients and *C difficile* multilocus sequence typing genotype. The resolution of the model was enhanced by incorporating all recorded patient movements between wards to trace the spread of *C difficile* 027 within the hospital. The investigators were able to identify 32 transmission events including 21 ward-based transmission events and 11 directional transmission events within and between specific wards. The majority of transmission events (60%) occurred within specific wards except the infectious disease/isolation wards with stringent infection control practices in place. *C difficile* was spread between wards in 22% of events. Highly contagious donors of *C difficile* with the potential of having been "super-spreaders" were identified in the acute medicine assessment unit (AMAU) and were responsible for spreading infection throughout the hospital. The relatively short infectious period of super-spreaders suggest a brief but highly contagious state.

**N. M. Khardori, MD, PhD**

*Reference*

1. He M, Miyajima F, Roberts P, et al. Emergence and global spread of epidemic healthcare-associated *Clostridium difficile*. *Nat Genet*. 2013;45:109-113.

# 23 New Antibiotics

**Alternating antibiotic treatments constrain evolutionary paths to multidrug resistance**

Kim S, Lieberman TD, Kishony R (Harvard Med School, Boston, MA)

*Proc Natl Acad Sci U S A* 111:14494-14499, 2014

Alternating antibiotic therapy, in which pairs of drugs are cycled during treatment, has been suggested as a means to inhibit the evolution of de novo resistance while avoiding the toxicity associated with more traditional combination therapy. However, it remains unclear under which conditions and by what means such alternating treatments impede the evolution of resistance. Here, we tracked multistep evolution of resistance in replicate populations of Staphylococcus aureus during 22 d of continuously increasing single-, mixed-, and alternating-drug treatment. In all three tested drug pairs, the alternating treatment reduced the overall rate of resistance by slowing the acquisition of resistance to one of the two component drugs, sometimes as effectively as mixed treatment. This slower rate of evolution is reflected in the genomewide mutational profiles; under alternating treatments, bacteria acquire mutations in different genes than under corresponding single-drug treatments. To test whether this observed constraint on adaptive paths reflects trade-offs in which resistance to one drug is accompanied by sensitivity to a second drug, we profiled many single-step mutants for cross-resistance. Indeed, the average cross-resistance of single-step mutants can help predict whether or not evolution was slower in alternating drugs. Together, these results show that despite the complex evolutionary landscape of multidrug resistance, alternating-drug therapy can slow evolution by constraining the mutational paths toward resistance.

▶ Antibiotic cycling or rotation (ie, selected agents used for defined periods of time in a systematic manner in entire hospital wards) has been used and debated as a tool to reduce development of resistance.[1] In a recent study, *Escherichia coli* cells with a mutation conferring resistance to 1 drug and collateral sensitivity to a second drug (negative cross-resistance) were shown to be outcompeted by wild-type cells in the presence of the second drug, suggesting that acquisition of resistance may be slowed by cycling.[2] Alternating antibiotic regimens avoids the cost, toxicity, and risk of antagonism associated with traditional combination therapy. Also how such treatments affect adaptive mutational paths to resistance is the crucial question.

In this study, the rate of evolution of resistance in *Staphylococcus aureus* in the presence of single, mixed (combination) and alternating antimicrobial drugs was characterized. The drugs chosen for the study are neomycin (representing aminoglycosides), ciprofloxacin (representing fluoroquinolones), and trimethoprim (representing a commonly prescribed combination of trimethoprim and sulfamethoxazole). These agents were chosen based on their 3 different mechanisms of antibacterial activity. The evolved population after exposure were sequenced to understand genotypic adaptation in single and multiple drug environments. The cross-resistance profiles of a separate set of single step mutants exposed to each of the 3 drugs were determined to explore whether the effectiveness of alternating drugs is associated with diminished selection for resistance mutations to 1 drug, but increased sensitivity to the other. Using whole-genome sequencing and experimental evolution of antibiotic resistance, the researchers present evidence that alternating drugs slows the rate of increase in resistance compared with same-drug treatment. The underlying mechanism is by constraining resistance mutations with trade-off in resistance to a second drug even when the drugs are not used simultaneously. The authors speculate that in addition to the effect on de novo mutations, alternating therapy may also impede horizontal acquisition of antibiotic resistance by increasing the likelihood that bacteria with the acquired mechanism would be inhibited by at least 1 antibiotic.

**N. M. Khardori, MD, PhD**

*References*

1. Brown EM, Nathwani D. Antibiotic cycling or rotation: a systematic review of the evidence of efficacy. *J Antimicrob Chemother.* 2005;55:6-9.
2. Imamovic L, Sommer MOA. Use of collateral sensitivity networks to design drug cycling protocols that avoid resistance development. *Sci Transl Med.* 2013;5: ra132.

---

**Microbiology: Phage therapy redux – What is to be done?**

Young R, Gill JJ (Texas A&M Univ, College Station)

*Science* 350:1163-1164, 2015

---

*Background.*—Phage therapy is the use of viruses that infect and replicate in a bacterium to treat pathogenic bacteria. Although the approach was proposed many years ago, it was discarded in the 1940s because of a poor understanding of what phages were and how they functioned compared to the chemical antibiotics that were being developed. With the global crisis in antibiotic-resistant microorganisms and a better appreciation of the human microbiota, interest in phage therapy is resurging for not just bacterial infections but also as a way to modulate microbiota.

*New Focus.*—The tailed phages, or *Caudovirales,* are the most numerous and diverse biological entities in the biosphere and have a head, a tail, and usually tail fibers. The phage makes specific contacts with receptors on the bacterial target using the tail or tail fibers. Once the DNA is injected into the cell through the tail, the phage follows a replicative cycle that ends with host lysis, which frees hundreds of progeny virions. Some phages can also become stable components of the host genome, forming dormant prophages; these are called temperate or lysogenic phages.

Just as in classic phage therapy, the technique relies on the isolation and use of naturally occurring phages found in the environment. Phages are isolated, screened for host ranges among pathogenic bacterial strains, and then assessed in vitro or in vivo in animal models.

Lysins or muralytic enzymes are used by phages to penetrate DNA through the cell envelope and in the host lysis process. These enzymes rapidly kill Gram-positive bacteria, demonstrate genus-level specificity, and have not yet generated resistant organisms.

Tailocins are phage tail-like bacteriocins or headless phages. Once adsorbed to a receptor, the tailocin particle lethally damages the host cell envelop. Engineered tailocins can be retargeted to heterologous hosts, can be deployed even in the absence of the environmental release of recombinant DNA, and can be given in a defined dose.

*Uses and Regulation.*—All three of the phage-based strategies are being pursued commercially and are in various preclinical stages. The most attention is being directed toward bacterial pathogens that are already hard to manage with conventional antibiotics, including *Pseudomonas aeruginosa, Staphylococcus aureus,* and *Clostridium difficile.* Phage products for controlling food-borne pathogens are already being used.

Before proceeding further, researchers need to establish some phage-specific rules. Examples include prohibiting the use of lysogenic phages because they usually carry genes that alter the pathogenic potential of their hosts and establishing the identity of the host receptor for all phages proposed for therapeutic use. Standardizing phage collections and using phages consistently across studies would further development in this area. In addition, many phages require interactions with other host components to complete their life cycles. These interactions must be better understood, as should the transport of phages into the niches where their targets reside, interactions with bacteria in their normal physiological state, and possible surprises that may arise.

*Conclusions.*—Phage therapy offers the possibility of using biological entities with a wide diversity and adaptability to address difficult bacterial infections. However, the use of phages to support human health should be pursued with caution, diligence, rigor, and patience to avoid too many surprises.

► The short life of bacteriophage therapy ended in the mid-20th century as a result of the development of antimicrobial chemotherapeutic agents and critical reports from the American Medical Association.[1] With the recognition of significance of preservation of individual human microbiota and the realities of the global resistance of pathogenic bacteria to antimicrobial agents, there is a resurgence of interest in phage therapy. In 2015, a meeting on phage-based therapeutics was hosted by the US National Institute of Allergy and Infectious Diseases. In addition to phage biologists, the participants included public and governmental research organizations, clinicians, private companies, and the federal regulatory community. Despite differences of opinion among groups, there was consensus about the potential of phage therapy and therefore appropriate investigation.

The renewed focus on this form of therapy is based on the recognition of the tailed phages, aka *caudovirales*. These are the most numerous and diverse biological entities in the biosphere.[2] They have a head containing a linear double-stranded DNA molecule of 15 to 500 kilo-base pairs, a tail, and in most cases tail fibers. They make specific contacts with the receptors of their bacterial host using the tail or tail fibers or both. The phage undergoes a replicative cycle (following the injection of DNA) resulting in host/bacterial cell lysis and liberation of hundreds of virions ready to infect more bacterial cells. The temperate or lysogenic *caudovirales* phage form dormant prophages inside the bacterial host. For potential therapeutic use, phages are isolated, screened for their host ranges, evaluated in vitro and in animal models, and sometimes formulated in mixture to cover a broad host range similar to what is done for chemotherapeutic antimicrobial agents. The 2 other emerging phage-related potential therapeutic options are muralytic enzymes or lysins and tailocins. Lysins are used by phages during the penetration of DNA and in the phage lysis process and able to rapidly kill Gram-positive bacteria. Tailocins or phage tail-like bacteriocins or headless phages cause a single-hit lethality by damage to the host cell envelope. To produce "ideal" killer phages, both the good news and the potential of surprise in store need to be considered. The majority of phage genes are of unknown function, and phages have incredible diversity and adaptability.

**N. M. Khardori, MD, PhD**

*References*

1. Summers WC. Bacteriophage therapy. *Annu Rev Microbiol.* 2001;55:437.
2. Brussow H, Hendrix RW. Phage genomics: small is beautiful. *Cell.* 2002;108: 13-16.

---

**Antibiotics: Homed to the hideout**

Hardt W-D (ETH Zürich, Switzerland)
*Nature* 527:309-310, 2015

---

*Background.*—Antibiotics are the basis for much of modern medicine, but the worldwide spread of antibiotic-resistant genes makes it difficult to treat some infections, such as those caused by *Staphylococcus aureus*. However, even strains of *S aureus* that lack resistance genes can be difficult to eradicate with current antibiotics because the bacteria can "hide" inside host cells and take on a "persistent" lifestyle. A construct has been developed in which an antibiotic is linked to an antibody that binds to the surface of the pathogenic bacterium, creating a "prodrug." It is inactive by itself, but when the prodrug-coated bacteria enter host cells, enzymes trigger the release of the antibiotic. Mouse trials have indicated that this approach is measurably more potent than standard antibiotic agents.

*Prodrug Strategy.*—Researchers generated a rifampicin derivative (rifalogue) with modified physicochemical properties that is active against *S aureus* cells that have switched to a persistent lifestyle and are resistant to antibiotics. Then they identified an antibody that binds tightly to the sugar structures on the surface of all the *S aureus* strains that were considered. These were covalently bonded using a chemical bridge that breaks when exposed to protease enzymes in the intracellular sites where *S aureus* is believed to be hiding. This antibody-antibiotic conjugate (AAC) reduced pathogen loads more effectively than two conventional antibiotics used against resistant *S aureus*.

*Efficacy.*—The efficacy of the AAC approach is greater than that of standard antibiotics for a number of possible reasons. First, the rifalogue is more efficient than rifampicin in killing persistent *S aureus* cells. Second, its fusion with the antibody appears to produce more favorable kinetics of drug distribution, excretion, and inactivation. Third, coating the bacterial cells with the prodrug and antibiotic may steer the bacteria into intracellular compartments with high levels of the enzymes required to release the antibiotic. Fourth, an accumulation of the AAC on the pathogen's surface may yield high local concentrations of the bacteria in the intracellular site.

*Conclusions.*—Reminiscent of antibody-targeted prodrug therapies used against cancer, this targeted AAC approach offers promise in the fight against resistant intracellular pathogens such as *S aureus*. It is likely that this approach will reduce the emergence of antibiotic resistance and any disruption of the body's normal microbial communities. Researchers may also be able to use older antibiotics that weren't developed further because of unfavorable pharmacokinetics or toxicity. Finally, this is just one alternative strategy to address antibiotic resistance. Other approaches include antibiotics targeted to specific persistent cells, agents that will stimulate the host's antimicrobial defenses to buoy up the antibiotic treatment, or harmless "biocontrol" agents that colonize the host and inhibit the growth of pathogens.

► It has been known for more than 5 decades that *Staphylococcus aureus* is able to invade and survive inside mammalian cells including the phagocytic cells responsible for killing the bacteria.[1] Incomplete clearance of *S aureus* inside phagocytes allows these infected cell to act as Trojan horses for dissemination away from the initial site of infection. There is evidence that patients with normal neutrophil counts may be more susceptible to disseminated disease than those with reduced counts.[2] Once delivered "live" by neutrophils to the tissues, *S aureus* invades nonphagocytic tissue cells leading to chronic or recurrent infection. Intracellular *S aureus*, in addition, induces destruction of neutrophils further undermining innate immune responses.[3,4] Taken together, these data point to ablation of intracellular *S aureus* as the key to clinical success.

This study provides evidence for this hypothesis that so far has not been tested directly. First, the data show that *S aureus* sequestered inside murine macrophages were not killed by vancomycin, daptomycin, or linezolid when exposed to clinically achievable concentrations of these agents. Second, intracellular

*S aureus* sequestered inside mouse peritoneal neutrophils and macrophages infected mice with higher bacterial burdens in the kidneys, brains, osteoblast, and many other cell types in the presence of vancomycin treatment. Intracellular growth of *S aureus* occurred in many cell types despite ongoing antibiotic therapy. Third, they developed a novel therapeutic agent (AAC) that is activated specifically inside mammalian cells with sequestered *S aureus*. AAC, the antibody-antibiotic conjugate consists of an anti–*S aureus* antibody (TH10MAB) covalently linked to a highly efficacious antibiotic using a cathepsin-cleavable linker containing a novel quaternary ammonium salt. The designed AAC has no direct antibacterial activity and does not diffused into mammalian cells due to the size of the antibody molecule. Once AAC opsonized bacteria are taken up by the host cells, intracellular proteases cleave the linker and release the active antibiotic. A sufficient concentration of free antibiotic within the phagosome is released to cause bacterial killing. Fourth, the AAC was shown to specifically target intracellular *S aureus* and prevent cell-to-cell transfer of bacteria. Treatment with a single dose of AAC eliminated the bacteria that had escaped vancomycin treatment and were able to colonize the brain. Fifth, the effect of AAC on the sequestered bacteria was superior to that of vancomycin, antibody alone, or unconjugated antibiotic (a rifalogue). The release of the antibiotic from the AAC was essential for efficacy. This rifalogue is able to kill nonreplicating bacteria and antibiotic resistant persister cells.

**N. M. Khardori, MD, PhD**

*References*


1. Gresham HD, Lowrance JH, Caver TE, Wilson BS, Cheung AL, Lindberg FP. Survival of Staphylococcus aureus inside neutrophils contributes to infection. *J Immunol.* 2000;164:3713-3722.
2. Velasco E, Byington R, Martins CA, Schirmer M, Dias LM, Gonçalves VM. Comparative study of clinical characteristics of neurtopenic and non-neutropenic adult cancer patiens with bloodstream infections. *Eur J Clin Microbial Infect Dis.* 2006;25:1-7.
3. Greenlee-Wacker MC, Rigby KM, Kobayashi SD, Porter AR, DeLeo FR, Nauseef WM. Phagocytosis of Staphylocossus aureus by human neutrophils prevents macrophage efferocytosis and induces programmed necrosis. *J Immunol.* 2014;192:4709-4717.
4. KIobayashi SD, Braughton KR, Palazzolo-Ballance AM, et al. Rapid neutrophil destruction following phagocytosis of *Staphylococcus aureus. J Innate Immun.* 2010;2:2560-2575.


## A Phase 2 Trial of Oral Solithromycin 1200 mg or 1000 mg as Single-Dose Oral Therapy for Uncomplicated Gonorrhea

Hook EW III, Golden M, Jamieson BD, et al (Univ of Alabama at Birmingham; Univ of Washington, Seattle; Cempra Inc, Chapel Hill, NC)

*Clin Infect Dis* 61:1043-1048, 2015

*Background.*—Progressive resistance to antimicrobial agents has reduced options for gonorrhea therapy worldwide. Solithromycin (CEM-101) is a novel oral fluoroketolide antimicrobial with substantial in vitro activity against *Neisseria gonorrhoeae.*

*Methods.*—We conducted a phase 2 trial of 2 oral doses of solithromycin (1200 and 1000 mg) for treatment of uncomplicated gonorrhea.

*Results.*—A total of 59 participants were enrolled and treated in this trial; 28 participants received 1200 mg of solithromycin and 31 received 1000 mg. Forty-six (78%) participants had positive cultures for *N. gonorrhoeae* at the time of enrollment: 24 of the 28 persons (86%) who received 1200 mg of oral solithromycin, and 22 of 31 (71%) who received 1000 mg. In addition, 8 participants had positive pharyngeal gonococcal cultures, and 4 had positive rectal cultures. All patients with positive cultures for *N. gonorrhoeae* were cured at all sites of infection. *Chlamydia trachomatis and Mycoplasma genitalium* coinfections were evaluated using nucleic acid amplification tests and were negative at 1 week of follow-up in 9 of 11 (82%) participants positive for *C. trachomatis* and 7 of 10 (70%) participants positive for *M. genitalium.* Mild dose-related gastrointestinal side effects (nausea, loose stools, vomiting) were common but did not limit therapy.

*Conclusions.*—Oral single-dose solithromycin, in doses of 1000 mg and 1200 mg, was 100% effective for treatment of culture-proven gonorrhea at genital, oral, and rectal sites of infection and is a promising new agent for gonorrhea treatment.

*Clinical Trials Registration.*—NCT01591447.

► In the recent years, the ongoing resistance and dwindling number of antibiotics available for treatment of gonorrhea has become a global public health problem. The US Centers for Disease Control and Prevention recently narrowed the recommended therapy for gonorrhea to a single regimen consisting of an injectable cephalosporin, ceftriaxone (250 mg), administered concomitantly with a single 1 g oral dose of azithromycin.[1] Given the documented progressive decline in susceptibility of *Neisseria gonorrhoeae* to cephalosporins and 10% US population reporting allergy to beta-lactam antibiotics, alternate antibiotic classes are needed for treatment and control of gonorrhea.

In this study, solithromycin, a novel oral fluoroketolide antimicrobial agent with excellent in vitro activity against *N gonorrhoeae*, was used to treat uncomplicated gonorrhea in a phase II clinical trial. Of the 59 patients enrolled, 46 had positive genital cultures for *N gonorrhoeae*, 8 had positive pharyngeal cultures, and 6 had positive rectal cultures. In addition, 11 and 10 patients, respectively, showed evidence of *Chlamydia trachomatis* and *Mycoplasma genitalium* coinfections diagnosed by nucleic acid amplification tests. All patients received the experimental drug, 1200 mg for 28 and 1000 mg for 31 patients, respectively.

In vitro antimicrobial susceptibility testing on 47 pretreatment *N gonorrhoeae* isolates show minimum inhibitory concentrations of <0.008 to 0.125 μg/mL. The most common treatment-associated (dose-related) adverse events were gastrointestinal in nature. There were no adverse events limiting medication use. A microbiological cure was documented in all patients with positive cultures at all sites of infection including the harder to treat extra-genital sites indicating a

100% efficacy. The highly sensitive nucleic acid amplification tests were negative for *C trachomatis* in 82% and for *M genitalium* in 70% at 1-week follow-up. The activity of a single oral dose of solithromycin for *N gonorrhoeae* and concomitant *C trachomatis* and *M genitalium* infection in this study is highly promising.

**N. M. Khardori, MD, PhD**

*Reference*

1. Centers for Disease Control and Prevention. Update to CDC's sexually transmitted diseases treatment guidelines, 2010: oral cephalosporins no longer a recommended treatment for gonococcal infections. *MMWR Morb Mortal Wkly Rep*. 2012;61: 590-594.

**PART THREE**

# KIDNEY, WATER, AND ELECTROLYTES

RENEE GARRICK, MD

# Introduction

*Mediators and Modifiers of Kidney Disease*

Attention continues to focus on factors which may allow early identification of, or mediate or modify, renal injury. Plasma levels of soluble urokinase receptor-type plasminogen activator receptor (suPAR), have been associated with certain types of glomerular injury. New data demonstrate that elevated levels of suPAR are independently associated with incident CKD and with an accelerated decline in estimated GFR (eGFR). The findings suggest suPAR may be a new biomarker that can be used to identify those patients at greatest risk for the development and progression of CKD. Other novel studies this year demonstrated that obstructive sleep apnea is associated with higher mortality, a higher risk of incident CKD, and with a more rapid decline in renal function. The SYNERGY trial demonstrated that treatment with pre-and pro-biotics can alter gut microbiota and can potentially favorably influence both kidney disease progression and the development of renal related cardiovascular disease. Another interesting trial suggested that plant (as compared to animal) protein intake is associated with a lower all-cause mortality in patients with an estimated GFR (eGFR) of less than 60 mL/min/1.73 $m^2$

*Acute Kidney Injury*

Acute kidney injury has stimulated a great deal of interest because even a single episode of AKI is associated with both increased mortality and an increased risk of the development of progressive CKD.

This year's selections teach us that in addition to the typical markers of severe sepsis, (serum lactate levels, central venous pressure, mechanical ventilation, etc.), low systemic oxygen delivery (measured as $DO_2I$), and hypotension are independently associated with the progression to a more serious level of AKI. These findings should help us identify clinically useful and relevant parameters that can be readily applied to the care of patients with sepsis. Cardiac surgery is frequently associated with acute kidney injury. Studies this year focused on agents that may (Levosimendan) or may not (Atorvastin), protect against the development of AKI in patients undergoing cardiac surgery. The last selection focuses on the results of the SPILT trial which found that infusion of buffered crystalloid did not reduce the risk of AKI as compared to the use of saline-based resuscitation fluids.

*Selected Topics in Clinical Nephrology*

The first selection confirms the validity of the urine albumin to creatinine ratio as compared to a 24 hour urine collection for staging albumin excretion rates. These data are drawn from over 7,600 patients from two well-defined trials, and are a welcome addition to clinical care pathways. Blood-pressure control continues to be a critically important and somewhat controversial area for individuals at risk for progressive renal disease. The SPRINT trial demonstrated that in non-diabetics at high risk for cardiovascular disease, a systolic pressure target of under 120 mm Hg, as compared to 140 mm Hg, yields a reduced rate of fatal and nonfatal major cardiovascular events and death, but is associated with a greater rate of some adverse events such as hypotension and certain electrolyte abnormalities. The lower target range seemed to be most useful in non-diabetics with underlying CKD. In those without baseline CKD, a fall in the eGFR of 30% or more (to under 60 mL/min/1.73 $m^2$) occurred more often in the intensive-treatment group than in the standard-treatment group (1.21% per year vs. 0.35% per year). Certainly more related publications will be forthcoming and we will continue to follow this literature. Other studies focusing on blood-pressure control included the PATHWAY-2 trial which demonstrated that Spironolactone is an effective, well tolerated add-on drug for the treatment of resistant hypertension. Wang and colleagues investigated the frequency and effectiveness of the implementation of treatment guidelines into routine clinical practice. Current practice guidelines suggest that eligible post- myocardial infarction patients, over the age of 65 with an ejection fraction of less than 40%, be treated with both an aldosterone antagonist, and either an ACEi or ARB. They discovered that both these treatment regimens are often not implemented, and that their use was associated with an increased risk of hyperkalemia and acute kidney injury. The findings remind us that the "real- world" implementation of practice guidelines derived from carefully structured study protocols can reveal unexpected adverse events and close clinical follow-up is typically required.

The next selections highlight polycystic kidney disease which is the most common inherited cause of kidney disease and include the new Pro PKD scoring system which can be used to predict renal survival in autosomal dominant PKD. The other topics in clinical nephrology remind us that elective supra-renal endovascular aneurysm repair is associated with a significant decline in renal function, which is more marked than that seen with open repair. The decline is greatest, but not limited to the first post-operative year. The next selections focus on the presentation of clinically important kidney disease in patients with sickle cell (SS and SC) disease, the risk of vitamin C supplementation and incident kidney stones in men, and the final selection reviews the long–term clinical outcomes of kidney donation in donor candidates.

*Chronic Kidney Disease*

This year a number of selections relate to the care of patients with chronic kidney disease. The first three selections focus on medication use in patients with CKD. An important article by Hung and colleagues calls attention to the fact that metformin use in patients with advanced (approximately stage 5) CKD is associated with increased risk of all cause mortality, and the authors warn against its use in these patients. On a more positive note, new data suggest that, as compared with warfarin, individuals with CKD may be safely and adequately treated with the new novel oral anticoagulants without an increased risk in major bleeding. Data from the REVOKE trial suggest that treatment with intravenous iron therapy in non-dialyzed patients with CKD (stage 3 and 4) is associated with an increased risk of cardiovascular events and infections. Use of such therapy in these patients should be judicious and reserved for individuals who have definitively failed more conservative forms of iron supplementation.

Roughly 40% of patients with type II diabetes will develop either albuminuria or a reduced GFR, both of which are indicators of chronic kidney disease. The search continues for indicators to help determine those patients at greatest risk for CKD. Studies by Dunkler and colleagues suggest that albuminuria and the eGFR can predict the onset and progression of early CKD in patients with type II diabetes. Other studies from the AMD-Annals Study Group found that in type II diabetics, a mild increase in the serum uric acid is associated with an increased risk of CKD. The incidence of an eGFR of under 60 mls/min/1.73 $m^2$ tracked in parallel with the uric acid quintile. Interestingly, this change in serum uric acid was only significantly associated with albuminuria when the eGFR was under 60 mls/min/1.73 $m^2$.

The next series of selections informs us that among patients with CKD, mortality risk can be predicted by changes in a resting 12 lead EKG, and that mortality risk is increased by smoking, increased glycated hemoglobin A1 C levels (in non-diabetic CKD patients) and independently by both social deprivation and elevated levels of serum phosphate. The final selections teach us that the presence of retinopathy in non-diabetics with CKD predicts the occurrence of future cardiovascular events, and that the presence of peripheral arterial disease in patients with underlying CKD is associated with a marked increase in both morbidity and mortality as compared to individuals with normal renal function. The final selection shares the early findings of the Brain in Kidney Disease (BRINK) Cohort Study and reminds us that cognitive function is significantly impaired in individuals with CKD, and these limitations must be considered when instructing patients about their medications and clinical care regimens.

*Hemodialysis*

Patients with dialysis dependent renal disease are a particularly vulnerable population and their care must be evidence-based and strategically individualized. It is well-known that patients with advanced kidney disease are at high risk for both atrial fibrillation and stroke. Lee and colleagues evaluated warfarin use in approximately 9500 dialysis patients and found that its use was associated with a higher risk of hemorrhagic stroke, but not with an increase in overall mortality. The data from Clark and colleagues demonstrate that sepsis and septic shock are common among chronic dialysis patients. Both the sites of infection and the causative organisms are unique and clinicians need to appreciate these issues when choosing initial empiric antibiotic regimens. The next selection points out that preventative dental care can mitigate the risk of early death associated with poor dental hygiene. The final selection reminds us that frailty and global cognitive dysfunction are extremely prevalent in patients with ESRD, and to be effective our care plans must identify and appropriately address these functional limitations.

**Renee Garrick, MD**

# 24 Mediators and Modifiers of Kidney Disease

---

**Soluble Urokinase Receptor and Chronic Kidney Disease**

Hayek SS, Sever S, Ko Y-A, et al (Emory Univ School of Medicine, Atlanta, GA; Emory Univ, Atlanta, GA; et al)

*N Engl J Med* 373:1916-1925, 2015

---

*Background.*—Relatively high plasma levels of soluble urokinase-type plasminogen activator receptor (suPAR) have been associated with focal segmental glomerulosclerosis and poor clinical outcomes in patients with various conditions. It is unknown whether elevated suPAR levels in patients with normal kidney function are associated with future decline in the estimated glomerular filtration rate (eGFR) and with incident chronic kidney disease.

*Methods.*—We measured plasma suPAR levels in 3683 persons enrolled in the Emory Cardiovascular Biobank (mean age, 63 years; 65% men; median suPAR level, 3040 pg per milliliter) and determined renal function at enrollment and at subsequent visits in 2292 persons. The relationship between suPAR levels and the eGFR at baseline, the change in the eGFR over time, and the development of chronic kidney disease (eGFR <60 ml per minute per 1.73 $m^2$ of body-surface area) were analyzed with the use of linear mixed models and Cox regression after adjustment for demographic and clinical variables.

*Results.*—A higher suPAR level at baseline was associated with a greater decline in the eGFR during follow-up; the annual change in the eGFR was −0.9 ml per minute per 1.73 $m^2$ among participants in the lowest quartile of suPAR levels as compared with −4.2 ml per minute per 1.73 $m^2$ among participants in the highest quartile ($P < 0.001$). The 921 participants with a normal eGFR (≥90 ml per minute per 1.73 $m^2$) at baseline had the largest suPAR-related decline in the eGFR. In 1335 participants with a baseline eGFR of at least 60 ml per minute per 1.73 $m^2$, the risk of progression to chronic kidney disease in the highest quartile of suPAR levels was 3.13 times as high (95% confidence interval, 2.11 to 4.65) as that in the lowest quartile.

*Conclusions.*—An elevated level of suPAR was independently associated with incident chronic kidney disease and an accelerated decline in the eGFR in the groups studied. (Funded by the Abraham J. and Phyllis Katz Foundation and others.)

▶ Identification of this receptor may represent a true breakthrough in the care of patients at risk for progressive kidney disease. Chronic kidney disease (CKD) affects more than 10% of the US population and is an independent risk factor for mortality and cardiovascular disease.[1] As a progressive disease, early identification and treatment of the underlying disease process are pivotal to slowing progression. The available indicators of renal function, such as the serum creatinine and proteinuria, are relatively insensitive markers of early renal injury and/or risk of for disease progression. A more useful biomarker is one that would is reliably detect early kidney injury and delineate those at greatest risk for progressive disease.

SuPAR (soluble urokinase type plasminogen activator receptor) is expressed in a variety of cells including endothelial cells and renal glomerular podocytes. Utilizing the Emory Cardiovascular Bio Bank, the investigators designed a prospective cohort study that included measuring plasma suPAR levels in approximately 3700 patients. Baseline and follow-up renal function were measured in 2292 patients (median follow-up 3.6 years), and proteinuria was measured at baseline in 1147 patients and at subsequent follow-up in 815 patients. Patients with possible AKI were excluded from analysis.

The results (based on the quartiles) demonstrated that higher suPAR levels at baseline were associated with a greater decline in the estimated glomerular filtration rate (eGFR) at follow-up. The annual eGFR change was −0.9 mL/minute in patients with lowest quartile of suPAR levels compared with −4.2 mL/minute among patients with highest quartile ($P < .001$).

Moreover, the risk of incident CKD among patients in the highest quartile of suPAR was 3.13 times as high as the risk among those in the lowest quartile.

The authors note that suPAR meets many of the requirements of biomarker for chronic kidney disease. Most important, the levels were stable in plasma, and therefore it can be reliably measured. The biomarker was found to be increased before any detectable change in the serum creatinine, and therefore it can detect incident disease. In addition, higher levels of suPAR at baseline were associated with a faster decline in eGFR, and therefore the biomarker may have predictive value for risk of progression to more advanced levels of CKD. Finally, the validity of the biomarker was not affected by racial background.

This study has many strengths, including the size of the cohort studied and the additional validation steps that were performed, which included testing different isoforms of suPAR, and validating the marker in a subgroup of patients with HIV.

Thus, in this cohort of adult patients with cardiovascular disease and a normal baseline serum creatinine, an elevated plasma suPAR level was associated with a decline in glomerular filtration rate and with progression to more advanced stages of CKD. The association was independent of other conventional risk factors for kidney and cardiovascular disease.

If validated in additional populations, this biomarker will be clinically powerful. It could allow us to identify the presence of renal disease and the risk for progression with greater sensitivity than currently possible, and it could greatly enhance our ability to strategically test therapeutic interventions.

**S. Chugh, MD**

*Reference*

1. Chronic Kidney Disease Issue Brief. Centers for Disease Control and Prevention. http://www.cdc.gov/diabetes/programs/initiatives/ckd_overview.html. Accessed May 3, 2016.

---

**Association of incident obstructive sleep apnoea with outcomes in a large cohort of US veterans**

Molnar MZ, Mucsi I, Novak M, et al (Univ of Tennessee Health Science Ctr, Memphis; Univ of Toronto, Canada; Semmelweis Univ, Budapest, Hungary; et al)

*Thorax* 70:888-895, 2015

---

*Rationale.*—There is a paucity of large cohort studies examining the association of obstructive sleep apnoea (OSA) with clinical outcomes including all-cause mortality, coronary heart disease (CHD), strokes and chronic kidney disease (CKD).

*Objectives.*—We hypothesised that a diagnosis of incident OSA is associated with higher risks of these adverse clinical outcomes.

*Methods, Measurements.*—In a nationally representative cohort of over 3 million (n=3 079 514) US veterans (93% male) with baseline estimated glomerular filtration rate (eGFR) ≥60 mL/min/1.73 m$^2$, we examined the association between the diagnosis of incident OSA, treated and untreated with CPAP, and: (1) all-cause mortality, (2) incident CHD, (3) incident strokes, (4) incident CKD defined as eGFR <60 mL/min/1.73 m$^2$, and (5) slopes of eGFR.

*Main Results.*—Compared with OSA-negative patients, untreated and treated OSA was associated with 86% higher mortality risk, (adjusted HR and 95% CI 1.86 (1.81 to 1.91) and 35% (1.35 (1.21 to 1.51)), respectively. Similarly, untreated and treated OSA was associated with 3.5 times (3.54 (3.40 to 3.69)) and 3 times (3.06 (2.62 to 3.56)) higher risk of incident CHD; 3.5 times higher risk of incident strokes (3.48 (3.28 to 3.64) and 3.50 (2.92 to 4.19)) for untreated and treated OSA, respectively. The risk of incident CKD was also significantly higher in untreated (2.27 (2.19 to 2.36)) and treated (2.79 (2.48 to 3.13)) patients with OSA. The median (IQR) of the eGFR slope was −0.41 (−2.01 to 0.99), −0.61 (−2.69 to 0.93) and −0.87 (−3.00 to 0.70) mL/min/1.73 m$^2$ in OSA-negative patients, untreated OSA-positive patients and treated OSA-positive patients, respectively.

*Conclusions.*—In this large and contemporary cohort of more than 3 million US veterans, a diagnosis of incident OSA was associated with higher mortality, incident CHD, stroke and CKD and with faster kidney function decline.

▶ Individuals who live with people who snore have certainly long wondered whether the consequences of snoring affect both parties equally. This cohort study included more than 3 million veterans (93% male) with a baseline estimated glomerular filtration rate (eGFR) $>60\ mL/min/1.73\ m^2$. The investigators studied the association between the diagnosis of incident obstructive sleep apnea (OSA), both treated and untreated, and mortality as well as incident chronic kidney disease (CKD; eGFR $<60$), stroke, and coronary heart disease.

The data show that within this population, the risk of incident CKD is increased 2.3 and 2.8 times in patients with untreated and treated OSA. Presumably, the incidence of CKD was higher in treated patients because they were clinically more symptomatic (perhaps indicative of more significant underlying disease), and they therefore sought OSA treatment and the renal disease was detected. OSA has been linked with renal hyperfiltration[1] and has been associated with an increased risk of cardiac and cerebral vascular disease.[2,3] This is the first study to show an association of the diagnosis of incident OSA with incident CKD and to demonstrate that this, in turn, is linked to a faster decline of renal function. Whether the etiology of this association is linked to underlying cardiovascular disease or other factors remains to be determined, as does the possible impact of OSA treatment on the development and progression of CKD. The veterans database findings suggest that OSA may be an independent risk factor for the development of CKD and are similar to the recent findings of Chen and colleagues based on data from the Taiwanese National Health Insurance Research Database.[4] These findings open new horizons for clinical studies and could help unveil a new, nontraditional risk factor for CKD.

**R. Garrick, MD**

*References*

1. Kinebuchi S, Kazama JJ, Satoh M, et al. Short-term use of continuous positive airway pressure ameliorates glomerular hyperfiltration in patients with obstructive sleep apnoea syndrome. *Clin Sci (Lond).* 2004;107:317-322.
2. Seicean S, Strohl KP, Seicean A, et al. Sleep disordered breathing as a risk of cardiac events in subjects with diabetes mellitus and normal exercise echocardiographic findings. *Am J Cardiol.* 2013;111:1214-1220.
3. Redline S, Yenokyan G, Gottlieb DJ, et al. Obstructive sleep apnea-hypopnea and incident stroke: the sleep heart health study. *Am J Respir Crit Care Med.* 2010; 182:269-277.
4. Chu H, Shih C-J, Ou S-M, et al. Association of sleep apnoea with chronic kidney disease in a large cohort from Taiwan. *Respirology.* 2016;21:754-760.

**Synbiotics Easing Renal Failure by Improving Gut Microbiology (SYNERGY): A Randomized Trial**

Rossi M, Johnson DW, Morrison M, et al (The Univ of Queensland, Brisbane, Australia; Translational Res Inst, Brisbane, Queensland, Australia; et al)

*Clin J Am Soc Nephrol* 11:223-231, 2016

*Background and Objectives.*—The generation of key uremic nephrovascular toxins, indoxyl sulfate (IS), and p-cresyl sulfate (PCS), is attributed to the dysbiotic gut microbiota in CKD. The aim of our study was to evaluate whether synbiotic (pre- and probiotic) therapy alters the gut microbiota and reduces serum concentrations of microbiome–generated uremic toxins, IS and PCS, in patients with CKD.

*Design, Setting, Participants, & Measurements.*—Predialysis adult participants with CKD(eGFR = 10–30 ml/min per 1.73 $m^2$) were recruited between January 5, 2013 and November 12, 2013 to a randomized, double–blind, placebo–controlled, crossover trial of synbiotic therapy over 6 weeks (4-week washout). The primary outcome was serum IS. Secondary outcomes included serum PCS, stool microbiota profile, eGFR, proteinuria-albuminuria, urinary kidney injury molecule-1, serum inflammatory biomarkers (IL-1$\beta$, IL-6, IL-10, and TNF-$\alpha$), serum oxidative stress biomarkers ($F_2$-isoprostanes and glutathione peroxidase), serum LPS, patient-reported health, Gastrointestinal Symptom Score, and dietary intake. A prespecified subgroup analysis explored the effect of antibiotic use on treatment effect.

*Results.*—Of 37 individuals randomized (age = 69 ± 10 years old; 57% men; eGFR = 24 ± 8 ml/min per 1.73 $m^2$), 31 completed the study. Synbiotic therapy did not significantly reduce serum IS (−2 μmol/L; 95% confidence interval [95% CI], −5 to 1 μmol/L) but did significantly reduce serum PCS (−14 μmol/L; 95% CI, −27 to −2 μmol/L). Decreases in both PCS and IS concentrations were more pronounced in patients who did not receive antibiotics during the study ($n = 21$; serum PCS, −25 μmol/L; 95% CI, −38 to −12 μmol/L; serum IS, −5 μmol/L; 95% CI, −8 to −1 μmol/L). Synbiotics also altered the stool microbiome, particularly with enrichment of *Bifidobacterium* and depletion of *Ruminococcaceae*. Except for an increase in albuminuria of 38 mg/24 h ($P = 0.03$) in the synbiotic arm, no changes were observed in the other secondary outcomes.

*Conclusion.*—In patients with CKD, synbiotics did not significantly reduce serum IS but did decrease serum PCS and favorably modified the stool microbiome. Large–scale clinical trials are justified.

▶ We included this trial in the YEAR BOOK because it is a relatively new and extremely interesting area of research. The intestinal microbiome has been referred to as the "second human genome" and is known to play important role in both health and disease.[1,2] Changes in the intestinal flora, and the metabolic products created by that new biome, can be induced by the uremic state. These new flora and their end-metabolic products, in turn, serve to further contribute to, and exacerbate, kidney injury and perhaps cardiovascular injury as well.[3] Increased concentrations of urea, which drive ammonia metabolism, and other retained metabolic compounds, as well as the dietary restrictions and substitutions initiated as part of the care of patients with chronic kidney disease (CKD) are believed to fuel the changes that have been detected in the gut biome.

The Synbiotics Easing Renal Failure by Improving Gut Microbiology was designed to evaluate the generation of uremic vascular toxins such as indoxyl-sulfate (IS) and p-cresyl sulfate (PCS) and to determine whether specific prebiotic and probiotic (synbiotic) therapy can effectively alter the gut microbiota and, in turn, alter the production of these toxins. This randomized double-blind placebo-controlled crossover trial included patients with stage 4 and 5 CKD who had no known underlying independent gastrointestinal disorders. Prebiotic therapy consisted of a mixture of inulin and fructo- and galacto-oligosaccharides. The probiotic component was a mixture of several types of *Lactobacillus*, *Bifidobacteria*, and *Streptococcus* species. Patients were encouraged to remain on their usual diet and medications during the study period and maintained a dietary log. Stool samples were used to evaluate the microbiota of gut was evaluated at the various stages of the study.

Compared with placebo, synbiotic therapy resulted in a significant mean reduction in the concentration of PCS but not IS (the primary outcome). However, when adjusted for the antibiotic exposure, which occurred in some participants, both serum free and total IS levels were reduced. Stool content of *Bifidobacterium* increased, whereas *Ruminococcaceae* levels were reduced. These changes are in accord with the alteration in serum PCS levels.

Treatment had no effect on eGFR and a variety of other markers, and although the urine albumin excretion did increase, the significance of this is not yet known; longer term studies will be required to determine whether manipulation of the gut microbiome can favorably alter the uremic milieu and related renal and perhaps cardiovascular outcomes.

**R. Garrick, MD**

*References*

1. Ali Ramezani A, Massy Z, Meijers B, et al. Role of the gut microbiome in uremia: a potential therapeutic target. *Am J Kidney Dis*. 2016;67:483-498.
2. Vaziri ND. Effect of synbiotic therapy on gut-derived uremic toxins and the intestinal microbiome in patients with CKD. *Clin J Am Soc Nephrol*. 2016;11:199-201.
3. Lin CJ, Pan CF, Chuang CK, et al. P-cresyl sulfate is a valuable predictor of clinical outcomes in pre-ESRD patients. *BioMed Res Int*. 2014;2014:526932.

---

**The Associations of Plant Protein Intake With All-Cause Mortality in CKD**

Chen X, Wei G, Jalili T, et al (Univ of Utah School of Medicine, Salt Lake City; et al)

*Am J Kidney Dis* 67:423-430, 2016

---

*Background.*—Plant protein intake is associated with lower production of uremic toxins and lower serum phosphorus levels. Therefore, at a given total protein intake, a higher proportion of dietary protein from plant sources might be associated with lower mortality in chronic kidney disease.

*Study Design.*—Observational study.

*Settings & Participants.*—14,866 NHANES III participants 20 years or older without missing data for plant and animal protein intake and mortality.

*Predictors.*—Plant protein to total protein ratio and total plant protein intake. Patients were stratified by estimated glomerular filtration rate (eGFR) < 60 or ≥60 mL/min/1.73 $m^2$.

*Outcomes.*—All-cause mortality.

*Measurements.*—Plant and total protein intakes were estimated from 24-hour dietary recalls. Mortality was ascertained by probabilistic linkage with National Death Index records through December 31, 2000.

*Results.*—Mean values for plant protein intake and plant protein to total protein ratio were 24.6 ± 13.2 (SD) g/d and 33.0% ± 14.0%, respectively. The prevalence of eGFRs < 60 mL/min/1.73 $m^2$ was 4.9%. There were 2,163 deaths over an average follow-up of 8.4 years. Adjusted for demographics, smoking, alcohol use, comorbid conditions, body mass index, calorie and total protein intake, and physical inactivity, each 33% increase in plant protein to total protein ratio was not associated with mortality (HR, 0.88; 95% CI, 0.74-1.04) in the eGFR ≥ 60 mL/min/1.73 $m^2$ subpopulation, but was associated with lower mortality risk (HR, 0.77; 95% CI, 0.61-0.96) in the eGFR < 60 mL/min/1.73 $m^2$ subpopulation. In sensitivity analyses, results were similar in those with eGFR < 60 mL/min/1.73 $m^2$ defined by serum cystatin C level.

*Limitations.*—Whether results are related to plant protein itself or to other factors associated with more plant-based diets is difficult to establish.

*Conclusions.*—A diet with a higher proportion of protein from plant sources is associated with lower mortality in those with eGFR < 60 mL/min/1.73 $m^2$. Future studies are warranted to determine the causal role of plant protein intake in reducing mortality in those with eGFR < 60 mL/min/1.73 $m^2$.

► It is estimated that approximately 14% of the population (about 26 million people) have some element of chronic kidney disease (CKD).[1] The mortality rates among patients with more advanced stages of CKD (estimated glomerular filtration rate [eGFR] < 30 mL/min/1.73 $m^2$) are increased compared with those observed in the general population. Thus, much attention has been focused on the population of patients with moderate CKD (typically defined as eGFR between 30 and 60 ml/min/1.73 $m^2$) to both mitigate disease progression and reduce mortality risk. With this in mind, the data of Chen and colleagues are particularly interesting. The researchers evaluated the plant and total protein intake of more than 14 800 participants in the NHANESIII health and nutrition survey. They were stratified based on the eGFR rate ( < 60 or ≥60 mL/min/1.73 $m^2$), and dietary recall of plant and animal protein was assessed. After adjusting for demographics and multiple comorbidities, the researchers noted that every 33% increase in the ratio of plant protein to total protein consumed resulted in a 23% reduction in mortality. These findings were not evident in the population of patients with an eGFR of > 60 mL/min/1.73 $m^2$ nor among those with a urinary albumin/creatinine ratio of > 30 mg/g.

There are a few obvious caveats here. The first of the studies was based on dietary recall which, even at its best, is subject to error. Second, the findings are observational and therefore offer no direct insight as to the physiological mechanisms responsible for the effects observed. It is tempting to speculate that the effects were related to a lower intake of meat-rich phosphate, leading to a favorable effect on FGF-23 levels or to a lower daily net acid load as associated with plant versus animal protein intake, or that plant protein reduced the intake of certain amino acids and the production of uremic toxins. However, definitive diet-matched controlled trials will be needed to sort out the causal mechanisms. In the meantime, most CKD patients are typically advised to limit their protein intake to about 0.8 g/kg body weight per day, and although the mechanisms for mortality reduction associated with plant-protein intake are being delineated, it seems prudent to counsel patients with moderate CKD about the potential impact of plant versus animal proteins on mortality.

**R. Garrick, MD**

*Reference*

1. Collins AJ, Foley RN, Chavers B, et al. US renal data system 2013 annual data report. *Am J Kidney Dis*. 2014;63:e1-e420.

# 25 Acute Kidney Injury

**Low Systemic Oxygen Delivery and BP and Risk of Progression of Early AKI**

Raimundo M, Crichton S, Syed Y, et al (King's College London, UK)

*Clin J Am Soc Nephrol* 10:1340-1349, 2015

*Background and Objectives.*—The optimal hemodynamic management of patients with early AKI is unknown. This study aimed to investigate the association between hemodynamic parameters in early AKI and progression to severe AKI and hospital mortality.

*Design, Setting, Participants, & Measurements.*—This study retrospectively analyzed the data of all patients admitted to the adult intensive care unit in a tertiary care center between July 2007 and June 2009 and identified those with stage 1AKI (AKI I) per the AKI Network classification. In patients in whom hemodynamic monitoring was performed within 12 hours of AKI I, hemodynamic parameters in the first 12 hours of AKI I and on the day of AKI III (if AKI III developed) or 72 hours after AKI I (if AKI III did not develop) were recorded. Risk factors for AKI III and mortality were identified using univariate and multivariate logistic regression analyses.

*Results.*—Among 790 patients with AKI I, 210 (median age 70 years; 138 men) had hemodynamic monitoring within 12 hours of AKI I; 85 patients (41.5%) progressed to AKI III and 91 (43%) died in the hospital. AKI progressors had a significantly higher Sequential Organ Failure Assessment score (8.0 versus 9.6; $P < 0.001$), lower indexed systemic oxygen delivery ($DO_2I$) (median 325 versus 405 ml/min per $m^2$; $P < 0.001$), higher central venous pressure (16 versus 13; $P = 0.02$), and lower mean arterial blood pressure (MAP) (median 71 versus 74 mm Hg; $P = 0.01$) in the first 12 hours of AKI I compared with nonprogressors. Multivariate analysis confirmed that raised lactate, central venous pressure, and Sequential Organ Failure Assessment score as well as mechanical ventilation were independently associated with progression to AKI III; higher $DO_2I$ and MAP were independently associated with a lower risk of AKI III but not survival. The associations were independent of sepsis, heart disease, recent cardiac surgery, or chronic hypertension.

*Conclusions.*—Higher $DO_2I$ and MAP in early AKI were independently associated with a lower risk of progression.

► Acute kidney injury (AKI) among hospitalized patients is extremely common, with a recent study suggesting that AKI occurs in 1 in 5 adults hospitalized with an acute illness. AKI is associated with an increased risk of both death and end-stage renal disease (ESRD) and substantially adds to the annual cost of health care. Steps to mitigate the development of AKI will certainly benefit both our patients and the health care system.[1-3]

It has been suggested that maintaining global blood flow, via the use of fluid and/or drugs in patients undergoing surgery, may mitigate AKI, and the recent KIDIGO guidelines recommend that hemodynamic monitoring be considered in patients at risk for AKI.[3,4] However, the best hemodynamic indictors and targets to mitigate against AKI remain uncertain.

This single-center, retrospective study investigated the association between hemodynamics in early AKI and progression to severe AKI and hospital mortality. Of approximately 790 patients with AKI, aggressive hemodynamic monitoring had been initiated in 210 patients within the first 12 hours of development of early AKI (serum creatinine increase of 0.3 mg/dL or by 50% from baseline in 48 hours). Patients were then divided into nonprogressors and progressors based on progression (by AKIN criteria) from stage I to stage III AKI within 72 hours of diagnosis.

Progressors had significantly higher Sequential Organ Failure Assessment Score (SOFA; 8% vs 9.6%; $P < .001$) and central venous pressure (CVP; 16 vs 13) and lower indexed systemic oxygen delivery ($DO_2I$; $DO_2I = 1.34 \times Hb \times SO_2 \times$ cardiac index) and mean arterial blood pressure (MAP) in first 12 hours. Multivariable analysis confirmed that markers of perfusion and illness severity (increased lactate, CVP and SOFA score) were independently associated with progression. Higher $DO_2I$ and MAP were independently associated with lower AKI risk but not with survival. These finding were not influenced by the presence of sepsis, cardiac disease, recent cardiac surgery, or chronic hypotension.

There are limitations to this retrospective, single-center study. Patients were not matched for comorbidities, and the decision to provide hemodynamic monitoring was the purview of the clinical care team, which may have introduced unknown variables into the data. Nonetheless, the findings are of clinical interest. The impact of $DO_2I$ was most marked when the $DO_2I$ was normal before the onset of AKI. Increasing $DO_2I$ more than 12 hours after the onset of AKI did not improve AKI progression. Interesting, a rise in MAP by at least 5 mm Hg after the initial 12-hour AKI window did reduce the likelihood of progression, whereas volume expansion (increase in cumulative fluid balance by $\geq$1 L) after the onset of AKI was associated with an odds ratio of AKI III of 6.09 (95% confidence interval 2.39-15.52).

The kidney normally receives 20% of the cardiac output and is highly susceptible to hypoxic injury. Hypotension and low cardiac output are deleterious to renal function, and this study, in keeping with others,[5] suggests that volume management significantly influences AKI progression. The current observational study demonstrates that maintenance of perfusion in patients at risk for AKI, and the application of readily available bedside indicators may help mitigate AKI progression. The findings also highlight the need for well-controlled studies aimed at defining the optimal hemodynamic targets to best defend against AKI.

**V. Buddharaju, MD**

*References*

1. Rewa O, Bagshaw SM. Acute kidney injury—epidemiology, outcomes and economics. *Nat Rev Nephrol.* 2014;10:193-207.
2. Kerr M, Bedford M, Matthews B, O'Donoghue D. The economic impact of acute kidney injury in England. *Nephrol Dial Transplant.* 2014;29:1362-1368.
3. Grocott MP, Dushianthan A, Hamilton MA, et al. Optimisation Systematic Review Steering Group: Perioperative increase in global blood flow to explicit defined goals and outcomes following surgery. *Cochrane Database Syst Rev.* 2012;(11):CD004082.
4. Kidney Disease: Improving Global Outcomes (KDIGO) Acute Kidney Injury Work Group. KDIGO clinical practice guideline for acute kidney injury. *Kidney Inter Suppl.* 2012;2:1-138.
5. Grams ME, Estrella MM, Coresh J, et al. National Heart, Lung, and Blood Institute Acute Respiratory Distress Syndrome Network: fluid balance, diuretic use, and mortality in acute kidney injury. *Clin J Am Soc Nephrol.* 2011;6:966-973.

**Levosimendan for Prevention of Acute Kidney Injury After Cardiac Surgery: A Meta-analysis of Randomized Controlled Trials**

Zhou C, Gong J, Chen D, et al (Chinese Academy of Med Sciences and Peking Union Med College, Beijing, China; et al)

*Am J Kidney Dis* 67:408-416, 2016

*Background.*—Levosimendan has been shown to confer direct renoprotection in renal endotoxemic and ischemia-reperfusion injury and could increase renal blood flow in patients with low-cardiac-output heart failure. Results from clinical trials of levosimendan on acute kidney injury (AKI) following cardiac surgery are controversial.

*Study Design.*—A random-effect meta-analysis was conducted based on evidence from PubMed, EMBASE, and Cochrane Library.

*Settings & Population.*—Adult patients undergoing cardiac surgery.

*Selection Criteria for Studies.*—Randomized controlled trials comparing the renal effect of levosimendan versus placebo or other inotropic drugs during cardiac surgery.

*Intervention.*—Perioperative levosimendan continuous infusion at a rate of 0.1 to 0.2 μg/kg/min following a loading dose (6-24 μg/kg) for 24 hours or only 1 loading dose (24 μg/kg) within 1 hour.

*Outcomes.*—AKI, need for renal replacement therapy, mechanical ventilation duration, intensive care unit stay during hospitalization, and postoperative mortality (in-hospital or within 30 days).

*Results.*—13 trials with a total of 1,345 study patients were selected. Compared with controls, levosimendan reduced the incidence of postoperative AKI (40/460 vs 78/499; OR, 0.51; 95% CI, 0.34-0.76; $P = 0.001$; $I^2 = 0.0\%$), renal replacement therapy (22/492 vs 49/491; OR, 0.43; 95% CI, 0.25-0.76; $P = 0.002$; $I^2 = 0.0\%$), postoperative mortality (35/658 vs 94/657; OR, 0.41; 95% CI, 0.27-0.62; $P < 0.001$; $I^2 = 0.0\%$), mechanical ventilation duration (in days; n = 235; weighted mean difference, −0.34; 95% CI, −0.58 to −0.09; $P = 0.007$), and intensive care unit stay (in days; n = 500; weighted mean difference, −2.2; 95% CI, −4.21 to −0.13; $P = 0.04$).

*Limitations.*—Different definitions for AKI among studies. Small sample size for some trials.

*Conclusions.*—Perioperative administration of levosimendan in patients undergoing cardiac surgery may reduce complications. Future trials are needed to determine the dose effect of levosimendan in improving outcomes, especially in patients with decreased baseline kidney function.

▶ Acute kidney injury (AKI) is independently associated with higher mortality and morbidity in patients with heart failure or those undergoing cardiac surgery.[1,2] Many drugs have been evaluated for the prevention of AKI, but to date none have been shown to be definitively effective. With the failure of nesiritide,[3] focus shifted to levosimendan, a calcium sensitizer that has been approved for acute decompensated heart failure.

This random effects meta-analysis was designed to evaluate the perioperative renoprotective effects of levosimendan compared with placebo or other inotropic agents in patients undergoing cardiac surgery. The hard end points were incidence of postoperative AKI, use of renal replacement therapy (RRT), duration on mechanical ventilation, intensive care unit stay, and in-hospital or 30-day mortality. Out of 87 potential studies, 13 trials, totaling 1345 patients, met criteria for inclusion. The odds ratio and mean difference were calculated, and of 128 patients with AKI, the odds of developing AKI was 0.51 and the odds of requiring RRT was 0.43, in patients treated with levosimendan compared with the control group (which included patients treated with placebo, dobutamine and milrinone), respectively. The overall risk of mortality was also reduced in levosimendan group with an odds ratio of 0.41. The mean length of stay in the hospital and days requiring mechanical ventilation were reduced by 2.2 and 0.34 days, respectively.

These results are encouraging. However, there are some limitations of the study. First, there was no uniform definition of AKI, and the dose of levosimendan was not standardized. This is important because high doses ( > 12 μg/kg) or rapid infusion ( < 10 minutes) can lead to hypotension, which can counteract any positive renal effects of the drug. Also, there is no patient-specific data included, so the effects of other confounders (heart failure, preexisting renal failure), cannot be determined, nor is it possible to definitively determine whether treatment affords a long-term survival advantage. Even with these limitations in mind, this meta-analysis suggests a role for this agent in the prevention of cardiac surgery—associated AKI. An intervention trial evaluating the renoprotective effect of levosimendan in sepsis is now underway and is expected to be completed in 2017.[4] This may shed additional light on the application of this drug. While awaiting these results, it would seem reasonable to consider using this drug preoperatively in high-risk cardiac surgery patients.

**S. Chugh, MD**

*References*

1. Lassnigg A, Schmidlin D, Mouhieddine M, et al. Minimal changes of serum creatinine predict prognosis in patients after cardiothoracic surgery: a prospective cohort study. *J Am Soc Nephrol.* 2004;15:1597-1605.
2. Chertow GM, Burdick E, Honour M, et al. Acute kidney injury, mortality, length of stay, and costs in hospitalized patients. *J Am Soc Nephrol.* 2005;16:3365-3370.
3. O'Connor CM, Starling RC, Hernandez AF, et al. Effect of nesiritide in patients with acute decompensated heart failure. *N Engl J Med.* 2011;365:32-43.
4. Orme RML, Perkins GD, McAuley DF, et al. An efficacy and mechanism evaluation study of Levosimendan for the Prevention of Acute Organ Dysfunction in Sepsis (LeoPARDS): protocol for a randomized controlled trial. *Trials.* 2014;15:199.

**High-Dose Perioperative Atorvastatin and Acute Kidney Injury Following Cardiac Surgery: A Randomized Clinical Trial**

Billings FT, Hendricks PA, Schildcrout JS, et al (Vanderbilt Univ School of Medicine, Nashville, TN; et al)

*JAMA* 315:877-888, 2016

*Importance.*—Statins affect several mechanisms underlying acute kidney injury (AKI).

*Objective.*—To test the hypothesis that short-term high-dose perioperative atorvastatin would reduce AKI following cardiac surgery.

*Design, Setting, and Participants.*—Double-blinded, placebo-controlled, randomized clinical trial of adult cardiac surgery patients conducted from November 2009 to October 2014 at Vanderbilt University Medical Center.

*Interventions.*—Patients naive to statin treatment (n = 199) were randomly assigned 80 mg of atorvastatin the day before surgery, 40 mg of atorvastatin the morning of surgery, and 40 mg of atorvastatin daily following surgery (n = 102) or matching placebo (n = 97). Patients already taking a statin prior to study enrollment (n = 416) continued taking the preenrollment statin until the day of surgery, were randomly assigned 80 mg of atorvastatin the morning of surgery and 40 mg of atorvastatin the morning after (n = 206) or matching placebo (n = 210), and resumed taking the previously prescribed statin on postoperative day 2.

*Main Outcomes and Measures.*—Acute kidney injury defined as an increase of 0.3 mg/dL in serum creatinine concentration within 48 hours of surgery (Acute Kidney Injury Network criteria).

*Results.*—The data and safety monitoring board recommended stopping the group naive to statin treatment due to increased AKI among these participants with chronic kidney disease (estimated glomerular filtration rate <60 mL/min/1.73 m$^2$) receiving atorvastatin. The board later recommended stopping for futility after 615 participants (median age, 67 years; 188 [30.6%] were women; 202 [32.8%] had diabetes) completed the study. Among all participants (n = 615), AKI occurred in 64 of 308 (20.8%) in the atorvastatin group vs 60 of 307 (19.5%) in the placebo group (relative risk [RR], 1.06 [95%CI, 0.78 to 1.46]; $P$ = .75). Among patients naive to statin treatment (n = 199), AKI occurred in 22 of 102 (21.6%) in the atorvastatin group vs 13 of 97 (13.4%) in the placebo group (RR, 1.61 [0.86 to 3.01]; $P = .15$) and serum creatinine concentration increased by a median of 0.11mg/dL (10th-90th percentile, −0.11 to 0.56 mg/dL) in the atorvastatin group vs by a median of 0.05 mg/dL (10th-90th percentile, −0.12 to 0.33 mg/dL) in the placebo group (mean difference, 0.08 mg/dL [95% CI, 0.01 to 0.15 mg/dL]; $P = .007$). Among patients already taking a statin (n = 416), AKI occurred in 42 of 206 (20.4%) in the atorvastatin group vs 47 of 210 (22.4%) in the placebo group (RR, 0.91 [0.63 to 1.32]; $P = .63$).

*Conclusions and Relevance.*—Among patients undergoing cardiac surgery, high-dose perioperative atorvastatin treatment compared with placebo did not reduce the risk of AKI overall, among patients naive to treatment with statins, or in patients already taking a statin. These results do not support the initiation of statin therapy to prevent AKI following cardiac surgery.

*Trial Registration.*—clinicaltrials.gov Identifier: NCT00791648.

▶ This single-center randomized double-blind placebo-controlled trial was initiated in an attempt to answer the vexing question as to whether statins should be given to prevent acute kidney injury (AKI) before cardiac surgery. Prior observational studies have demonstrated conflicting results.[1,2] The study design evaluated the effects of short-term, high-dose perioperative atorvastatin on kidney function. AKI was defined by the Acute Kidney Injury Network (AKIN) criteria, which define stage 1 AKI as an increase of 0.3 mg/dL in serum creatinine or by 50% within 48 hours of surgery, stage 2 as a 100% increase, and stage 3 as a 200% increase or initiation of renal replacement therapy. The baseline creatinine concentration was the most recent preoperative serum creatinine. A number of predefined subgroup analyses were included: (1) patients who were naive to statins, (2) patients who were taking statins preoperatively, and (3) patients with chronic kidney disease CKD who were either naive to (group 4) or already on (group 5) a statin treatment. Patients on dialysis and those requiring emergency surgery were excluded, as were patients with acute coronary syndrome, hepatic disease, and those on CYP 3A4 inhibitors. The baseline demographic characteristics were thoroughly defined, and patients underwent coronary artery bypass grafting (50% of patients), valve surgery (two-thirds of patients), or ascending aortic surgery. The mean serum low-density lipid cholesterol concentration in the group that received preoperative (presurgical) statin therapy was significantly lower (by 8.1 mg/dL) than in the placebo group.

The results are quite informative. Contrary to their hypothesis, initiation of statin therapy in naive patients did not reduce the incidence of AKI. Rather, among naive patients, high-dose atorvastatin therapy increased the serum creatinine concentration, and in statin-naive CKD patients, high-dose statin therapy may increase the incidence of AKI. The latter possibility was not definitively established because the number of CKD patients naive to statin therapy was small.

The results call attention to the importance of performing randomized controlled trials to test the validity of observational data. Thus, their data demonstrate that there is no indication to initiate statin therapy to prevent AKI in patients undergoing cardiac surgery. However, it is important also to note that among patients with normal renal function already taking a statin, the incidence of AKI did not differ between the atorvastatin and the placebo groups. This is clinically important because other studies have demonstrated that withholding statins in patients undergoing percutaneous coronary intervention may increase myocardial injury.[3] The mechanisms responsible for these outcomes will require additional study, and because the protocol included only a brief perioperative period, the results cannot be generalized to different dosing regimens, nor can and conclusions be drawn regarding the long-term renal outcomes.

**R. Garrick, MD**

*References*

1. Layton JB, Kshirsagar AV, Simpson RJ Jr, et al. Effect of statin use on acute kidney injury risk following coronary artery bypass grafting. *Am J Cardiol.* 2013;111: 823-828.
2. Argalious M, Xu M, Sun Z, Smedira N, Koch CG. Preoperative statin therapy is not associated with a reduced incidence of postoperative acute kidney injury after cardiac surgery. *Anesth Analg.* 2010;111:324-330.
3. Heeschen C, Hamm CW, Laufs U, et al. Platelet Receptor Inhibition in Ischemic Syndrome Management (PRISM) Investigators. Withdrawal of statins increases event rates in patients with acute coronary syndromes. *Circulation.* 2002;105: 1446-1452.

---

**Effect of a Buffered Crystalloid Solution vs Saline on Acute Kidney Injury Among Patients in the Intensive Care Unit: The SPLIT Randomized Clinical Trial**

Young P, for the SPLIT Investigators and the ANZICS CTG (Med Res Inst of New Zealand, Wellington; et al)
*JAMA* 314:1701-1710, 2015

---

*Importance.*—Saline (0.9% sodium chloride) is the most commonly administered intravenous fluid; however, its use may be associated with acute kidney injury (AKI) and increased mortality.

*Objective.*—To determine the effect of a buffered crystalloid compared with saline on renal complications in patients admitted to the intensive care unit (ICU).

*Design and Setting.*—Double-blind, cluster randomized, double-crossover trial conducted in 4 ICUs in New Zealand from April 2014 through October 2014. Three ICUs were general medical and surgical ICUs; 1 ICU had a predominance of cardiothoracic and vascular surgical patients.

*Participants.*—All patients admitted to the ICU requiring crystalloid fluid therapy were eligible for inclusion. Patients with established AKI requiring renal replacement therapy (RRT) were excluded. All 2278 eligible patients were enrolled; 1152 of 1162 patients (99.1%) receiving buffered crystalloid and 1110 of 1116 patients (99.5%) receiving saline were analyzed.

*Interventions.*—Participating ICUs were assigned a masked study fluid, either saline or a buffered crystalloid, for alternating 7-week treatment blocks. Two ICUs commenced using 1 fluid and the other 2 commenced using the alternative fluid. Two crossovers occurred so that each ICU used each fluid twice over the 28 weeks of the study. The treating clinician determined the rate and frequency of fluid administration.

*Main Outcomes and Measures.*—The primary outcome was proportion of patients with AKI (defined as a rise in serum creatinine level of at least 2-fold or a serum creatinine level of ≥3.96 mg/dL with an increase of ≥0.5 mg/dL); main secondary outcomes were incidence of RRT use and in-hospital mortality.

*Results.*—In the buffered crystalloid group, 102 of 1067 patients (9.6%) developed AKI within 90 days after enrollment compared with 94 of 1025 patients (9.2%) in the saline group (absolute difference, 0.4% [95% CI, −2.1% to 2.9%]; relative risk [RR], 1.04 [95% CI, 0.80 to 1.36]; $P=.77$). In the buffered crystalloid group, RRT was used in 38 of 1152 patients (3.3%) compared with 38 of 1110 patients (3.4%) in the saline group (absolute difference, −0.1% [95% CI, −1.6% to 1.4%]; RR, 0.96 [95% CI, 0.62 to 1.50]; $P=.91$). Overall, 87 of 1152 patients (7.6%) in the buffered crystalloid group and 95 of 1110 patients (8.6%) in the saline group died in the hospital (absolute difference, −1.0% [95% CI, −3.3% to 1.2%]; RR, 0.88 [95% CI, 0.67 to 1.17]; $P=.40$).

*Conclusions and Relevance.*—Among patients receiving crystalloid fluid therapy in the ICU, use of a buffered crystalloid compared with saline did not reduce the risk of AKI. Further large randomized clinical trials are needed to assess efficacy in higher-risk populations and to measure clinical outcomes such as mortality.

*Trial Registration.*—clinicaltrials.gov Identifier: ACTRN12613001370796.

▶ Controversy remains over which is the safest solution for intravenous (IV) rehydration, buffered crystalloid (BC) or normal saline (NS). Uncontrolled studies suggest that NS increases the risk of acute kidney injury (AKI),[1] but no well-designed randomized trials have been conducted to verify this finding for the broad range of patients seen in an intensive care unit (ICU).

Young et al prospectively assessed the effect of NS versus BC on the incidence of AKI in ICU patients. They employed a double-blind cluster randomized crossover trial in 4 ICUs at 2 hospitals. Over a 28-week period, all patients were assigned on admission to receive either NS or BC (Plasmalyte) for alternating 7-day periods with 2 crossovers, such that by the end of the trial, each ICU used solution twice. This netted more than 2000 patients who received either NS or BC. The final evaluation included 1067 who received BC and 1025 who received NS. Only those already near or at dialysis and those admitted for palliative care were excluded.

After the treatment period, the investigators assessed the incidence of negative renal effects using the RIFLE criteria[2] to quantify the incidence of kidney injury, failure, loss, and end-stage effects. Pre-enrollment APACHE scores were used to account for differences in severity of the presenting illness, which might have contributed to the primary outcome AKI, independent of the study fluid used.

They found that 9.6% of the BC group had negative renal outcomes compared with 9.2% in the NS group. This was considered to be not statistically significant. Nor were the secondary outcomes of in-hospital mortality (7.6% vs 8.6%) and dialysis use (3.3% vs 3.4%) found to be statistically different. Interestingly, there was no increase in severe metabolic acidosis (pH <7.2) in the NS group, although two-thirds of the treating physicians were able to guess the fluid that was used, presumably by noting some degree of change in chloride and bicarbonate.

This study adds some convincing evidence that the adequacy of rehydration may be more important than the actual choice of a specific IV solution in an unselected population of ICU patients.

**M. Klein, MD, JD**

*References*

1. Yunos NM, Bellomo R, Hegarty C, Story D, Ho L, Bailey M. Association between a chloride-liberal vs chloride-restrictive intravenous fluid administration strategy and kidney injury in critically ill adults. *JAMA*. 2012;308:1566-1572.
2. Ricci Z, Cruz D, Ronco C. The RIFLE criteria and mortality in acute kidney injury: a systematic review. *Kidney Int*. 2008;73:538-546.

# 26 Selected Topics in Clinical Nephrology

**Urine Albumin-Creatinine Ratio Versus Albumin Excretion for Albuminuria Staging: A Prospective Longitudinal Cohort Study**

Vart P, on behalf of the PREVEND Study Group and the RENAAL Investigators (Univ of Groningen, the Netherlands)

*Am J Kidney Dis* 67:70-78, 2016

*Background.*—New guidelines advocate the use of albumin-creatinine ratio (ACR) in a urine sample instead of 24-hour urinary albumin excretion (UAE) for staging albuminuria. Concern has been expressed that this may result in misclassification for reasons including interindividual differences in urinary creatinine excretion.

*Study Design.*—Prospective longitudinal cohort study.

*Setting & Participants.*—We examined 7,623 participants of the PREVEND and RENAAL studies for reclassified when using ACR instead of 24-hour UAE, the characteristics of reclassified participants, and their outcomes. Albuminuria was categorized into 3 ACR and UAE categories: <30, 30 to 300, and >300 mg/g or mg/24 h, respectively.

*Predictors.*—Baseline ACR and 24-hour UAE.

*Outcomes.*—Cardiovascular (CV) morbidity and mortality and all-cause mortality.

*Results.*—When using ACR in the early morning void instead of 24-hour UAE, 88% of participants were classified in corresponding albuminuria categories. 307 (4.0%) participants were reclassified to a higher, and 603 (7.9%), to a lower category. Participants who were reclassified to a higher ACR category in general had a worse CV risk profile compared with nonreclassified participants, whereas the reverse was true for participants reclassified to a lower ACR category. Similarly, Cox proportional hazards regression analyses showed that reclassification to a higher ACR category was associated with a tendency for increased risk for CV morbidity and mortality and all-cause mortality, whereas reclassification to a lower ACR category was associated with a tendency for lower risk. Net reclassification improvement, adjusted for age, sex, and duration of follow-up, was 0.107 ($P = 0.002$) for CV events and 0.089 ($P < 0.001$) for all-cause mortality.

*Limitations.*—Early morning void urine collection instead of spot urine collection.

*Conclusions.*—Our results indicate that there is high agreement between early morning void ACR and 24-hour UAE categories. Reclassification is therefore limited, but when present, is generally indicative of the presence of CV risk factors and prognosis.

▶ Albumin excretion rates (AER) have a high positive correlation with adverse cardiovascular (CV) outcomes.[1] Measurement of AER can be cumbersome when relying on 24-hour collections for urine albumin excretion (UAE), which are often subject to collection error. Early morning albumin/creatinine ratios (ACR) are also presumed imperfect due to disparate interpatient creatinine excretion and circadian variations in protein excretion. Although imperfect, spot urine ACR are easier to obtain and less subject to user error. Hence, validating the predictive value of ACR would be clinically useful.

Vart et al have attempted to verify the correlation of spot ACR with 24-hour UAE using data from the PREVEND and RENAAL trials. Looking at more than 7500 subjects, they determined the frequency of reclassified AER following ACR, which differed from the 24-hour collections. Albuminuria was classified as $<30$ (mild), 30-300 (moderate), and $>300$ (severe) mg/g for ACR or mg/24 h for UAE.[2] A $3 \times 3$ array was used to determine frequency of reclassification.

There was 95.3% correlation in the mild cases and 84.8% correlation in the severe cases. There were very small numbers of subjects that were reclassified upward or downward by more than 1 category. Only 0.1% was reclassified from mild to severe and vice versa. They then evaluated the effect that reclassification, although infrequent, had on actual CV morbidity/mortality risk. They found that reclassifications to higher or lower degrees of albuminuria seem to have significant positive and negative predictive value respectively for CV risk.

This study suggests that despite the inherent inaccuracies in ACR assessments, they seem to correlate relatively well with 24-hour UAE rates and, compared with 24-hour UAE, may have higher positive and negative predictive values for CV morbidity and mortality, thereby bolstering the validity of this relatively simple test.

**M. Klein, MD, JD**

*References*

1. Gerstein HC, Mann JF, Yi Q, et al. HOPE Study Investigators. Albuminuria and risk of cardiovascular events, death, and heart failure in diabetic and nondiabetic individuals. *JAMA*. 2001;286:421-426.
2. KDIGO 2012 clinical practice guideline for the evaluation and management of chronic kidney disease. *Kidney Int Suppl*. 2013;3:5-14.

**A Randomized Trial of Intensive versus Standard Blood-Pressure Control**
The SPRINT Research Group (Case Western Reserve Univ, Cleveland, OH; Louis Stokes Cleveland Veterans Affairs (VA) Med Ctr, OH; et al)
*N Engl J Med* 373:2103-2116, 2015

*Background.*—The most appropriate targets for systolic blood pressure to reduce cardiovascular morbidity and mortality among persons without diabetes remain uncertain.

*Methods.*—We randomly assigned 9361 persons with a systolic blood pressure of 130 mm Hg or higher and an increased cardiovascular risk, but without diabetes, to a systolic blood-pressure target of less than 120 mm Hg (intensive treatment) or a target of less than 140 mm Hg (standard treatment). The primary composite outcome was myocardial infarction, other acute coronary syndromes, stroke, heart failure, or death from cardiovascular causes.

*Results.*—At 1 year, the mean systolic blood pressure was 121.4 mm Hg in the intensive-treatment group and 136.2 mm Hg in the standard-treatment group. The intervention was stopped early after a median follow-up of 3.26 years owing to a significantly lower rate of the primary composite outcome in the intensive-treatment group than in the standard-treatment group (1.65% per year vs. 2.19% per year; hazard ratio with intensive treatment, 0.75; 95% confidence interval [CI], 0.64 to 0.89; $P < 0.001$). All-cause mortality was also significantly lower in the intensive-treatment group (hazard ratio, 0.73; 95% CI, 0.60 to 0.90; $P = 0.003$). Rates of serious adverse events of hypotension, syncope, electrolyte abnormalities, and acute kidney injury or failure, but not of injurious falls, were higher in the intensive-treatment group than in the standard-treatment group.

*Conclusions.*—Among patients at high risk for cardiovascular events but without diabetes, targeting a systolic blood pressure of less than 120 mm Hg, as compared with less than 140 mm Hg, resulted in lower rates of fatal and nonfatal major cardiovascular events and death from any cause, although significantly higher rates of some adverse events were observed in the intensive-treatment group. (Funded by the National Institutes of Health; ClinicalTrials.gov number, NCT01206062.)

▶ Systolic hypertension (SHTN) is the most common form of hypertension after age 50, and it is a leading cause of death and disability. Many trials have successfully shown that treatment of hypertension significantly reduces the risk of cardiovascular disease (CVD). However, blood pressure (BP) is a continuous variable, and the patient populations involved have both distinct and overlapping etiologies and risk factors. As such, the optimal systolic blood pressure (SBP) required to achieve the maximum cardiovascular benefit, remains a topic of debate. The National Institutes of Health (NIH)-sponsored ACCORD trial studied more than 4000 diabetic patients[1] and found that targeting an SBP of <120 mm Hg compared with a recommended pressure of <140 mm Hg did not conclusively reduce the overall risk of a major cardiovascular event, although the lower BP level was associated with a reduced risk of stroke.

The NIH-sponsored randomized, multicenter, controlled, open-label SPRINT trial was designed to determine the optimal systolic BP target in nondiabetics with cardiovascular risk factors, aged 50 years and older. Patients with diabetes, a prior history of stroke, and polycystic kidney disease and with > 1 g of proteinuria or > 600 mg of albuminuria were excluded. Inclusion criteria included an estimated glomerular filtration rate (eGFR) between 20 and 60 mL/min/1.73 $m^2$ a 10-year Framingham risk score of > 15%, clinical or subclinical cardiovascular disease, or age over 75 years (28% of patients). The key question was whether intensive control of hypertension (< 120 mm Hg) is better at preventing hypertension-related complications compared with the recommended target of < 140 mm Hg.

More than 65% of patients had SBP more than 145 mm Hg at the time of enrollment. All the patients were encouraged to use 3 first-line antihypertensive medications (chlorthalidone as first line then angiotensin-converting enzyme inhibitor/angiotensin receptor blocker and calcium channel blockade) to achieve the desired BP (< 120 mm Hg in the intensive and < 140 mm Hg in standard group). The study was stopped before the planned 2018 completion date (mean follow-up of 3.3 years) because the occurrence rate of the primary composite outcome of cardiovascular events (myocardial infarction [MI], acute coronary syndrome not resulting in MI, stroke, acute decompensated heart failure, or death from cardiovascular disease) was reduced by 30%, and all-cause mortality was reduced by nearly 25% in the intensive-target arm compared with the standard arm.

The overall adverse events were not statistically increased (38% vs 37%), but the incidence of hypotension, syncope, acute kidney injury (AKI), and electrolyte imbalance was higher in the intensive group. Surprisingly, orthostatic hypotensive episodes (assessed during office follow-up visits) were slightly more common in the standard arm, but the number of falls was not different between the groups. As the authors note, the significance of (and potential to mitigate against) these adverse events must be weighed against the benefits seen in cardiovascular events and death with more intensive control of systolic BP.

With regard to kidney disease patients, the incidence of AKI was higher in the intensive group. In patients with no chronic kidney disease at initiation, a greater number in the intensive target group experienced a reduction in eGFR to ≤60 mL/min/1.73 $m^2$. The authors note these findings will require additional scrutiny.

So where does this leave us? The 2014 Eighth Joint National Committee (JNC8) guidelines relaxed the target BP to 150/90 in patients ≥60 years old and to 140/90 mm Hg in essentially everybody else.[2] The findings from SPRINT suggest that at least some higher risk patients will benefit from tighter control. Since its publication, the SPRINT trial has been contrasted with the findings of the ACCORD trial and the recommendations of JNC8. Although ACCORD and SPRINT shared similar BP targets, the populations enrolled, the inclusion criteria, patient age, underlying medical conditions, and patient number (ACCORD n = 4733; SPRINT n = 9361) were distinctly different, and it is not possible to reasonably fully generalize the results of one study to the other. With regard to

JNC8, the current recommendations suggest that if a patient over age 60 years has achieved a BP of <150/90 and is tolerating the medications without difficulty that there is no indication to reduce the dosage.

If detailed analysis of the end points of SPRINT sustain the initial findings (and there is no reason to believe otherwise), the results of SPRINT will need to be incorporated into our treatment guidelines and into our therapeutic approach to systolic hypertension. On the basis of the current results, should clinicians choose more intensive therapy for some patients, the SPRINT findings do indicate the need to monitor renal function and electrolyte balance both acutely and long term and to serially assess patients for the occurrence of other adverse events such as hypotension and syncope.

**S. Chugh, MD**

*References*

1. Cushman WC, Evans GW, Byington RP, et al. for the ACCORD Study Group. Effects of intensive blood-pressure control in type 2 diabetes mellitus. *N Engl J Med.* 2010;362:1575-1585.
2. James PA, Oparil S, Carter BL, et al. for the writing group. 2014 evidence-based guideline for the management of high blood pressure in adults report from the panel members appointed to the eighth joint national committee (JNC 8). *JAMA.* 2014;311:507-520.

---

**Spironolactone versus placebo, bisoprolol, and doxazosin to determine the optimal treatment for drug-resistant hypertension (PATHWAY-2): a randomised, double-blind, crossover trial**

Williams B, for The British Hypertension Society's PATHWAY Studies Group (Natl Inst for Health Res (NIHR) UCL/UCL Hosps Biomedical Rese Centre, London, UK; et al)

*Lancet* 386:2059-2068, 2015

---

*Background.*—Optimal drug treatment for patients with resistant hypertension is undefined. We aimed to test the hypotheses that resistant hypertension is most often caused by excessive sodium retention, and that spironolactone would therefore be superior to non-diuretic add-on drugs at lowering blood pressure.

*Methods.*—In this double-blind, placebo-controlled, crossover trial, we enrolled patients aged 18–79 years with seated clinic systolic blood pressure 140 mm Hg or greater (or ≥135 mm Hg for patients with diabetes) and home systolic blood pressure (18 readings over 4 days) 130 mm Hg or greater, despite treatment for at least 3 months with maximally tolerated doses of three drugs, from 12 secondary and two primary care sites in the UK. Patients rotated, in a preassigned, randomised order, through 12 weeks of once daily treatment with each of spironolactone (25–50 mg), bisoprolol (5–10 mg), doxazosin modified release (4–8 mg), and placebo, in addition to their baseline blood pressure drugs. Random assignment was done via a central computer system. Investigators and patients were masked to the identity of drugs, and to their sequence allocation. The dose was doubled after 6 weeks of each cycle. The hierarchical primary end points were the difference in averaged home systolic blood pressure between spironolactone and placebo, followed (if significant) by the difference in home systolic blood pressure between spironolactone and the average of the other two active drugs, followed by the difference in home systolic blood pressure between spironolactone and each of the other two drugs. Analysis was by intention to treat. The trial is registered with EudraCT number 2008-007149-30, and ClinicalTrials.gov number, NCT02369081.

*Findings.*—Between May 15, 2009, and July 8, 2014, we screened 436 patients, of whom 335 were randomly assigned. After 21 were excluded, 285 patients received spironolactone, 282 doxazosin, 285 bisoprolol, and 274 placebo; 230 patients completed all treatment cycles. The average reduction in home systolic blood pressure by spironolactone was superior to placebo (−870 mm Hg [95% CI −972 to −769]; $p < 00001$), superior to the mean of the other two active treatments (doxazosin and bisoprolol; −426 [−513 to −338]; $p < 00001$), and superior when compared with the individual treatments; versus doxazosin (−403 [−504 to −302]; $p < 00001$) and versus bisoprolol (−448 [−550 to −346]; $p < 00001$). Spironolactone was the most effective blood pressure-lowering treatment, throughout the distribution of baseline plasma renin; but its margin of superiority and likelihood of being the best drug for the individual patient were many-fold greater in the lower than higher ends of the distribution. All treatments were well tolerated. In six of the 285 patients who received spironolactone, serum potassium exceeded 60 mmol/L on one occasion.

*Interpretation.*—Spironolactone was the most effective add-on drug for the treatment of resistant hypertension. The superiority of spironolactone supports a primary role of sodium retention in this condition.

▶ The PATHWAY-2 trial investigated the optimal treatment for Resistant Hypertension (RHTN). According to the American Heart Association, approximately 80 million people in the United States are hypertensive. About 20% of those have resistant hypertension (RHTN), which is defined as suboptimal blood pressure control despite using 3 "first-line" agents, which are typically renin–angiotensin–aldosterone system inhibitors (A), calcium channel blockers (C), and diuretics (D), typically of thiazide class. Recently, after initial optimism, renal denervation proved unsuccessful in the treatment of RHTN,[1] which renewed interest in a purely pharmacological approach. However, the pathophysiology of resistant hypertension is poorly understood. Although some studies have suggested the superiority of spironolactone for this condition,[2] there have been no prior studies investigating the head-to-head superiority of spironolactone versus other additive agents.

To address this gap, PATHWAY-2, a double blind, placebo-controlled, crossover trial, was designed to determine whether spironolactone, doxazosin, or bisoprolol is most effective as an additive treatment for RHTN. Patients with systolic blood pressure over 140 mm Hg (or ≥135 mm Hg for patients with diabetes) and with home systolic blood pressure of 130 mm Hg or greater, despite treatment for at least 3 months with maximally tolerated doses of 3 drugs, were eligible for inclusion. The protocol involved a 1-month single-blind placebo run-in, followed by 4 cycles (without a washout) of 12-week duration with (1) spironolactone (25-50 mg), (2) doxazosin (4-8 mg), (3) bisoprolol (5-10 mg), and (4) placebo. Hierarchically defined primary end points were prespecified.

The results were quite convincing. Spironolactone was superior to placebo (−8.7 mm Hg with 95% confidence interval [CI] −9.72 to −7.69), mean of the other 2 drugs (95% CI −5.13 to −3.38) and to both doxazosin (−4.03, 95% CI −5.04 to −3.02) and bisoprolol (−4.48 with 95% CI −5.50 to −3.46). Interestingly, spironolactone was superior across all ranges of plasma renin levels. However, its superiority was most marked among those with low renin levels, which suggests that a high salt/low renin hypertensive pathophysiology is present among this population.

Hyperkalemia (serum potassium > 6.0), occurred in approximately 2% of the patients, and estimated glomerular filtration rate (eGFR) was reduced with all of the regimens (by about 10 mL/minute).

This was a well-conducted randomized controlled trial that is unequivocal in its support for spironolactone in resistant hypertension, but there are some caveats. First, patients with an eGFR less than 45 mL/minute were excluded from the study. Thus, great care should be taken before these results are generalized to patients with more serious renal disease in whom a higher incidence of spironolactone-associated hyperkalemia has been reported.[3] Second, other disorders associated with increase of the risk of progressive renal injury or hyperkalemia, such as diabetes, were underrepresented. Additionally, there was no washout between the cycles, and each cycle only lasted 12 weeks. However, the cycle length was likely long enough to both correct for any residual drug overlap between the cycles and to have detected any escape from blood pressure (B/P) control. The determination of whether the B/P lowering effect of spironolactone indicates a role for primary hyperaldosteronism in the pathophysiology of resistant hypertension or reflects the effect of diuretics to improve a salt-sensitive state will require additional studies with additional agents. In the meantime, in the population studied, the available data support the addition of the aldosterone antagonist spironolactone as additive agent in the treatment of RHTN.

**S. Chugh, MD**

*References*

1. Bhatt DL, Kandzari DE, O'Neill WW, et al. SYMPLICITY HTN-3 Investigators. A controlled trial of renal denervation for resistant hypertension. *N Engl J Med.* 2014;370:1393-1401.
2. Dahal K, Kunwar S, Rijal J, et al. The effects of aldosterone antagonists in patients with resistant hypertension: a meta-analysis of randomised and non-randomised studies. *Am J Hypertens.* 2015;28:1376-1385.
3. Khosla N, Kalaitzidis R, Bakris GL. Predictors of hyperkalemia risk following hypertension control with aldosterone blockade. *Am J Nephrol.* 2009;30:418-424.

## Effectiveness and Safety of Aldosterone Antagonist Therapy Use Among Older Patients With Reduced Ejection Fraction After Acute Myocardial Infarction

Wang TY, Vora AN, Peng SA, et al (Duke Univ Med Ctr, Durham, NC)
*J Am Heart Assoc* 5:e002612, 2016

*Background.*—While aldosterone antagonists have proven benefit among post-myocardial infarction (MI) patients with low ejection fraction (EF), how this treatment is used among older MI patients in routine practice is not well described.

*Methods and Results.*—Using ACTION Registry-GWTG linked to Medicare data, we examined 12 080 MI patients ≥65 years with EF ≤40% who were indicated for aldosterone antagonist therapy per current guidelines and without documented contraindications. Of these, 11% (n = 1310) were prescribed aldosterone antagonists at discharge. Notably, 10% of patients prescribed an aldosterone antagonist were eligible for, but not concurrently treated with, an angiotensin-converting enzyme inhibitor/angiotensin receptor blocker. Spironolactone was the predominantly prescribed aldosterone antagonist. At 2-year follow-up, aldosterone antagonist use was not associated with lower mortality (unadjusted 39% versus 38%; HR 0.99, 95% CI 0.88−1.33 using inverse probability weighted propensity adjustment) except in symptomatic HF patients (HR 0.84, 95% CI 0.72−0.99, $P_{interaction} = 0.009$). Risks of hyperkalemia were low at 30 days, but significantly higher among patients prescribed aldosterone antagonists (unadjusted 2.3% versus 1.5%; adjusted HR 2.04, 95% CI 1.16−3.60), as was 2-year risk of acute renal failure (unadjusted 6.7% versus 4.8%; adjusted HR 1.39, 95% CI 1.01−1.92) compared with patients not prescribed aldosterone antagonists.

*Conclusions.*—Aldosterone antagonist use among eligible older MI patients in routine clinical practice was not associated with lower mortality except in patients with HF symptoms, but was associated with increased risks of hyperkalemia and acute renal failure. These results underscore the importance of close post-discharge monitoring of this patient population.

▶ A post hoc analysis of the well-controlled Eplerenone Postacute Myocardial Infarction and Survival Study (EPHESUS) demonstrated a small risk of hyperkalemia (6% risk overall; 4.4% with $K^+$ > 5.5 meq/Land 1.6% with $K^+$ ≥6 meq/L), without an increase in mortality.[1] However, as the authors point out, elderly patients are often underrepresented in clinical trials. To better assess the risk of untoward medication effects in the elderly, in the current study the researchers aligned the ACTION—Get with the Guidelines registry and Medicare administrative databases to evaluate both guideline compliance and the impact of treatment with aldosterone antagonists in a population of patients ≥65 years old with a prior myocardial infarction and a reduced ejection fraction ( < 40%). Per the American Heart Association/American College of Cardiology guidelines, approximately 12 100 patients were eligible to receive treatment with aldosterone antagonist. However, within this real-world cohort, only 11% of eligible patients received an aldosterone antagonist (primarily spironolactone). Per the guidelines, approximately 10% were also eligible, but did not receive, concomitant treatment with either an angiotensin-converting enzyme inhibitor (ACEI) or and angiotensin receptor blocker (ARB). Other studies on the use of aldosterone antagonists have also highlighted that the findings observed during well-controlled clinical trials may differ from those observed with widespread clinical use.[2,3]

Within this population of elderly patients with reduced ejection fraction, approximately 3% of the population developed hyperkalemia, and there was a 2-fold risk of rehospitalization for hyperkalemia within 30 days. In addition to the risk of hyperkalemia, among the aldosterone-antagonist treated group, there was approximately a 40% increased risk of hospitalization for acute renal failure at 2 years. Specific analyses, stratified by age, sex, baseline renal function, and concurrent ACEI/ARB therapy did not demonstrate any particular risk factors for the development of hyperkalemia. Of note, regarding improved cardiac status, use of aldosterone antagonists was not associated with significant differences in mortality or improved cardiac rehospitalization risk among patients ≥65 years except in those with symptomatic heart failure.

Because this is a registry study, there are of course some limitations. For example, the submitted data may have failed to include the development of hyperkalemia or acute kidney injury/chronic kidney disease, so the actual incidence may be underreported. Also, registry data may not discern whether a treatment was withheld for well-founded clinical reasons that were simply not well documented.

The data suggest that "best-practice" indications for the use of aldosterone antagonists in the elderly with cardiac disease may require some refinement. The findings are interesting both because of the lack of compliance with the guidelines and also because of the observed risk of hyperkalemia within this elderly population. The combination of these findings is noteworthy; had the guidelines been more rigorously applied, the incidence of hyperkalemia would perhaps been even higher. Taken together, the findings suggest that when elderly patients with reduced ejection fractions are treated with aldosterone antagonists, with or without the addition of ACEi/ARB, serum potassium, and renal function should be closely monitored.

**R. Garrick, MD**

*References*

1. Pitt B, Bakris G, Ruilope LM, et al. EPHESUS Investigators. Serum potassium and clinical outcomes in the eplerenone post-acute myocardial infarction heart failure efficacy and survival study (EPHESUS). *Circulation.* 2008;118:1643-1650.
2. Juurlink DN, Mamdani MM, Lee DS, et al. Rates of hyperkalemia after publication of the randomized aldactone evaluation study. *N Engl J Med.* 2004;351: 543-551.
3. Bozkurt B, Agoston I, Knowlton AA. Complications of inappropriate use of spironolactone in heart failure: when an old medicine spirals out of new guidelines. *J Am Coll Cardiol.* 2003;41:211-214.

### New-onset Atrial Fibrillation is Associated With Polycystic Kidney Disease: A Nationwide Population-based Cohort Study

Yu T-M, Chuang Y-W, Yu M-C, et al (China Med Univ, Taiwan; Taichung Veterans General Hosp, Taiwan; Chang Gung Univ College of Medicine, Taoyuan, Taiwan; et al)
*Medicine* 95:e2623, 2016

Cardiovascular complications remain the major problems contributing to morbidity and mortality in patients with polycystic kidney disease (PKD).

Therefore, the authors hypothesized that atrial fibrillation (AF) is closely associated with PKD. The authors conducted a nationwide population-based cohort study to investigate the risk of AF in patients with PKD.

Using data from inpatient claims, the authors enrolled 7203 patients aged over 20 years who were diagnosed with PKD from 1998 to 2010 with no history of AF as the PKD cohort. They randomly selected 28,739 people without PKD as controls and frequency matched them with patients with PKD according to their age, sex, and baseline comorbidity.

In total, 247 PKD patients were diagnosed with AF, representing an incidence of 7.08 per 1000 person-years, whereas 807 cases of AF occurred in the comparison cohort, yielding an incidence of 4.98 per 1000 person-years, with an adjusted HR(aHR) of 1.31 (95% CI = 1.14–1.51). The risk of AF increased from an aHR of 1.59 (95% CI = 1.15–2.21) to 3.64 (95% CI = 1.93–6.85) when the number of risk factors increased from 1 to more than 5 in comparison with patients without risk factors.

A remarkably high incidence rate and risk was observed in patients with PKD when multiple risk factors were combined. A high index of suspicion should be maintained when examining PKD patients with irregular betas. Early prophylactic therapy is warranted in these patients.

▶ Atrial fibrillation is the most common cardiac arrhythmia, and cardiovascular complications are quite common in patients with polycystic kidney disease (PKD). These researchers used Taiwan's national health care insurance research database to evaluate the intersection of these 2 conditions. Investigators randomly selected 28 739 patients without PKD or atrial fibrillation as controls and compared the incidence of atrial fibrillation against patients with known polycystic kidney disease.

The majority the patients with PKD were older than age 65 years, and more than half were women. Overall, patients with PKD had a 31% increased risk of atrial fibrillation. The risk was greatest in patients aged 50 to 64 and persisted in the absence of comorbidities, leading the researchers to suggest that atrial fibrillation is associated with the "presence of PKD itself," rather than with other concomitant comorbidities. The incidence of atrial fibrillation was close to 7 per 1000 in the patients with PKD compared with approximate 5 per 1000 person-years in the control cohort.

However, when other comorbidities were present, the risk of atrial fibrillation was even more marked, such that patients with 1 risk factor had approximatly a

60% increase in atrial fibrillation, and the risk increased to 67% in patients with 3 risk factors. The highest risk occurred in PKD patients with congestive heart failure and abnormal renal function, where the hazard ratio was 6.09 (95% confidence interval 1.94—19.1). The presence of atrial fibrillation also increased mortality, and the odds of dying from atrial fibrillation were approximately 70% higher in patients with PKD than in the comparison cohort.

A strength of the study is its control population-based design and careful peer review applied to the Taiwanese governmental insurance base, which supports the reliability of the PKD classification code. A weakness of the study is the lack of information regarding structural heart disease, which can occur in patients with PKD and may increase the risk of atrial fibrillation[1,2] and the absence of information regarding the underlying status of the sympathetic nervous system and the renin-angiotensin system both of which are altered in patients with PKD[3,4] and can influence the risk of atrial fibrillation. Additionally, limited information on some (chronic obstructive pulmonary disease, coronary disease, stroke), but not other comorbid risk factors (thyroid disease, alcohol use, smoking), was available.

It is interesting to speculate that the observed increased incidence of atrial fibrillation is somehow linked to an effect of polycystin-2 on the myocyte calcium channel, similar to its reported effect at the level of the kidney.[5] However, those speculations will require further controlled investigations, and the observations from this database certainly support the need for further studies regarding the links between atrial fibrillation and PKD. Clinically, this large population study is the first to demonstrate that autosomal dominant PKD is an independent risk factor for atrial fibrillation, and this should be considered as we care for and counsel our PKD patients.

**R. Garrick, MD**

*References*

1. Chapman AB, Johnson AM, Rainguet S, et al. Left ventricular hypertrophy in autosomal dominant polycystic kidney disease. *J Am Soc Nephrol.* 1997;8: 1292-1297.
2. Martinez-Vea A, Valero FA, Bardaji A, et al. Left ventricular hypertrophy in hypertensive patients with autosomal dominant polycystic kidney disease: influence of blood pressure and humoral and neurohormonal factors. *Am J Nephrol.* 2000; 20:193-200.
3. Schrier RW. Renal volume, renin-angiotensin-aldosterone system, hypertension, and left ventricular hypertrophy in patients with autosomal dominant polycystic kidney disease. *J Am Soc Nephrol.* 2009;20:1888-1893.
4. Cerasola G, Vecchi M, Mule G, et al. Sympathetic activity and blood pressure pattern in autosomal dominant polycystic kidney disease hypertensives. *Am J Nephrol.* 1998;18:391-398.
5. Paavola J, Schliffke S, Rossetti S, et al. Polycystin-2 mutations lead to impaired calcium cycling in the heart and predispose to dilated cardiomyopathy. *J Mol Cell Cardiol.* 2013;58:199-208.

**The PROPKD Score: A New Algorithm to Predict Renal Survival in Autosomal Dominant Polycystic Kidney Disease**

Cornec-Le Gall E, Audrézet M-P, Rousseau A, et al (Univ Hosp, Brest, France; Natl Inst of Health and Med Sciences, Brest, France; Univ Hosp, Limoges, France; et al)

*J Am Soc Nephrol* 27:942-951, 2016

The course of autosomal dominant polycystic kidney disease (ADPKD) varies among individuals, with some reaching ESRD before 40 years of age and others never requiring RRT. In this study, we developed a prognostic model to predict renal outcomes in patients with ADPKD on the basis of genetic and clinical data. We conducted a cross-sectional study of 1341 patients from the Genkyst cohort and evaluated the influence of clinical and genetic factors on renal survival. Multivariate survival analysis identified four variables that were significantly associated with age at ESRD onset, and a scoring system from 0 to 9 was developed as follows: being male: 1 point; hypertension before 35 years of age: 2 points; first urologic event before 35 years of age: 2 points; *PKD2* mutation: 0 points; nontruncating *PKD1* mutation: 2 points; and truncating *PKD1* mutation: 4 points. Three risk categories were subsequently defined as low risk (0-3 points), intermediate risk (4-6 points), and high risk (7-9 points) of progression to ESRD, with corresponding median ages for ESRD onset of 70.6, 56.9, and 49 years, respectively. Whereas a score ≤3 eliminates evolution to ESRD before 60 years of age with a negative predictive value of 81.4%, a score >6 forecasts ESRD onset before 60 years of age with a positive predictive value of 90.9%. This newprognostic score accurately predicts renal outcomes in patients with ADPKD and may enable the personalization of therapeutic management of ADPKD.

▶ Autosomal dominant polycystic kidney disease (ADPKD), the most common inherited cause of kidney failure, has multiple genotypic etiologies and outcomes.[1] There is much heterogeneity in the age of onset, rapidity of progression, associated abnormalities, and responses to therapy.[2]

Cornec-le Gall et al have derived a useful scoring system for ADPKD based on a novel algorithm that accurately predicts renal outcomes in these patients.

They conducted a cross-sectional study of more than 1300 patients from 913 pedigrees for which molecular genetic analysis was completed. Using both multivariate and univariate analyses, they made some interesting observations. They found that early-onset hypertension (HTN; < age 35 years), early onset of urological symptoms (hematuria, cyst infection, or flank pain), and *PKD1* mutations, especially truncated ones, all yielded worse renal outcomes. Truncated *PKD1* mutations were particularly ominous for males. Smoking or multiparity did not have any effect in univariate analysis.

After multivariate analysis of 973 patients, these 4 independent predictors of progression remained. These features were then assigned weightings based on the observed hazard ratios (HR). Specifically, male sex (HR 1.55), the presence of truncated *PKD1* mutations (HR 4.75), early onset of HTN (HR 2.11), and early first urological symptoms (HR 1.73) all predicted the worst renal outcomes.

A summation of these weightings was called the PORPKD score. The PROPKD score was used to delineate 3 overall risk categories; point totals 0 to 3, 4 to 6, and 7 to 9 designated low risk, intermediate risk, and high risk, respectively.

The accuracy of these assignments by score was high. By age 60, the Kaplan-Meier probabilities of end-stage renal disease (ESRD) were 19.3%, 60.8%, and 91.9% in the low-, intermediate-, and high-risk groups, respectively. These risk categories also accurately predicted the median age of ESRD onset (70.6, 56.9, and 49, respectively), and the rates of renal function decline (2.0, 3.4, and 4.4 mL/min/year respectively).

This scoring system could be helpful in counseling patients for treatment, as well as life and family planning purposes. This accurate and reproducible scoring system could also be helpful for research purposes in assessing the efficacy of new treatments.

**M. Klein, MD, JD**

*References*


1. Harris PC, Hopp K. The mutation, a key determinant of phenotype in ADPKD. *J Am Soc Nephrol.* 2013;24:868-870.
2. Schrier RW, Brosnahan G, Cadnapaphornchai MA, et al. Predictors of autosomal dominant polycystic kidney disease progression. *J Am Soc Nephrol.* 2014;25:2399-2418.


---

**Long-Term Renal Function after Endovascular Aneurysm Repair**

Saratzis A, Bath MF, Harrison S, et al (Leicester NIHR Cardiovascular Biomedical Res Unit, UK; et al)

*Clin J Am Soc Nephrol* 10:1930-1936, 2015

---

*Background and Objectives.*—Endovascular repair (EVAR) is a common treatment for abdominal aortic aneurysm (AAA). However, its long-term effects on renal function remain unclear. We aimed to assess long-term renal dysfunction after EVAR using a contemporary estimate of GFR and to compare long-term renal outcomes in patients after EVAR with open aneurysm repair (OAR) and in patients without an AAA.

*Design, Settings, Participants, & Measurements.*—We performed a nested case-matched analysis of 726 patients (using a prospectively maintained database for repairs that took place between January 2000 and May 2010 in a tertiary center): 121 patients undergoing OAR (with data at baseline and 5 years postrepair) were case matched (age, sex, smoking, diabetes, baseline eGFR) to patients undergoing suprarenal and infrarenal fixation EVAR (242 in each group) and to 121 patients undergoing carotid endarterectomy (CEA) without AAA. Changes in eGFR were compared (1 and 5 years).

*Results.*—The OAR patients lost an average of 7.4 ml/min per 1.73 $m^2$ at 5 years (95% confidence interval [95% CI], 4.8 to 10.6), compared with

8.2 ml/min per 1.73 $m^2$ (95% CI, 6.5 to 10.8; $P < 0.001$) for infrarenal-fixation EVAR, 16.9 ml/min per 1.73 $m^2$ (95% CI, 13.0 to 21.9, $P < 0.001$) for suprarenal-fixation EVAR, and 5.4 ml/min per 1.73 $m^2$ (95% CI, 1.7 to 7.5; $P < 0.001$) for CEA. The decrease in eGFR was steeper during the first postoperative year, with each group losing −2.2 ml/min per 1.73 $m^2$ (infrarenal-fixation EVAR), −10.7 ml/min per 1.73 $m^2$ (suprarenal-fixation EVAR), and −4.6 ml/min per 1.73 $m^2$ (OAR), compared with −1.9 ml/min per 1.73 $m^2$ for CEA.

*Conclusions.*—Elective EVAR is associated with a significant decline in eGFR after 5 years, which is steeper in the first postoperative year and more pronounced compared with a similar population with atherosclerotic disease.

▶ In last year's edition, we reviewed data demonstrating the underreporting of renal complications after endovascular abdominal aortic aneurysm repair (EVAR),[1] which is considered the first-line treatment modality for abdominal aortic aneurysm (AAA) because both medium-term morbidity and mortality are superior to open aneurysm repair (OAR). However, both techniques may adversely affect renal function, and a prior meta-analysis demonstrated that during the first postoperative year, the serum creatinine increases by about 30% in approximately 18% of EVAR patients.[1]

Much of our understanding of the risk of EVAR comes from retrospective reviews. To better delineate the short-term and long-term renal impact of EVAR and OAR, the authors use a prospectively maintained database to perform a nested case-matched analysis of renal complications among individuals undergoing these repairs. Patients with leaking, and/or infected aneurysms, those requiring emergency surgery, or those requiring presurgical renal replacement therapy were excluded. The 5-year change in estimated glomerular filtration rate (eGFR) among these patients was compared another high-risk vascular group comprising patients undergoing carotid endarterectomy (without AAA repair). The main outcome measure was a change in eGFR derived from Chronic Kidney Disease Epidemiology Collaboration (CKD-EPI).

This study is the first attempt to compare long-term renal outcomes among a defined matched population of patients undergoing EVAR and OAR aneurysm repair, and the results are both interesting and somewhat surprising. As demonstrated in Fig 1 of the original article, the initial and long-term renal outcome of suprarenal EVAR was inferior to that of other techniques, and in all cases, over the same timeframe, renal function declined more significantly after AAA than in another high-risk population (patients undergoing carotid endarterectomy).

Multivariate linear regression assessed use of angiotensin-converting enzyme inhibitors ($P = .10$), development of AKI ($P = .06$), history of cardiovascular disease ($P = .52$), and baseline eGFR ($P = .03$). The regression results confirmed that treatment group was significantly associated with a change in eGFR at 5 years, after adjusting for other covariates ($P = .04$).

The results are clinically important. Abdominal aortic aneurysms are present between 2% and 8% of men over the age of 65 and aneurysmal repair is a common surgical procedure. EVAR patients, who presumably did well at the time of surgery, remain at risk for a significant loss of renal function over time. This risk is most marked in those undergoing suprarenal EVAR repair, was steepest in the first postoperative year, and continued over the entire five-year follow-up. The extent of renal injury seen is noteworthy. Until specific risk factors can be more definitively identified, the findings suggest that long-term renal surveillance is required and that both peri-operative (hydration, ischemia reduction and medication management strategies) and long-term reno-protective strategies are rational considerations.

**R. Ledesma, MD**

*Reference*

1. Karthikesalingam A, Bahia SS, Patel SR, et al. A systematic review and meta-analysis indicates underreporting of renal dysfunction following endovascular aneurysm repair. *Kidney Int.* 2015;87:442-445.

---

**Kidney Disease among Patients with Sickle Cell Disease, Hemoglobin SS and SC**

Drawz P, Ayyappan S, Nouraie M, et al (Univ of Minnesota, Minneapolis; Case Western Reserve Univ, Cleveland, OH; Howard Univ, Washington, DC; et al)
*Clin J Am Soc Nephrol* 11:207-215, 2016

---

*Background and Objectives.*—Sickle cell disease (SCD) is an inherited anemia that afflicts millions worldwide. Kidney disease is a major contributor to its morbidity and mortality. We examined contemporary and historical SCD populations to understand how renal disease behaved in hemoglobin SS (HbSS) compared with HbSC.

*Design, Setting, Participants, & Measurements.*—Kidney function was examined in the multicentered Treatment of Pulmonary Hypertension and Sickle Cell Disease with Sildenafil Therapy (Walk-PHaSST) Trial (HbSS = 463; HbSC = 127; years 2007–2009) and historical comparator populations from the Cooperative Study of Sickle Cell Disease (CSSCD; HbSS = 708) and the Multicenter Study of Hydroxyurea in Sickle Cell Disease (MSH; HbSS = 299).

*Results.*—In adults with SCD, eGFR was lower among older individuals: −1.78 ml/min per 1.73 $m^2$ per year of age (95% confidence interval [95% CI], −2.06 to −1.50; Walk-PHaSST Trial), −1.75 ml/min per 1.73 $m^2$ per year of age (95% CI, −2.05 to −1.44; MSH), and −1.69 ml/min per 1.73 $m^2$ per year of age (95% CI, −2.00 to −1.38; CSSCD) in HbSS compared with −1.09 ml/min per 1.73 $m^2$ per year of age (95% CI, −1.39 to −0.75) in HbSC (Walk-PHaSST Trial). Macroalbuminuria was seen in 20% of participants with SCD (HbSS or HbSC; $P = 0.45$; Walk-PHaSST Trial), but microalbuminuria was more prevalent in HbSS (44% versus 23% in HbSC; $P < 0.002$). In the Walk-PHaSST Trial, albuminuria was associated with hemolysis (higher lactate dehydrogenase, $P < 0.001$; higher absolute reticulocyte count, $P < 0.02$; and lower Hb, $P = 0.07$) and elevated systolic BP ($P < 0.001$) in HbSS. One half of all participants with HbSS (20 of 39) versus one fifth without (41 of 228) elevated tricuspid regurgitant jet velocity (≥3 m/s; adverse prognostic indicator in SCD) had macroalbuminuria ($P < 0.001$). In the CSSCD, overt proteinuria, detected (less sensitively) by urine dipstick, associated with higher 3-year mortality (odds ratio, 2.48; 95% CI, 1.07 to 5.77). Serum bicarbonate was lower in HbSS (23.8 versus 24.8 mEq/dl in HbSC; $P < 0.05$) and associated with reticulocytopenic anemia and decreased renal function.

*Conclusions.*—In SCD, albuminuria or proteinuria was highly prevalent, in HbSS more than in HbSC. Proteinuria associated with mortality in HbSS. Older individuals had a lower than expected eGFR, and this was more prominent in HbSS. Current management does not routinely address renal complications in SCD, which could plausibly reduce morbidity and mortality.

▶ We are very accustomed to encountering the bone, pulmonary, and cardiovascular complications of sickle cell disease (SCD); however sometimes the extent and severity of the renal involvement in SCD goes unrecognized. Inherited as an autosomal mutation in the beta-globin chain of adult hemoglobin (HbA; $\alpha_2\beta_2$), homozygous HbSS ($\alpha_2\beta^S{}_2$) is most common alteration. However, up to 30% of adults have HbSC ($\alpha_2\beta^s\beta^c$) or sickle C disease. Although HbSS is more severe, both genetic patterns can be associated with renal disease.[1] Characterized by early mortality, the morbidity of HbSS includes hemolytic anemia, painful vaso-occlusive episodes, and pulmonary and bone disease, that latter of which can include avascular bone necrosis. HbSC is typically associated with retinopathy, avascular necrosis of the bones, and chronic pain. Although kidney disease is seen in most adults with SCD and can affect all areas of the kidney (glomeruli, tubules, and interstitial and vascular structures), the details regarding the severity and extent of renal involvement have not been fully characterized.

The current study examined the kidney function in patients from a well-defined population in the multicentered Treatment of Pulmonary Hypertension and Sickle Cell Disease with Sildenafil Therapy (Walk-PHaSST) trial, which included 463 patients with HbSS and 127 with HbSC. The objective of this study was to evaluate renal function and acid-base complications in HbSS and HbSC as they related to erythroid reserve, hemolysis, and mortality.

Their findings are clinically useful. The estimated glomerular filtration rate (eGFR) was significantly lower among older individuals with SCD, most prominently in HbSS compared with HbSC (−1.78 vs −1.09 mL/min per 1.73 $m^2$ per year of age; $P < .001$). Microalbuminuria was present by age 30 in about 40% of patients with HbSS and in a similar number of HbSc patients over the age of 50. Macroalbuminuria was most prevalent in patients with HbSS and correlated with cardiac abnormalities, especially echocardiographic assessment of tricuspid regurgitant jet velocity. Overall, unlike eGFR, proteinuria was associated with greater hemolysis. With regard to tubular abnormalities, serum bicarbonate was lower in patients with HbSS ($P = .004$) compared with those with HbSC. This change correlated with the eGFR as well, and 25.4% of participants with

HbSS had a serum bicarbonate of less than 22 mEq/dl. Serum potassium was significantly higher in HbSS compared with HbSC ($P < .001$).

The study highlights clinical issues that can directly affect the care of these patients; for example, monitoring the bicarbonate and correcting acidemia in HbSS may reduce sickling risk by improving the oxygen dissociation curve. Albuminuria is more prevalent in HbSS and was associated with hemolysis and more overt cardiovascular disease, such as a higher systolic blood pressure, and appreciation of these associations might improve patient outcome. Both overt proteinuria and eGFR in HbSS disease were associated with a higher mortality risk, and these findings can also help prioritize our therapeutic efforts. The results in this well-defined population are clinically useful. They better define the clinical phenotype of renal disease and demonstrate that, although more subtle in patients with HbSC, all forms of SCD are at risk of renal injury and are associated with clinical factors, such as hypertension and proteinuria, that may improve with intervention.

**R. Pawar, MD**

*Reference*

1. Lionnet F, Hammoudi N, Stojanovic KS, et al. Hemoglobin SC disease complications: a clinical study of 179 cases. *Haematologica*. 2012;97:1136-1141.

---

**Total, Dietary, and Supplemental Vitamin C Intake and Risk of Incident Kidney Stones**

Ferraro PM, Curhan GC, Gambaro G, et al (Catholic Univ of the Sacred Heart, Rome, Italy; Harvard Med School, Boston, MA; et al)
*Am J Kidney Dis* 67:400-407, 2016

---

*Background.*—Previous studies of vitamin C and kidney stones were conducted mostly in men and either reported disparate results for supplemental and dietary vitamin C or did not examine dietary vitamin C.

*Study Design.*—Prospective cohort analysis.

*Setting & Participants.*—156,735 women in the Nurses' Health Study (NHS) I and II and 40,536 men in the Health Professionals Follow-up Study (HPFS).

*Predictor.*—Total, dietary, and supplemental vitamin C intake, adjusted for age, body mass index, thiazide use, and dietary factors.

*Outcomes.*—Incident kidney stones.

*Results.*—During a median follow-up of 11.3 to 11.7 years, 6,245 incident kidney stones were identified. After multivariable adjustment, total vitamin C intake (<90 [reference], 90-249, 250-499, 500-999, and ≥1,000 mg/d) was not significantly associated with risk for kidney stones among women, but was among men (HRs of 1.00 [reference], 1.19 [95% CI, 0.99-1.46], 1.15 [95% CI, 0.93-1.42], 1.29 [95% CI, 1.04-1.60], and 1.43 [95% CI, 1.15-1.79], respectively; $P$ for trend = 0.005). Median total vitamin C intake for the 500- to 999-mg/d category was ~700 mg/d. Supplemental vitamin C intake (no use [reference], <500, 500-999, and

≥1,000 mg/d) was not significantly associated with risk for kidney stones among women, but was among men (HR, 1.19 [95% CI, 1.01-1.40] for ≥1,000 mg/d; *P* for trend = 0.001). Dietary vitamin C intake was not associated with stones among men or women, although few participants had dietary intakes >700 mg/d.

*Limitations.*—Nutrient intakes derived from food-frequency questionnaires, lack of data on stone composition for all cases.

*Conclusions.*—Total and supplemental vitamin C intake was significantly associated with higher risk for incident kidney stones in men, but not in women.

▶ Kidney stones are common with a lifetime of prevalence of ~10% in the US population, and diet is thought to play an important role in its development. Ascorbic acid (vitamin C) is an essential nutrient and a cofactor in several enzymatic pathways. Dietary vitamin C is partly converted to oxalate and excreted in urine and thus potentially increases the risk of calcium oxalate stone formation. Two previous studies looked at the risk of kidney stones in relationship to vitamin C intake. In the Health Professionals Follow-up Study (HPFS), ≥1000 mg/day of total vitamin C intake was associated with a 41% higher risk for stones compared with ≤90 mg/day.[1] A second study, among 23 355 Swedish men, reported a positive association between vitamin C intake and kidney stones; the adjusted relative risk associated with supplemental vitamin C use was double compared with no use.[2] To date, selective vitamin C–induced stone risk in women has only been evaluated in the Nurses' Health Study (NHS) I cohort, which found no association between vitamin C intake and the risk for stones.[3]

The current prospective cohort analysis examined the independent associations of total, supplemental, and dietary vitamin C intake and risk of kidney stones in the 156 735 women in the NHS I and II,[4] and 40 536 men in the HPFS. Participants were asked to complete biennial questionnaires with information on medical history, lifestyle, and medications.

During a median follow-up of 11.7 years for NHS I, 11.5 years for NHS II, and 11.3 years for HPFS, 6245 incident kidney stone events occurred. In all the cohorts, no association was found between dietary vitamin C intake and incident kidney stones: the multivariable-adjusted hazard ratio (HR) for dietary vitamin C intake ≥250 compared with < 90 mg/day was 0.92 (95% CI, 0.68-1.24; *P* for trend = .3) in the NHS cohort and 0.95 (95% CI, 0.75-1.19; *P* for trend = 0.7) in the HPFS cohort.

However, unlike dietary intake, the authors found a higher risk of stone disease among men with higher total and supplemental vitamin C intakes. Among women, supplemental vitamin C intake in the ranges studied did not increase the risk of stone formation. Importantly, the dietary C intake was under 700 mg in most patients, and thus it is possible that the results may not be generalizable to populations of women with higher intakes of vitamin C. Additionally, the uncertainties intrinsic to dietary recall and the lack of urinary measurements also limit the strength of these observations. With these limitations in mind, it is reasonable to advise male patients with oxalate-related stone disease to limit their intake of supplemental vitamin C. In woman, neither supplemental or dietary vitamin C intake in the amounts studied appear to increase the risk of oxalate-related stone disease.

**R. Pawar, MD**

*References*


1. Taylor EN, Stampfer MJ, Curhan GC. Dietary factors and the risk of incident kidney stones in men: new insights after 14 years of follow-up. *J Am Soc Nephrol.* 2004;15:3225-3232.
2. Thomas LDK, Elinder C-G, Tiselius H-G, Wolk A, Akesson A. Ascorbic acid supplements and kidney stone incidence among men: a prospective study. *JAMA Intern Med.* 2013;173:386-388.
3. Curhan GC, Willett WC, Speizer FE, Stampfer MJ. Intake of vitamins B6 and C and the risk of kidney stones in women. *J Am Soc Nephrol.* 1999;10:840-845.
4. Curhan GC, Willett WC, Knight EL, Stampfer MJ. Dietary factors and the risk of incident kidney stones in younger women: Nurses' Health Study II. *Arch Intern Med.* 2004;164:885-891.


---

**Kidney-Failure Risk Projection for the Living Kidney-Donor Candidate**

Grams ME, for the Chronic Kidney Disease Prognosis Consortium (Johns Hopkins Univ School of Medicine, Baltimore, MD; et al)

*N Engl J Med* 374:411-421, 2016

---

*Background.*—Evaluation of candidates to serve as living kidney donors relies on screening for individual risk factors for end-stage renal disease (ESRD). To support an empirical approach to donor selection, we developed a tool that simultaneously incorporates multiple health characteristics to estimate a person's probable long-term risk of ESRD if that person does not donate a kidney.

*Methods.*—We used risk associations from a meta-analysis of seven general population cohorts, calibrated to the population-level incidence of ESRD and mortality in the United States, to project the estimated long-term incidence of ESRD among persons who do not donate a kidney, according to 10 demographic and health characteristics. We then compared 15-year projections with the observed risk among 52,998 living kidney donors in the United States.

*Results.*—A total of 4,933,314 participants from seven cohorts were followed for a median of 4 to 16 years. For a 40-year-old person with health characteristics that were similar to those of age-matched kidney donors, the 15-year projections of the risk of ESRD in the absence of donation varied according to race and sex; the risk was 0.24% among black men, 0.15% among black women, 0.06% among white men, and 0.04% among white women. Risk projections were higher in the presence of a lower estimated glomerular filtration rate, higher albuminuria, hypertension, current or former smoking, diabetes, and obesity. In the model-based lifetime projections, the risk of ESRD was highest among persons in the youngest age group, particularly among young blacks. The 15-year observed risks after donation among kidney donors in the United

States were 3.5 to 5.3 times as high as the projected risks in the absence of donation.

*Conclusions.*—Multiple demographic and health characteristics may be used together to estimate the projected long-term risk of ESRD among living kidney-donor candidates and to inform acceptance criteria for kidney donors. (Funded by the National Institute of Diabetes and Digestive and Kidney Diseases and others.)

▶ Kidney donation is a voluntary gift, so physicians must provide accurate predictive information regarding the attendant risks and benefits. Although the short-term donor risks are acceptably low,[1] recent studies suggest that the long-term consequences may not be as benign as once assumed.[2]

Grams et al devised a tool that may be helpful to clinicians and patients in making informed decisions on this matter. They evaluated nearly 5 million participants from 7 cohorts followed from 4 to 16 years for long-term risks of end-stage renal disease. They leveraged more than 31 million person-years of follow-up, during which they assessed demographics and health characteristics to help derive a predictive formula for the incidence of end-stage renal disease (ESRD) in the healthy nondonor population. They found that the 15-year predonation risk of ESRD varied with age, sex, and race. The highest risks were among middle-aged black men (ie, projected risks 0.32% vs 0.08% for 60-year-old black men and white women, respectively). The lifetime projected risk was obviously higher but was less than 2% for all scenarios.

They then applied these risk formulas to the US donor population and found that 94% had a projected 15-year ESRD risk of less than 1%. Unfortunately, the actual observed 15-year risk among donors was higher. For instance, the projected risk for an average black male eligible donor was 0.21%, but the actual observed risk after donation was 0.96%—a 3.5- to 5.3-fold increased risk. This risk is low, to be sure, but it is significantly higher than in the nondonors.

Interestingly, due to shorter average years of remaining life, the older subjects had a lower lifetime incidence of ESRD then the younger subjects, even in the presence of known risk factors for poorer renal outcomes. The outcomes for the recipients from older kidneys are quite good as well.[3]

This study validates a useful tool that can help quantify the small but significant 15-year projected risk of ESRD in kidney donors. It can help clinicians fulfill their ethical obligations of providing accurate risk assessments during the informed consent process.

**M. Klein, MD, JD**

*References*

1. Mjøen G, Øyen O, Holdaas H, Midtvedt K, Line PD. Morbidity and mortality in 1022 consecutive living donor nephrectomies: benefits of a living donor registry. *Transplantation.* 2009;88:1273-1279.
2. Muzaale AD, Massie AB, Wang MC, et al. Risk of end-stage renal disease following live kidney donation. *JAMA.* 2014;311:579-586.
3. Englum BR, Schechter MA, Irish WD, et al. Outcomes in kidney transplant recipients from older living donors. *Transplantation.* 2015;99:309-315.

# 27 Chronic Kidney Disease

**Metformin use and mortality in patients with advanced chronic kidney disease: national, retrospective, observational, cohort study**

Hung S-C, Chang Y-K, Liu J-S, et al (Tzu Chi Univ, Hualien, Taiwan; Natl Health Rese Insts, Zhunan, Taiwan; et al)

*Lancet Diabetes Endocrinol* 3:605-614, 2015

*Background.*—Metformin is recommended as a first-line treatment for patients with type 2 diabetes. However, use of this drug has been contraindicated in individuals with impaired kidney function because of the perceived risk of lactic acidosis. Evidence now supports cautious use of metformin in people with mild-to-moderate chronic kidney disease. However, studies examining the use of metformin in patients with advanced chronic kidney disease are lacking. We aimed to assess the safety of metformin in patients with type 2 diabetes and advanced (approximately stage 5) chronic kidney disease.

*Methods.*—We did a retrospective, observational, cohort study of patients with type 2 diabetes who were enrolled prospectively in Taiwan's national health insurance research database between Jan 1, 2000, and June 30, 2009, and had follow-up data until Dec 31, 2009. We included individuals with a serum creatinine concentration greater than 530 μmol/L, which is approximately equivalent to stage 5 chronic kidney disease. From a consecutive sample of 12 350 patients with type 2 diabetes and chronic kidney disease, 1005 used metformin and 11 345 were non-users. We matched users and non-users of metformin by propensity score in a 1:3 ratio. Our primary outcome was all-cause mortality.

*Findings.*—813 metformin users were matched by propensity score to 2439 non-users. The two groups of patients did not differ significantly by 30 baseline clinical and socioeconomic variables. Median follow-up in the matched cohort was 21 years (range 03–98). All-cause mortality was reported in 434 (53%) of 813 metformin users and in 1012 (41%) of 2439 non-users. After multivariate adjustment, metformin use was an independent risk factor for mortality (adjusted hazard ratio 135, 95% CI 120–151; $p < 00001$). The increased mortality risk was dose-dependent and was consistent across all subgroup analyses. However, metformin use compared with no use was associated with a higher but non-significant risk of metabolic acidosis (16 *vs* 13 events per 100 patient-years; adjusted hazard ratio 130, 95% CI 088–193; $p = 019$).

*Interpretation.*—Use of metformin in people with type 2 diabetes and a serum creatinine concentration greater than 530 µmol/L is associated with a significantly increased risk of all-cause mortality compared with non-users. Metformin use should not be encouraged in this patient group.

▶ The warning "don't give a finger or they will want the whole hand" aptly applies to the use of metformin in the treatment of type II diabetes (DMII) in patients with chronic kidney disease (CKD). Metformin has long been the preferred agent for treatment of DMII because of its proven cardiovascular and mortality benefits.[1] Perpetually threatening, however, has been the risk of lactic acidosis, a rare but potentially fatal side effect of this medication. Due to its predominantly renal excretion, there has been concern that drug accumulation in CKD could increase the risk of this dreaded complication. Recent data, however, demonstrate that, at least in stages 1 to 3 of CKD, this risk is extremely low.[2] Consequently, many prescribers have become quite comfortable using metformin in this patient population.[3] Not surprisingly, with the drug's known efficacy and relative safety even in mild to moderate CKD, it has been tempting to extend its use to patients with higher stages of CKD. But, to date, safety and efficacy data have been lacking in this population.

Hung et al have shed some light on this question in this national observational study from Taiwan. The investigators accessed the National Health Service Research Database from which they pulled data on prevalent DMII and CKD with follow-up from 2000 to 2009, a period during which metformin was prescribed without regard to serum creatinine. A cohort of patients with CKD5 (creatinine > 530 mmol/L or 5.4 mg/dL) during this period were indirectly identified by noting reimbursement for ESA, which was covered only for anemic patients with at least CKD.[5] Comorbidity variables were determined from the ICD-9-CM codes, and the medications covered for the various comorbid diagnoses were similarly evaluated.

Although the primary outcome was the incidence of all-cause mortality, admissions coded as "acidosis" were also analyzed. In all, more than 12 000 patients were identified with both DMII and CKD.[5] After propensity matching 813 users and 2439 nonusers were identified. During 9 years of follow-up, 53% of users died versus 41% of nonusers. This represented a hazard ratio (HR) of 1.29. Higher doses accounted for much of the increased mortality in users. Metabolic acidosis occurred in 4% of both users and nonusers, which was not statistically significant, corroborating prior studies that found a minimal increase in this feared risk. Furthermore, users were statistically less likely than nonusers to require chronic dialysis, even when those who died before starting dialysis were excluded (HR 0.75).

Despite this being an observational study, the large sample size and the robustness of the data available make this a fairly strong argument against the practice of using metformin in more advanced stages of CKD. Indeed, the Food and Drug Administration issued a new recommendation reflecting caution in continuing metformin if GFR falls below 45 cc/min with an absolute contraindication for use if the GFR is less than 30 cc/min.[4] The reduced incidence of ESRD is outweighed by the increase in all cause mortality, even without significant increases in metabolic acidosis.

**M. Klein, MD, JD**

*References*

1. Effect of intensive blood-glucose control with Metformin on complications in overweight patients with type 2 diabetes (UKPDS 34). UK Prospective Diabetes Study (UKPDS) Group. *Lancet.* 1998;352:854-865.
2. Duong JK, Roberts DM, Furlong TJ, et al. Metformin therapy in patients with chronic kidney disease. *Diabetes Obes Metab.* 2012;14:963-965.
3. Holstein A, Nahrwold D, Hinze S, Egberts EH. Contra-indications to metformin therapy are largely disregarded. *Diabet Med.* 1999;16:692-696.
4. http://www.fda.gov/Safety/MedWatch/SafetyInformation/SafetyAlertsforHumanMedicalProducts/ucm494829.htm.

---

**Novel Oral Anticoagulants and the Risk of Major Hemorrhage in Elderly Patients With Chronic Kidney Disease: A Nested Case-Control Study**

Harel Z, Mamdani M, Juurlink DN, et al (Univ of Toronto, Ontario, Canada; Inst for Clinical Evaluative Sciences, Toronto, Ontario, Canada)

*Can J Cardiol* 32:986.e17-22, 2016

---

*Background.*—The novel oral anticoagulants, including dabigatran and rivaroxaban, differ in their degree of renal excretion.

*Methods.*—We conducted a population-based nested case-control study in patients 66 years and older with chronic kidney disease (CKD) (excluding patients undergoing chronic dialysis) who received an oral anticoagulant between April 2006 and March 2013. We calculated odds ratios for hospitalization with a major hemorrhagic event and receipt of dabigatran, rivaroxaban, or warfarin in the preceding 60 days. We also performed a sensitivity analysis to investigate whether a relationship exists between major hemorrhage and advanced age (age $< 80$ years or $\geq 80$ years).

*Results.*—We identified 237,409 patients with CKD, 4470 (1.9%) of whom experienced a major hemorrhage. We matched these patients to 14,460 controls. The use of dabigatran or rivaroxaban was not associated with a statistically significant elevated risk of hemorrhage compared with warfarin (adjusted odds ratio [aOR], 1.15; 95% confidence interval [CI], 0.91-1.45 for dabigatran; aOR, 1.22; 95% CI, 0.83-1.79 for rivaroxaban). Our sensitivity analysis found that older age was associated with an increased risk of hemorrhage for patients receiving dabigatran (aOR, 1.41; 95% CI, 1.06-1.88); results were similar but did not reach statistical significance for rivaroxaban (aOR, 1.57; 95% CI, 0.91-2.69).

*Conclusions.*—Among elderly patients with CKD, exposure to dabigatran or rivaroxaban was not associated with a statistically significant increased risk of major hemorrhagic events compared with exposure to warfarin.

▶ Warfarin anticoagulation (AC) has been the mainstay of therapy for atrial fibrillation and thromboembolic disorders. Because the safe use of warfarin requires careful and frequent monitoring as well as somewhat onerous dietary restrictions, alternative anticoagulants have been developed that circumvent many of these limitations. These novel anticoagulants are renally excreted to varying degrees,[1] and their safe use in patients with chronic kidney disease (CKD) has been questioned. Of these novel anticoagulants, only Apixaban is Food and Drug Administration approved for use in patients with stage 4 or higher CKD—an approval based solely on pharmacokinetic studies rather than on solid safety data.[2]

Harel et al, in this nested case-control study, examined the risk of major hemorrhage in elderly patients with CKD using either a novel anticoagulant or warfarin for various indications. They used national databases to identify more than 235 000 CKD cases over age 66. They included all CKD stages except end-stage renal disease on dialysis. The cases were the nearly 4500 subjects suffering major hemorrhagic events within 60 days of starting AC with warfarin, rivaroxaban, or dabigatran. These cases were compared with nearly 14 500 matched anticoagulated controls who suffered no such hemorrhagic events.

Although the vast majority (97%) used warfarin, the investigators found that the rates of major hemorrhage in those using warfarin were virtually identical to the rates in those using the novel agents rivaroxaban and dabigatran, dose variations notwithstanding. The adjusted odds ratios using warfarin as a reference were 1.15 and 1.22 for dabigatran and rivaroxaban, respectively. These were not statistically significant. Of note, age >86 conferred an independent risk for major hemorrhage in these patients.

This study provides some persuasive evidence that AC with these novel agents may provide predictable and effective therapy without significant increased risk of hemorrhage in patients with CKD. Caution is advised, however, in those over 86 years of age. Also unknown is whether this apparent non-inferiority to warfarin can be presumed in dialysis patients. Not addressed by this study, even if hemorrhagic risk is not enhanced, are other warfarin-related complications known to affect patients with advanced CKD (ie, calciphylaxis).[3] Further study is clearly needed.

**M. Klein, MD, JD**

*References*

1. Mueck W, Schwers S, Stampfuss J. Rivaroxaban and other novel oral anticoagulants: pharmacokinetics in healthy subjects, specific patient populations and relevance of coagulation monitoring. *Thromb J*. 2013;11:10.
2. http://packageinserts.bms.com/pi/pi_eliquis.pdf. Accessed May 3, 2016.
3. Nigwekar SU, Kroshinsky D, Nazarian RM, et al. Calciphylaxis: risk factors, diagnosis, and treatment. *Am J Kidney Dis*. 2015;66:133-146.

**A randomized trial of intravenous and oral iron in chronic kidney disease**

Agarwal R, Kusek JW, Pappas MK (Indiana Univ School of Medicine, Indianapolis; Natl Insts of Health, Bethesda, MD)

*Kidney Int* 88:905-914, 2015

Although iron is commonly used to correct iron deficiency anemia (IDA) in chronic kidney disease (CKD), its effect on kidney function is unclear. To assess this, we randomly assigned patients with stage 3 and 4 CKD and IDA to either open-label oral ferrous sulfate (69 patients to 325 mg three times daily for 8 weeks) or intravenous iron sucrose (67 patients to 200 mg every 2 weeks, total 1 g). The primary outcome was the between-group difference in slope of measured glomerular filtration rate (mGFR) change over two years. The trial was terminated early on the recommendation of an independent data and safety monitoring board based on little chance of finding differences in mGFR slopes, but a higher risk of serious adverse events in the intravenous iron treatment group. mGFR declined similarly over two years in both treatment groups (oral −3.6 ml/min per 1.73 $m^2$, intravenous −4.0 ml/min per 1.73 $m^2$, between-group difference −0.35 ml/min per 1.73 $m^2$; 95% confidence interval −2.9 to 2.3). There were 36 serious cardiovascular events among 19 participants assigned to the oral iron treatment group and 55 events among 17 participants of the intravenous iron group (adjusted incidence rate ratio 2.51 (1.56–4.04)). Infections resulting in hospitalizations had a significant adjusted incidence rate ratio of 2.12 (1.24–3.64). Thus, among non-dialyzed patients with CKD and IDA, intravenous iron therapy is associated with an increased risk of serious adverse events, including those from cardiovascular causes and infectious diseases.

► The REVOKE trial was designed to test whether intravenous iron might accelerate the decline in renal function more than oral therapy in patients with anemia of chronic kidney disease (CKD). The trial randomized 136 subjects with both iron deficiency and CKD to oral iron sulfate (325 mg three times daily) versus iron sucrose infusion.

Over the 2-year course of the trial, there were no significant intergroup differences noted in hemoglobin or in transferrin saturation, whereas markers of iron storage, total iron binding capacity (TIBC), and ferritin were significantly more affected by the intravenous therapy. Interestingly, the rate of renal function decline, the primary outcome, was identical between the 2 groups.

Although no significant difference was noted in the primary outcome, there was an unexpected increase in adverse cardiovascular and infectious events that warranted termination of the trial by the safety monitoring board. The investigators accepted these findings as plausible given the myriad data on iron, oxidative stress, and cardiovascular disease.[1]

What concerned the monitoring board were the rates of overall serious adverse events occurring with an adjusted incidence rate ratio (IRR) of 1.6, infectious adverse events occurring with an adjusted IRR of 2.1, and cardiovascular adverse events occurring with an adjusted IRR of 2.51. Notably, lung and skin infections increased 3- to 4-fold in the IV iron group compared with the oral group, whereas congestive heart failure and angina predominated the cardiovascular adverse incidents attributable to IV iron use.

This was not the first trial of IV versus oral iron repletion, but it was the longest. The FIND-CKD trial,[2] which compared IV ferric carboxymaltose (a different formulation) to a lower dose of oral iron (100 mg twice daily) demonstrated some benefit in hemoglobin response in the IV group that could be attributable to the relatively low-dose oral iron used rather than true superiority of IV therapy. The lack of an adverse safety signal could be attributed to the shorter duration (52 weeks) or the different iron formulation used.

Practitioners should be mindful that in our guideline-driven exuberance to reduce erythropoiesis stimulating agent (ESA) use via increased utilization of IV iron,[3] we may have been doing our patients a disservice. A more reasonable approach would be to reserve IV iron use for those patients who, even after an extended trial of high-dose oral iron, did not demonstrate sufficient improvement in hemoglobin or in ESA resistance. Often these patients have a nonhematological cause for inadequate responses that should always be carefully investigated. Iron formulations that improve absorption and tolerance should be investigated as well.

**M. Klein, MD, JD**

*References*

1. Ganguli A, Kohli HS, Khullar M, et al. Lipid peroxidation products formation with various intravenous iron preparations in chronic kidney disease. *Ren Fail.* 2009;31:106-110.
2. Macdougall IC, Bock AH, Carrera F, et al. FIND-CKD: a randomized trial of intravenous ferric carboxymaltose versus oral iron in patients with chronic kidney disease and iron deficiency anaemia. *Nephrol Dial Transplant.* 2014;29:2075-2084.
3. KDIGO Clinical Practice Guidelines. Use of iron to treat anemia in CKD. *Kidney Int Suppl.* 2012;2:292-298.

## Risk Prediction for Early CKD in Type 2 Diabetes

Dunkler D, on behalf of the ONTARGET and ORIGIN Investigators (Hamilton Health Sciences/McMaster Univ, Ontario, Canada; et al)
*Clin J Am Soc Nephrol* 10:1371-1379, 2015

*Background and Objectives.*—Quantitative data for prediction of incidence and progression of early CKD are scarce in individuals with type 2 diabetes. Therefore, two risk prediction models were developed for incidence and progression of CKD after 5.5 years and the relative effect of predictors were ascertained.

*Design, Setting, Participants, & Measurements.*—Baseline and prospective follow-up data of two randomized clinical trials, ONgoing Telmisartan Alone and in combination with Ramipril Global Endpoint Trial (ONTARGET) and Outcome Reduction with Initial Glargine Intervention (ORIGIN), were used as development and independent validation cohorts, respectively. Individuals aged ≥55 years with type 2 diabetes and normo- or microalbuminuria at baseline were included. Incidence or progression of CKD after 5.5 years was defined as new micro- or macroalbuminuria, doubling of creatinine, or ESRD. The competing risk of death was considered as an additional outcome state in the multinomial logistic models.

*Results.*—Of the 6766 ONTARGET participants with diabetes, 1079 (15.9%) experienced incidence or progression of CKD, and 1032 (15.3%) died. The well calibrated, parsimonious laboratory prediction model incorporating only baseline albuminuria, eGFR, sex, and age exhibited an externally validated c-statistic of 0.68 and an $R^2$ value of 10.6%. Albuminuria, modeled to depict the difference between baseline urinary albumin/creatinine ratio and the threshold for micro- or macroalbuminuria, was mostly responsible for the predictive performance. Inclusion of clinical predictors, such as glucose control, diabetes duration, number of prescribed antihypertensive drugs, previous vascular events, or vascular comorbidities, increased the externally validated c-statistic and $R^2$ value only to 0.69 and 12.1%, respectively. Explained variation was largely driven by renal and not clinical predictors.

*Conclusions.*—Albuminuria and eGFR were the most important factors to predict onset and progression of early CKD in individuals with type 2 diabetes. However, their predictive ability is modest. Inclusion of demographic, clinical, and other laboratory predictors barely improved predictive performance.

▶ Can the onset of microalbuminuria be used to predict the incidence or progression of type early 2 diabetic renal disease? Diabetes is the most common cause of end-stage renal disease (ESRD),[1] and dialysis, in turn, dramatically affects quality of life and expense of care, with a cost of approximately $88 000 per patient per year of ESRD treatment.[1] Thus, our ability to calculate the predictive risk of the occurrence and progression of chronic kidney disease (CKD) would be clinically useful and relevant. Drawn from the well-described cohorts of the ONTARGET and ORIGIN studies, the investigators sought to develop risk prediction models within diabetics aged ≥55 years of older with either normo- or micro-albuminuria at onset. Following 5.5 years of follow-up (with the competing risk of death separated as an additional outcome), the incidence or progression of CKD, as defined by levels of proteinuria, a doubling of serum creatinine, or progression to ESRD, was determined.

Two prediction models were developed: a laboratory model based on standard markers of kidney function, together with sex and age; and a second clinical model that used the same markers together with additional clinical comorbidities, such as atherosclerotic cardiac and cerebrovascular events retinopathy, peripheral arterial disease, diabetes duration, low-density lipoprotein, glucose, waist circumference, and presence in type of antihypertensive therapy.

The investigators developed a risk calculator (available online from http://www.meduniwien.ac.at/nephrogene/index.php/data), which performs risk stratification of patients with diabetes for incidence and progression of early CKD, and mortality. Interestingly, the urine albumin to creatinine ratio and estimated glomerular filtration rate (eGFR) were the most important factors predicting the incidence and progression of CKD. The addition of a variety of demographic, clinical, and laboratory data did not substantially improve the predictive model. The authors demonstrated that the eGFR was the most important predictor of death, whereas the urine albumin to creatinine ratio had a much greater effect on CKD.

The populations studied were at an early stage of CKD (within 5.5 years, CKD or death occurred in 16% and 15% of participants, respectively). The advantage of early prediction and treatment are readily apparent, and within the groups studied, these models may allow early identification of those at greatest risk for the development of nephropathy. However, even this encouraging news comes with a caveat. Despite the inclusion of a wide assortment of clinical and laboratory variables including eGFR and albuminuria, our ability to actually predict the incidence and progression of diabetic disease is still limited. Even the most robust model had a relatively modest statistical score, suggesting that other factors that will help identify those at risk must exist and remain to be determined.

**R. Garrick, MD**

*Reference*

1. United States Renal Data System. *2015 USRDS Annual Data Report: Epidemiology of Kidney Disease in the United States*. Bethesda, MD: National Institutes of Health, National Institute of Diabetes and Digestive and Kidney Diseases; 2015.

## Serum Uric Acid and Risk of CKD in Type 2 Diabetes

De Cosmo S, the AMD-Annals Study Group (Scientific Institute "Casa Sollievo della Sofferenza," San Giovanni Rotondo (FG), Italy)
*Clin J Am Soc Nephrol* 10:1921-1929, 2015

*Background and Objective.*—Serum uric acid may predict the onset and progression of kidney disease, but it is unclear whether uric acid is an independent risk factor for diabetic nephropathy. Our aim was to study the relationship between uric acid levels and the development of CKD components in patients with type 2 diabetes.

*Design, Setting, Participants, & Measurements.*—Longitudinal study of a cohort of patients with type 2 diabetes from the database of the Italian Association of Clinical Diabetologists network. From a total of 62,830 patients attending the diabetes centers between January 1, 2004, and June 30, 2008, we considered those with baseline eGFR values ≥60 ml/min per 1.73 $m^2$ and normal albumin excretion ($n = 20,142$). Urinary albumin excretion, GFR, and serumuric acid were available in 13,964 patients. We assessed the association of serum uric acid quintiles with onset of CKD components by multinomial logistic regression model adjusting for potential confounders. We calculated the relative risk ratios (RRRs) for eGFR <60 ml/min per 1.73 $m^2$, albuminuria, and their combination at 4 years.

*Results.*—At 4-year follow-up, 1109 (7.9%) patients developed GFR <60 ml/min per 1.73 $m^2$ with normoalbuminuria, 1968 (14.1%) had albuminuria with eGFR ≥60 ml/min per 1.73 $m^2$, and 286 (2.0%) had albuminuria with eGFR <60 ml/min per 1.73 $m^2$. The incidence of eGFR, <60 ml/min per 1.73 $m^2$ increased in parallel with uric acid quintiles: Compared with the lowest quintile, RRRs were 1.46 (95% confidence interval [CI], 1.14 to 1.88; $P = 0.003$), 1.44 (95% CI, 1.11 to 1.87; $P = 0.006$), 1.95 (95% CI, 1.48 to 2.58; $P < 0.001$), and 2.61 (95% CI, 1.98 to 3.42; $P < 0.001$) for second, third, fourth, and fifth quintiles, respectively. Serum uric acid was significantly associated with albuminuria only in presence of eGFR <60 ml/min per 1.73 $m^2$.

*Conclusions.*—Mild hyperuricemia is strongly associated with the risk of CKD in patients with type 2 diabetes.

▶ This is a very interesting study. Hyperuricemia is extremely common in patients with chronic kidney disease (CKD) and in patients with CKD and diabetes. The data regarding whether alterations in uric acid can reliably predict the occurrence or progression of CKD remain inconclusive.[1-3] The current study enrolled almost 64 000 patients with well-defined type II diabetes who had a normal estimated glomerular filtration rate (eGFR; > 60 mL/min/1.73 $m^2$) and normal albumin excretion. Incident CKD and new-onset albuminuria were defined outcome parameters. Serum uric acid quintiles and onset of CKD were evaluated by means of detailed and extensive multinomial logistic regression modeling was controlled for numerous demographics and comorbidities. After 4 years of follow-up, about 8% of patients had an eGFR under 60 mL/min/1.73 $m^2$ and that change in GFR tracked in parallel with uric acid quintiles. Compared with the lowest quintile, the relative risk ratio for the second to fifth quintile of uric acid were each statistically significant and ranged from 1.46 to 2.58. Interestingly, this change in serum uric acid only tracked with albuminuria in the setting of a reduced GFR.

This well-conceived observational study demonstrates that uric acid is an independent predictor of incident CKD in type 2 diabetics. This finding is reminiscent of the post hoc subgroup analysis done within the Reduction of Endpoints in Non-Insulin-Dependent Diabetes Mellitus With Angiotensin II Antagonist Losartan (RENAAL) trial, which noted that unfavorable renal outcomes were reduced 6% for every 0.5 mg/dL fall in serum uric acid levels.

Observational data cannot unravel physiological mechanisms, and it should be noted that the population studied was fairly homogenous and the serum uric acid levels occurred along with features of the metabolic syndrome, such as high BMI and increased triglycerides and hypertension. Nonetheless, these findings, performed on a large, carefully defined population are clinically applicable and significant. Microalbuminuria, hypertension, dyslipidemia, and glucose control have all been used to evaluate renal risk. The current observations suggest that baseline serum uric acid levels and the predictive risk for the subsequent development of renal damage may be particularly strong in patients with new-onset CKD (defined as eGFR < 60 mL/min/1.73 $m^2$). Remarkably, increased uric acid levels were associated with almost a 2-fold increased risk of developing diabetic kidney disease. On the basis of these findings, studies investigating whether pharmacologic manipulation of the uric acid level can mitigate disease progression will likely be forthcoming.

**R. Garrick, MD**

*References*

1. Johnson RJ, Nakagawa T, Jalal D, et al. Uric acid and chronic kidney disease: which is chasing which? *Nephrol Dial Transplant*. 2013;28:2221-2228.
2. Zoppini G, Targher G, Chonchol M, et al. Serum uric acid levels and incident chronic kidney disease in patients with type 2 diabetes and preserved kidney function. *Diabetes Care*. 2012;35:99-104.
3. Viazzi F, Leoncini G, Ratto E, et al. Mild hyperuricemia and subclinical renal damage in untreated primary hypertension. *Am J Hypertens*. 2007;20:1276-1282.

---

**Electrocardiographic Measures and Prediction of Cardiovascular and Noncardiovascular Death in CKD**

Deo R, Shou H, Soliman EZ, et al (Perelman School of Medicine at the Univ of Pennsylvania, Philadelphia; Wake Forest Univ School of Medicine, Winston Salem, NC; et al)

*J Am Soc Nephrol* 27:559-569, 2016

---

Limited studies have assessed the resting 12-lead electrocardiogram (ECG) as a screening test in intermediate risk populations. We evaluated whether a panel of common ECG parameters are independent predictors of mortality risk in a prospective cohort of participants with CKD. The Chronic Renal Insufficiency Cohort (CRIC) study enrolled 3939 participants with eGFR <70 ml/min per 1.73 $m^2$ from June 2003 to September 2008. Over a median follow-up of 7.5 years, 750 participants died. After adjudicating the initial 497 deaths, we identified 256 cardiovascular and 241 noncardiovascular deaths. ECG metrics were independent risk markers for cardiovascular death (hazard ratio, 95% confidence interval): PR interval ≥200 ms (1.62, 1.19–2.19); QRS interval 100–119 ms (1.64, 1.20–2.25) and ≥120 ms (1.75, 1.17–2.62); corrected QT (QTc) interval ≥450 ms in men or ≥460 ms in women (1.72, 1.19–2.49); and heart rate 60–90 beats perminute (1.21, 0.89–1.63) and ≥90 beats per minute (2.35, 1.03–5.33). Most ECG measures were stronger markers of risk for cardiovascular death than for all-cause mortality or noncardiovascular death. Adding these intervals to a comprehensive model of cardiorenal risk factors increased the C-statistic for cardiovascular death from 0.77 to 0.81 ($P < 0.001$). Furthermore, adding ECG metrics to the model adjusted for standard risk factors resulted in a net reclassification of 12.1% (95% confidence interval 8.1%–16.0%). These data suggest common ECG metrics are independent risk factors for cardiovascular death and enhance the ability to predict death events in a population with CKD.

▶ Electrocardiograms (ECGs) are not generally used to predict cardiovascular risk, especially in populations at low risk for cardiac disease. Using a sample of almost 3600 patients from the well-defined Chronic Renal Insufficiency Cohort (CRIC) study, investigators carefully identified patients who succumbed to cardiovascular and noncardiovascular disease. Specific electrocardiographic metrics were then identified as independent risk markers for cardiovascular death. The results are quite interesting. Simple determinants (PR interval, the corrected QTC interval, QRS duration) were shown to be strong markers for increased risk of cardiovascular death. Moreover, the addition of these factors to existing cardio-renal risk models improved the sensitivity of the model and improved our ability to predict cardiovascular events in patient with CKD.

The annual mortality rate within the multicenter CRIC cohort is approximately 3%, which is higher than among a normal standardized population. Among this group, increased heart rate associated with all-cause mortality and both cardiovascular and noncardiovascular death. Other, specific ECG determinants also stood apart as independent markers for cardiovascular death.

As always, data may not be readily generalized. Studies in the end-stage renal disease (ESRD) population, including the 4-D trial that examined the effect of statins in dialysis patients, suggested that several common ECG determinants (QT interval, heart rate, QRS duration) were not predictors of clinical events.[1] Thus, compared with patients with CKD, conflicting biochemical, structural, or hemodynamic modifiers may affect the ECG in the ESRD group.

Notwithstanding that caveat, the CRIC cohort is the largest CKD population to undergo such systematic ECG analysis. The predictive ability of these findings should prove clinically useful. Ultimately, the simple and readily available ECG may add a new dimension to our ability to preemptively identify, intervene, and possibly mitigate cardiovascular death among patients with CKD.

**R. Garrick, MD**

*Reference*

1. Krane V, Heinrich F, Meesmann M, et al. German Diabetes and Dialysis Study Investigators. Electrocardiography and outcome in patients with diabetes mellitus on maintenance hemodialysis. *Clin J Am Soc Nephrol.* 2009;4:394-400.

**Smoking increases the risk of all-cause and cardiovascular mortality in patients with chronic kidney disease**

Nakamura K, for the EPOCH—JAPAN Research Group (Hokkaido Univ Graduate School of Medicine, Sapporo, Japan; et al)

*Kidney Int* 88:1144-1152, 2015

Little is known about the magnitude and nature of the combined effect of chronic kidney disease (CKD) and smoking on cardiovascular diseases. We studied this in a Japanese population using a pooled analysis of 15,468 men and 19,154 women aged 40–89 years enrolled in 8 cohort studies. The risk of mortality from all-causes and cardiovascular disease was compared in 6 gender-specific categories of baseline CKD status (non-CKD or CKD) and smoking habits (lifelong never smoked, former smokers, or currently smoking). CKD was defined as a decreased level of estimated glomerular filtration rate (under 60 ml/min per 1.73 $m^2$) and/or dipstick proteinuria. Hazard ratios were estimated for each category, relative to never smokers without CKD. During the follow-up period (mean 14.8 years), there were 6771 deaths, 1975 of which were due to cardiovascular diseases. In both men and women, current or former smokers with CKD had the first or second highest crude mortality rates from all-cause and cardiovascular diseases among the 6 categories. After adjustment for age and other major cardiovascular risk factors, the hazard ratios in male and female current smokers with CKD were 2.26 (95% confidence interval, 1.95–2.63) and 1.78 (1.36–2.32) for all-causes, and 2.66 (2.04–3.47) and 1.71 (1.10–2.67) for cardiovascular diseases, respectively. Thus, coexistence of CKD and smoking may markedly increase the risk of all-cause and cardiovascular mortality.

▶ Intuitively, we would likely predict that a combination of smoking and kidney disease would be particularly hazardous. The data from Nakamura and colleagues show us the extent of this risk. Their data are drawn from a population of 34 622 men and women with a mean age of 57.5 years. Chronic kidney disease (CKD), defined as an estimated glomerular filtration rate (eGFR) of $< 60$ mL/min/1.73 $m^2$ or dipstick proteinuria, had a prevalence of 7% in men and 5.5% in women. The vast majority of women (90.8%) never smoked, and 7.2% were current smokers; almost 54% of the male cohort were current smokers, and 25.2% were former smokers. There was a total follow-up of almost 512 000 person-years over a follow-up period of approximately 14.8 years.

When grouped according to CKD and smoking habits, the crude mortality rates for all-cause and cardiovascular disease for current male smokers were 44.9 and 16/1000 patient-years, respectively. The adjusted hazard ratios were 2.26 and 2.66, respectively. The all-cause mortality was 3.91 among male smokers with CKD and proteinuria. Women fared only slightly better with adjusted hazard ratios of 1.78 for all cause mortality and 1.71 for cardiovascular mortality among current smokers. Looking specifically at coronary heart disease, the hazard ratio among current male smokers with CKD was 3.29 which was substantially greater than that found among individuals without CKD (1.56).

There are some limitations to this study. For example, smoking habits were not systematically reevaluated, and it is possible that an individual's smoking pattern changed over time. A strength of the study is its size and the fact that, to some extent, they were able to stratify patients by their smoking status, which allowed them to conclude that CKD and smoking independently affect cardiovascular risk. Smokers have many reasons to quit. For smokers with renal disease, the need to quit is even more urgent, and these data should be part of our standard counseling recommendations.

**R. Garrick, MD**

**Glycated Hemoglobin Level and Mortality in a Nondiabetic Population with CKD**

Trivin C, Eric Thervet on behalf of the NephroTest Study Group (Hôpital Européen G Pompidou, Paris, France)

*Clin J Am Soc Nephrol* 10:957-964, 2015

*Background and Objectives.*—Glycated hemoglobin ($HbA_{1c}$) is used to diagnose diabetes mellitus (DM) and guide its management. The association between higher $HbA_{1c}$ and progression to ESRD and mortality has been demonstrated in populations with DM. This study examined the association between $HbA_{1c}$ and these end points in a population with CKD and without DM.

*Design, Setting, Participants, & Measurements.*—In the hospital-based Nephro Test cohort study, measured GFR (mGFR) was taken by $^{51}$Cr-EDTA renal clearance and $HbA_{1c}$ in 1165 adults with nondialysis CKD stages 1–5 and without DM between January 2000 and December 2010. The median follow-up was 3.48 years (interquartile range, 1.94–5.82) for the competing events of ESRD and pre-ESRD mortality. Time-fixed and time-dependent Cox models were used to estimate hazard ratios (HRs) for ESRD and mortality according to $HbA_{1c}$, treated continuously or in tertiles.

*Results.*—At inclusion, the mean mGFR was 42.2 ± 19.9 ml/min per 1.73 $m^2$, and the mean $HbA_{1c}$ value was 5.5% ± 0.5%. During follow-up, 109 patients died, and 162 patients reached ESRD. Pre-ESRD mortality was significantly associated with $HbA_{1c}$ treated continuously: for every 1% higher $HbA_{1c}$, the crude HR was 2.16 (95% confidence interval [95% CI], 1.27 to 3.68), and it was 1.85 (95% CI, 1.05 to 3.24) after adjustment for mGFR and other risk factors of death. After excluding incident diabetes over time, the updated mean of $HbA_{1c}$ remained significantly associated with higher mortality risk: adjusted HR for the highest (5.7%–6.4%) versus the lowest tertile (<5.3%) was 2.62 (95% CI, 1.16 to 5.91). There was no association with ESRD risk after adjustment for risk factors of CKD progression.

*Conclusions.*—In a CKD cohort, $HbA_{1c}$ values in the prediabetes range are associated with mortality. Such values should be therefore included among the risk factors for negative outcomes in CKD populations.

▶ This is a very interesting construct. The authors sought to evaluate whether hemoglobin $A_{1c}$ values below those typically associated with the diabetic threshold level of 6.5% influence the development of end-stage renal disease (ESRD), or mortality, in patients with chronic kidney disease (CKD). Elevated glycated hemoglobin has been linked to progression of renal disease and to an increased risk of mortality in CKD populations with diabetes.[1,2] After exclusion criteria were met the NephroTest Cohort Study evaluated the measured glomerular filtration rate (GFR) (by chromium EDTA) and hemoglobin A1 in (baseline 5.5% ± 0.5%), in 1102 nondiabetic adults with stage 1–5 CKD (stage 1 is a GFR >90 mL/min/1.73 $m^2$ with hematuria, proteinuria, family history polycystic kidney disease, or renal imaging abnormalities). Renal function was tracked over time (mean follow-up 3.48 years), and patients were censored to for either ESRD or pre- ESRD mortality.

At enrollment, all patients were carefully screened to exclude the possibility of underlying, undiagnosed diabetes. Both hemoglobin $A_{1c}$ and GFR were measured at the time of enrollment in 490 patients, and, at both enrollment and during at least 1 follow-up visit, in 675 others. The data were adjusted for demographic characteristics (age, sex, ethnicity) and for traditional risk factors for CKD progression, including CVD, the use of angiotensin-converting enzyme inhibitors or angiotensin receptor blockers, smoking, hypertension ($>140/90$), and hypoalbuminemia. After exclusion of patients who developed diabetes during the follow-up period, hemoglobin $A_{1c}$ levels were significantly associated with both overall mortality and pre-ESRD mortality. The crude hazard risk of death was 2.16, and after adjustment for measured GFR and non-CKD risk factors, it was 1.85. Overall, even after adjustment for other known risk factors and independent of the baseline fasting glucose, patients with CKD and a hemoglobin $A_{1c}$ value greater than 5.7% had a higher risk of death than patients with lower values. Hemoglobin $A_{1c}$ values were not predictive of renal survival after adjustment for the most common predictive risk factors for CKD progression.

The findings are intriguing. A strength of this study is the size of the population and the use of a measured (rather than calculated) GFR; a weakness of the study is the lack of serial lab determinations in a substantial portion of the study population. Other studies in nondiabetic patients have noted that an abnormal response to a glycemic load (a marker of prediabetes), rather than particular hemoglobin $A_{1c}$ value was predictive of an increased risk of mortality.[3] However, these are the first available data in nondiabetic CKD patients analyzing the predictive risk of hemoglobin $A_{1c}$ against the measured GFR. The observation that mortality is increased in nondiabetic CKD patients with a hemoglobin $A_{1c}$ of greater than 5.7% suggests this measurement might need to be added to the list of clinical risk factors that already encumber this population.

**R. Garrick, MD**

*References*


1. Selvin E, Ning Y, Steffes MW, et al. Glycated hemoglobin and the risk of kidney disease and retinopathy in adults with and without diabetes. *Diabetes.* 2011;60:298-305.
2. Selvin E, Steffes MW, Zhu H, et al. Glycated hemoglobin, diabetes, and cardiovascular risk in nondiabetic adults. *N Engl J Med.* 2010;362:800-811.
3. Chonchol M, Katz R, Fried LF, et al. Glycosylated hemoglobin and the risk of death and cardiovascular mortality in the elderly. *Nutr Metab Cardiovasc Dis.* 2010;20:15-21.

**Serum phosphate and social deprivation independently predict all-cause mortality in chronic kidney disease**

Solbu MD, Thomson PC, Macpherson S, et al (Univ of Glasgow, UK)

*BMC Nephrol* 16:194, 2015

*Background.*—Hyperphosphataemia is linked to cardiovascular disease and mortality in chronic kidney disease (CKD). Outcome in CKD is also affected by socioeconomic status. The objective of this study was to assess the associations between serum phosphate, multiple deprivation and outcome in CKD patients.

*Methods.*—All adult patients currently not on renal replacement therapy (RRT), with first time attendance to the renal outpatient clinics in the Glasgow area between July 2010 and June 2014, were included in this prospective study. Area socioeconomic status was assessed as quintiles of the Scottish Index of Multiple Deprivation (SIMD). Outcomes were all-cause and cardiovascular mortality and commencement of RRT.

*Results.*—The cohort included 2950 patients with a median (interquartile range) age 67.6 (53.6–76.9) years. Median (interquartile range) eGFR was 38.1 (26.3–63.5) ml/min/1.73 $m^2$, mean ($\pm$standard deviation) phosphate was 1.13 ($\pm$0.24) mmol/L and 31.6 % belonged to the most deprived quintile (SIMD quintile I). During follow-up 375 patients died and 98 commenced RRT. Phosphate $\geq$1.50 mmol/L was associated with all-cause (hazard ratio (HR) 2.51; 95 % confidence interval (CI) 1.63-3.89) and cardiovascular (HR 5.05; 95 % CI 1.90–13.46) mortality when compared to phosphate 0.90–1.09 mmol/L in multivariable analyses. SIMD quintile I was independently associated with all-cause mortality. Phosphate did not weaken the association between deprivation index and mortality, and there was no interaction between phosphate and SIMD quintiles. Neither phosphate nor SIMD predicted commencement of RRT.

*Conclusions.*—Multiple deprivation and serum phosphate were strong, independent predictors of all-cause mortality in CKD and showed no interaction. Phosphate also predicted cardiovascular mortality. The results suggest that phosphate lowering should be pursued regardless of socioeconomic status.

▶ Earlier studies in other populations of patients with chronic kidney disease (CKD) have demonstrated a link between mortality and serum phosphorus levels. Interestingly, a previous VA trial demonstrated that a serum phosphate >3.5 mg/dL was associated with an increased risk of mortality.[1] The current cohort trial from Scotland evaluated almost 3,000 patients with CKD (median age 67.7; estimated glomerular filtration rate [eGFR] 38.1 mL/min/1.73 $m^2$). Multivariate analysis demonstrated an association between a phosphate level $\geq$1.5 mmol/L (4.64 mg/dL) and an increased risk of all cause and cardiovascular mortality compared with a phosphorus level of 0 .92 to 1.09 mmol/L (2.27–3.37 mg/dL). The increased serum phosphorus was associated with an increase in both all-cause and cardiovascular mortality hazard ratios.

In addition to serum phosphate, the investigators tracked socioeconomic status through the Scottish Index of Multiple Deprivation. Independent of serum phosphate, a low socioeconomic status was associated with an increased risk of mortality among patients with CKD. The authors note that the cause of death was not always available (which limited the cardiovascular data analysis), and information on other confounders such as tobacco use, medication use, antihypertensive agents, among others, was not uniformly available. However, despite these limitations, the findings are quite interesting. The data suggest that both low socioeconomic status and serum phosphate levels independently and collectively contribute to an increased risk of mortality in patients with CKD. The finding suggests that step should be taken to address both of these risk factors independently of the other.

**R. Garrick, MD**

*Reference*

1. Kestenbaum B, Sampson JN, Rudser KD, et al. Serum phosphate levels and mortality risk among people with chronic kidney disease. *J Am Soc Nephrol.* 2005;16: 520-528.

**Retinopathy and the Risk of Cardiovascular Disease in Patients With Chronic Kidney Disease (from the Chronic Renal Insufficiency Cohort Study)**

Grunwald JE, the CRIC Study Investigators (Univ of Pennsylvania Philadelphia; et al)

*Am J Cardiol* 116:1527-1533, 2015

Patients with chronic kidney disease (CKD) experience other diseases such as cardiovascular disease (CVD) and retinopathy. The purpose of this study was to assess whether retinopathy predicts future CVD events in a subgroup of the participants of the Chronic Renal Insufficiency Cohort (CRIC) study. In this ancillary investigation, 2,605 participants of the CRIC study were invited to participate, and nonmydriatic fundus photographs were obtained in 1,936 subjects. Using standard protocols, presence and severity of retinopathy (diabetic, hypertensive, or other) and vessel diameter caliber were assessed at a central photograph reading center by trained graders masked to study participant's information. Patients with a self-reported history of cardiovascular disease were excluded. Incident CVD events were adjudicated using medical records. Kidney function measurements, traditional and nontraditional risk factors, for CVD were obtained. Presence and severity of retinopathy were associated with increased risk of development of any CVD in this population of CKD patients, and these associations persisted after adjustment for traditional risk factors for CVD. We also found a direct relation between increased venular diameter and risk of development of CVD; however, the relation was not statistically significant after adjustment for traditional risk factors. In conclusion, the presence of retinopathy was associated

**with future CVD events, suggesting that retinovascular pathology may be indicative of macrovascular disease even after adjustment for renal dysfunction and traditional CVD risk factors. Assessment of retinal morphology may be valuable in assessing risk of CVD in patients with CKD, both clinically and in research settings.**

▶ Prior cohort studies from Australia demonstrated that retinopathy remained an independent predictor of coronary heart disease and death both in the presence and absence of diabetes.[1] The current study involves an ancillary subgroup from the Chronic Renal Insufficiency Cohort Trial (CRIC) and is the first study to evaluate the association between underlying retinopathy (both hypertensive and diabetic) and the development of an assortment of cardiovascular diseases. The power of the study draws from the fact that the patients have both well-defined renal function and underwent carefully defined and validated evaluations for retinopathy. The findings are noteworthy. Among patients with kidney disease, there is an association between retinopathy and the later development of any type of cardiovascular disease. The findings remained intact after evaluation for multiple comorbidities and established cardiovascular risk factors. Similar to earlier studies, the findings suggest that in patients with chronic kidney disease (CKD), retinopathy can help to independently predict the development of diseases in other vascular beds—most noteworthy the cerebral vascular bed, where the hazard ratio for stroke in patients with proliferative retinopathy was 9.09% (95% confidence interval 2.18—37.8).[2] Additionally, patients with proliferative retinopathy were also at increased risk of myocardial infarction (hazard ratio 5.4).

The clinical implications of these data among patients with kidney disease are quite significant. The results are based on data from a cohort of well-defined patients, which included a large number of African Americans, with a longitudinal follow-up of over 5 years. A limitation of the data is that the baseline evidence of underlying cardiovascular disease (which was an exclusion criteria) was based on the patients' self-provided history. Even with this in mind, the findings suggest that we may be able to earmark subgroups of patients with CKD who appear to be destined to develop later cardiovascular diseases. This population of patients, in turn, may benefit from more intensive, planned, longitudinal cardiovascular follow-up.

**R. Garrick, MD**

*References*

1. Liew G, Wong TY, Mitchell P, Cheung N, Wang JJ. Retinopathy predicts coronary heart disease mortality. *Heart*. 2009;95:391-394.
2. David Spence JD, Fraser A. Retinal vasculature a window on the brain. *Hypertension*. 2013;62:678-679.

**CKD and Acute and Long-Term Outcome of Patients with Peripheral Artery Disease and Critical Limb Ischemia**

Lüders F, Bunzemeier H, Engelbertz C, et al (Univ Hosp Muenster, Germany; et al)

*Clin J Am Soc Nephrol* 11:216-222, 2016

*Background and Objectives.*—Despite the many studies showing an association between CKD and a high risk of ischemic events and mortality, the association of CKD with peripheral arterial disease (PAD) still has not been well described.

*Design, Setting, Participants, & Measurements.*—This large cohort study assessed the association of CKD, even in the earlier stages, with morbidity, short- and long-term outcome, and costs among patients with PAD.

*Results.*—We identified 41,882 patients with PAD who had an index hospitalization between January 1, 2009, and December 31, 2011. Of these, 8470 (20.2%) also had CKD (CKD stage 2: $n=2158$ [26%]; stage 3: $n=3941$ [47%]; stage 4: $n=935$ [11%]; stage 5: $n=1436$ [17%]). The ratio of women to men was 1:1.2. Compared with patients without known CKD, those with CKD had higher frequencies of coronary artery disease (1.8-fold higher; $P<0.001$), chronic heart failure (3.3-fold higher; $P<0.001$), and Rutherford PAD categories 5 and 6 (1.8-fold higher; $P<0.001$); underwent significantly fewer revascularizations (0.9-fold fewer; $P<0.001$); had a nearly two-fold higher amputation rate ($P<0.001$); had higher frequencies of in-hospital infections (2.1-fold higher; $P<0.001$), acute renal failure (2.8-fold higher; $P<0.001$), and sepsis (1.9-fold higher; $P<0.001$); had a 2.5-fold higher frequency of myocardial infarction ($P<0.001$); and had a nearly three-fold higher in-hospital mortality rate ($P<0.001$). In an adjusted multivariable Cox regression model, CKD remained a significant predictor of long-term outcome of patients with PAD during follow-up for up to 4 years (until December 31, 2012; median, 775 days; 25th–75th percentiles, 469–1120 days); the hazard ratio was 2.59 (95% confidence interval, 2.21 to 2.78; $P<0.001$). The projected mortality rates after 4 years were 27% in patients without known CKD and 46%, 52%, 72%, and 78% in those with CKD stages 2, 3, 4, and 5, respectively. Lengths of hospital stay and reimbursement costs were on average nearly 1.4-fold higher ($P<0.001$) in patients who also had CKD.

*Conclusions.*—This analysis illustrates the significant and important association of CKD with in-hospital and long-term mortality, morbidity, amputation rates, duration and costs of hospitalization, in-hospital treatment, and complications in patients with PAD.

▶ Prior studies have identified the comorbid risk of peripheral arterial disease (PAD) mortality in patients with chronic kidney disease (CKD).[1,2] The current study evaluated almost 42 000 patients with peripheral arterial disease and provides a comprehensive analysis of the progressive risk and outcome of PAD in patients with underlying kidney disease. The prevalence of CKD-PAD was high (20% of patients with PAD had CKD), and compared with those without known CKD, patients with CKD were found to have a nearly 2-fold higher prevalence of ischemic ulcerations or gangrene. Interestingly, revascularization rates were lower and amputation rates higher among the CKD/PAD patients than among those with PAD without CKD. Multiple other risk parameters such as in-hospital infections, acute renal failure, and myocardial infarction were also greater in the PAD-CKD population, as was the overall risk of in hospital mortality, which was increased threefold. Overall, after adjustment for comorbidities, during a 4-year follow-up of patients with PAD, CKD remained a strongly stratified independent predictor of mortality. This effect was noted even in patients with stage 2 CKD (estimated glomerular filtration rate 60-90 mL/min/1.73 $m^2$) Not surprisingly, associated indicators such as number and length of hospital stays and associated costs were also influenced by the presence of CKD.

One potential drawback of the studies was the use of coded billing data. However, the *International Classification of Diseases*, 10th Revision, system has been in use in Europe for more than 10 years, and verification data suggest that the hard outcomes chosen (amputation myocardial infarction, stroke, and death) are usually correctly coded. The data are important. They illuminate and quantify the deleterious association of PAD and CKD and demonstrate that even mild degrees of renal insufficiency can influence the mortality rate of patients with PAD. The other striking findings were the high rates of in-hospital mortality and the high rate of limb loss among patients with combined CKD and PAD. Taken together, these data teach us that clinicians should be wary of the combination of CKD and PAD, and wherever possible, aggressive therapeutic initiatives and lifestyle modifications (smoking cessation, exercise, diet), should be undertaken.

**R. Garrick, MD**

*References*

1. Garimella PS, Hart PD, O'Hare A, et al. Peripheral artery disease and CKD: a focus on peripheral artery disease as a critical component of CKD care. *Am J Kidney Dis.* 2012;60:641-654.
2. Liew YP, Bartholomew JR, Demirjian S, et al. Combined effect of chronic kidney disease and peripheral arterial disease on all-cause mortality in a high-risk population. *Clin J Am Soc Nephrol.* 2008;3:1084-1089.

## The Brain in Kidney Disease (BRINK) Cohort Study: Design and Baseline Cognitive Function

Murray AM, Bell EJ, Tupper DE, et al (Hennepin County Med Ctr, Minneapolis, MN; et al)

*Am J Kidney Dis* 67:593-600, 2016

*Background.*—The Brain in Kidney Disease (BRINK) Study aims to identify mechanisms that contribute to increased risk for cognitive impairment in patients with chronic kidney disease (CKD). We describe the rationale, design, and methods of the study and report baseline recruitment and cognitive function results.

*Study Design.*—Longitudinal observational cohort study of the epidemiology of cognitive impairment in CKD. The primary aim is to characterize the association between (1) baseline and incident stroke, white matter disease, estimated glomerular filtration rate (eGFR), inflammation, microalbuminuria, and dialysis initiation and (2) cognitive decline over 3 years in a CKD cohort with a mean eGFR < 45 mL/min/1.73 $m^2$.

*Setting & Participants.*—Community-dwelling participants 45 years or older recruited from 4 health systems into 2 groups: reduced eGFR, defined as eGFR < 60 mL/min/1.73 $m^2$ (non–dialysis dependent), and control, defined as eGFR ≥ 60 mL/min/1.73 $m^2$.

*Predictor.*—eGFR group.

*Outcomes.*—Performance on cognitive function tests and structural brain magnetic resonance imaging.

*Measurements.*—Sequential cognitive and physical function testing, serum and urine biomarker measurement, and brain magnetic resonance images over 3 years.

*Results.*—Of 554 participants, mean age was 69.3 years; 333, 88, and 133 had eGFRs < 45 (non–dialysis dependent, nontransplantation), 45 to <60, and ≥60 (controls) mL/min/1.73 $m^2$, respectively. Mean eGFR in reduced-eGFR participants was 34.3 mL/min/1.73 $m^2$. Baseline cognitive performance was significantly associated with eGFR in all domains except language. Participants with eGFRs < 30 mL/min/1.73 $m^2$ performed significantly worse than those with eGFRs ≥ 30 mL/min/1.73 $m^2$ on tests of memory, processing speed, and executive function. Participants with reduced eGFRs overall scored worst on the Immediate Brief Visual-Spatial Memory Test-Revised.

*Limitations.*—Healthy cohort bias, competing risk for death versus cognitive decline.

*Conclusions.*—Cognitive function was significantly worse in participants with eGFRs < 30 mL/min/1.73 $m^2$. Future BRINK analyses will measure risk factors for cognitive decline using the longitudinal data.

▶ The BRINK trial is a longitudinal observational cohort study that is designed to evaluate brain function in patients with chronic kidney disease (CKD). The fact that patients with kidney disease have cognitive dysfunction is well recognized,[1,2] but the mechanisms responsible for this impairment are not well understood. Our limited understanding of the timing and progression of cognitive dysfunction impairs our ability to tailor our diagnostic and therapeutic approach. Patients with CKD are confronted by a number of complex therapeutic choices, are expected to manage complex medication regimens, and typically have many specialists and subspecialists involved in their care. A more complete understanding of the array of cognitive challenges confronted by these patients should help us improve the diagnostic and therapeutic specificity of our care.

The participants in the BRINK trial include community-dwelling patients 45 years or older with an estimated glomerular filtration rate (eGFR) of <45 or 45 to <60 mL/min/1.73 $m^2$. All patients complete a baseline cognitive and physical function evaluation and are then followed longitudinally over time. The study aims to characterize the association between baseline and incident stroke, white matter disease, eGFR, inflammation, proteinuria, and initiation dialysis therapy and cognitive decline.

Between 2011 and 2015, 2177 people were assessed and 554 enrolled. Full demographic data are available on each patient, and as expected, prevalence of diabetes, hypertension, and stroke were higher among patients with reduced eGFR than among controls. Overall individuals with an eGFR <30 mL/min/1.73 $m^2$ scored worse on object recall, verbal memory, image reproduction, and executive function and therefore met the criteria for mild cognitive impairment. The early BRINK data demonstrate that while an eGFR of under 45 mL/min/1.73 $m^2$ is an effective initial point to begin to identify cognitive impairment, individuals with an eGFR of <30 mL/min are at a substantially greater risk for cognitive dysfunction. The unique longitudinal design of the BRINK trial will help teach us how to identify and track cognitive dysfunction in patients with CKD. This should help guide our use of extra visual and auditory teaching aides and other techniques such as read-back and teach-back, which can help patients with CKD and cognitive impairment better understand their care plans and regimens.

**R. Garrick, MD**

*References*

1. Kurella-Tamura M, Wadley V, Yaffe K, et al. Kidney function and cognitive impairment in US adults: the Reasons for Geographic and Racial Differences in Stroke (REGARDS) Study. *Am J Kidney Dis.* 2008;52:227-234.
2. Elias MF, Elias PK, Seliger SL, Narsipur SS, Dore GA, Robbins MA. Chronic kidney disease, creatinine and cognitive functioning. *Nephrol Dial Transplant.* 2009;24:2446-2452.

# 28 Hemodialysis

**Warfarin Use and Risk of Stroke in Patients with Atrial Fibrillation Undergoing Hemodialysis: A Meta-Analysis**

Lee M, Saver JL, Hong K-S, et al (Chang Gung Univ College of Medicine, Puzi, Taiwan; Univ of California, Los Angeles; Inje Univ, Goyang, South Korea; et al)

*Medicine* 95:e2741, 2016

In spite of the substantial burden of atrial fibrillation and associated elevated ischemic stroke risk in patients undergoing hemodialysis, the role of warfarin in these high-risk patients remains uncertain. Our objective was to clarify the association between warfarin use and risk of stroke for patients with atrial fibrillation undergoing dialysis.

PubMed and Embase from January 1966 to January 2015 were searched to identify relevant studies. Inclusion criteria were cohort studies, patients with atrial fibrillation undergoing hemodialysis, and reported quantitative estimates of the multivariate adjusted relative risk (RR) and 95% confidence interval (CI) for future stroke associated with warfarin use. We identified 8 studies, with a total of 9539 participants and 706 stroke events. Three studies reported total stroke as primary endpoint and other studies reported ischemic stroke as primary endpoint. Pooling the results showed that warfarin use was associated with higher risk of any stroke (RR 1.50, 95% CI: 1.13–1.99). By stroke type, warfarin was not significantly linked to risk of ischemic stroke (RR 1.01, 95% CI: 0.65–1.57, $P = 0.97$), but was related to greater hemorrhagic stroke risk (RR 2.30, 95% CI: 1.62–3.27). Warfarin heightened overall bleeding risk (RR 1.27, 95% CI: 1.03–1.56), but not death (RR 0.67, 95% CI: 0.37–1.21).

Among patients with atrial fibrillation undergoing hemodialysis, use of warfarin is associated with a higher risk of hemorrhagic stroke, but did not increase overall mortality.

► Dialysis patients are at significantly elevated risk for both ischemic and hemorrhagic stroke.[1] In addition, the increased incidence of atrial fibrillation (AF) in dialysis patients, with its attendant increased risk of ischemic stroke, confers substantial additional morbidity to these patients.[2] Although warfarin anticoagulation is effective in reducing the stroke risk in AF,[3] its use has not been well studied in dialysis patients because most studies have excluded them from entry. The risk of embolism is high, but there are substantial risks in warfarin use due to platelet dysfunction, heparin use, vascular fragility, and fluctuations in blood pressure during the dialysis treatment. Evidence-based guidance is sorely needed to help physicians make rational treatment choices in these patients.

Lee et al identified studies that included a total of 9539 dialysis patients with atrial fibrillation and 705 stroke events. Their meta-analysis found that the overall stroke incidence was 50% higher in the patients on warfarin but, not surprisingly, most of this increase was due to hemorrhagic stroke. The effect on ischemic stroke seemed to be neutral at best. Overall bleeding risk was increased as well, but overall mortality was not increased by the use of warfarin. Of course, this was as meta-analysis of mostly retrospective observational studies, so the data may have many confounders.

These data provide some guidance to the clinician trying to make a rational decision on using warfarin in a dialysis patient with AF. This limited investigation would suggest that the risk of hemorrhage and hemorrhagic stroke may overwhelm any possible benefit in ischemic stroke prevention. Obviously, a large randomized trial would be needed for conclusive proof.

**M. Klein, MD, JD**

*References*


1. Wang HH, Hung SY, Sung JM, Hung KY, Wang JD. Risk of stroke in longtermdialysis patients compared with the general population. *Am J Kidney Dis.* 2014;63:604-611.
2. Zimmerman D, Sood MM, Rigatto C, Holden RM, Hiremath S, Clase CM. Systematic review and meta-analysis of incidence, prevalence and outcomes of atrial fibrillation in patients on dialysis. *Nephrol Dial Transplant.* 2012;27:3816-3822.
3. Hart RG, Pearce LA, Aguilar MI. Meta-analysis: antithrombotic therapy to prevent stroke in patients who have nonvalvular atrial fibrillation. *Ann Intern Med.* 2007;146:857-867.


**Septic shock in chronic dialysis patients: clinical characteristics, antimicrobial therapy and mortality**

Clark E, The Cooperative Antimicrobial Therapy of Septic Shock Database Research Group (Univ of Ottawa, Ontario, Canada; et al)

*Intensive Care Med* 42:222-232, 2016

*Objectives.*—To describe the clinical characteristics and inhospital mortality of chronic dialysis-dependent end-stage kidney disease patients with septic shock in comparison to septic shock patients not receiving chronic dialysis.

*Methods.*—Using an international, multicenter database, we conducted a retrospective analysis of data collected from 10,414 patients admitted to the intensive care unit (ICU) with septic shock from 1989 to 2013, of which 800 (7.7 %) were chronic dialysis patients. Data on demographic characteristics, sites of infection, microbial pathogens, antimicrobial usage patterns, and in-hospital mortality were aggregated and compared for chronic dialysis and non-dialysis patients. Multivariate time-varying Cox models with and without propensity score matching were constructed to determine the association between dialysis and in-hospital death.

*Results.*—Septic shock secondary to central venous catheter infection, peritonitis, ischemic bowel, and cellulitis was more frequent in chronic dialysis patients. The isolation of resistant organisms (10.7 vs. 7.1 %; $p = 0.005$) and delays in receiving antimicrobials (6.0 vs. 5.0 h) were more common in chronic dialysis patients than in non-dialysis patients. Delayed appropriate antimicrobial therapy was associated with an increased risk of death in chronic dialysis patients ($p < 0.0001$). In-hospital death occurred in 54.8 and 49.0 % of chronic dialysis and non-dialysis patients, respectively. After propensity score matching, there was no difference in overall survival between chronic dialysis and non-dialysis patients, but survival in chronic dialysis patients decreased over time compared to non-dialysis patients.

*Conclusions.*—The demographic and clinical characteristics of chronic dialysis patients with septic shock differ from those of similar non-dialysis patients. However, there was no significant difference in mortality between the chronic dialysis and non-dialysis patients with septic shock enrolled in this analysis (Figs 1 and 2).

▶ Infection is the leading cause of hospitalization and mortality among dialysis patients, and their risk of death from sepsis is as much as 300-fold higher than the general population. Multiple factors (recurrent venous needling, catheter use, relative immunosuppression), contribute to this risk.[1-3]

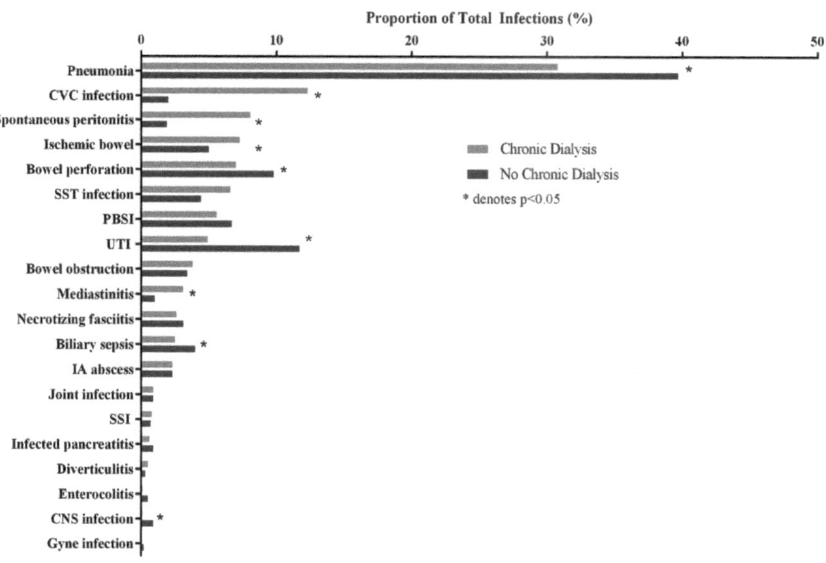


FIGURE 1.—Primary source of infection in chronic dialysis and non-dialysis patients with septic shock. *CVC* Central venous catheter, *SST* skin and soft tissue, *PBSI* primary blood stream infection, *UTI* urinary tract infection, *IA* intraabdominal, *SSI* surgical site infection, *CNS* central nervous system, *Gyne* gynecologic. (Reprinted from Clark E, The Cooperative Antimicrobial Therapy of Septic Shock Database Research Group. Septic shock in chronic dialysis patients: clinical characteristics, antimicrobial therapy and mortality. *Intensive Care Med.* 2016;42:222-232, with permission from Springer-Verlag Berlin Heidelberg and ESICM.)

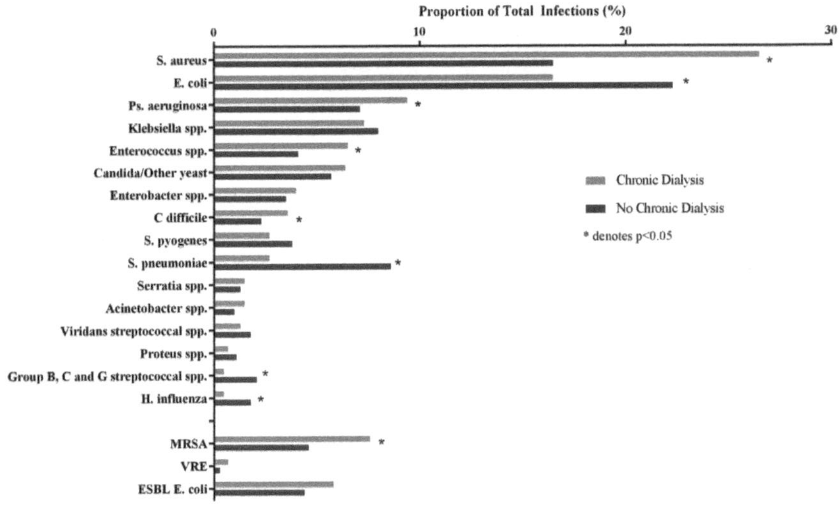


**FIGURE 2.**—Primary causative pathogens in chronic dialysis and non-dialysis patients with septic shock. *MRSA* Methicillin-resistant *Staphylococcus (S.) aureus*, *VRE* vancomycin-resistant enterococci, *ESBL E. coli* extended spectrum betalactamase *Escherichia coli, C. Clostridium, Ps. Pseudomonas, S. pyogenes, S. pneumoniae Streptococcus pyogenes, Streptococcus pneumoniae, H. Haemophilus.* (Reprinted from Clark E, The Cooperative Antimicrobial Therapy of Septic Shock Database Research Group. Septic shock in chronic dialysis patients: clinical characteristics, antimicrobial therapy and mortality. *Intensive Care Med.* 2016;42:222-232, with permission from Springer-Verlag Berlin Heidelberg and ESICM.)

The current international multicenter retrospective study improves our appreciation of the demographic and clinical characteristics of the patients at the greatest risk for sepsis and death.

Figs 1 and 2 define the underlying sites and organisms most associated with infection. Respiratory infections were the most common source of infection in both dialysis and nondialysis patients, whereas intravascular infections (especially linked to cardiovascular catheters), peritonitis, and ischemic bowel were more common in dialysis patients. *Staphylococcus aureus* (26.5%) was more common among dialysis patients, and *Escherichia coli* (22.3%) led the list in nondialysis patients. Chronic dialysis patients are more likely to be younger and to have multidrug resistant organisms such as methicillin-resistant S aureus, vancomycin-resistant *Enterococcus*, and extended-spectrum beta-lactamase. Although their white blood cell counts are usually higher, dialysis patients typically have a lower temperature, respiratory rate, and heart rate than nondialysis patients, but these changes were not associated with mortality risk.

After propensity score matching (for age, sex, comorbidities [cancer, immunocompromised state, congestive hear failure, coronary artery disease, elective or emergent surgery, chronic obstructive pulmonary disease, diabetes], and APACHE II score), there was no difference in the mortality rates in chronic dialysis compared with nondialysis patients. However, among the dialysis cohort, a delay in initiation of the appropriate antimicrobial was strongly associated with an increased mortality risk (adjusted odds ratio [OR] 1.07, 95% confidence interval 1.05–1.10 per hour delay; $P < .0001$)

This is the first, large international study to define the risks and demographic characteristic of sepsis and septic shock between dialysis and nondialysis patients. The data suggest that when treated promptly with appropriate antibiotics, the overall mortality risk between the groups is the same. Thus, the findings call into question the notion that the clinical outcomes will be worse in septic dialysis patients. Moreover, the findings support the development of specific diagnostic and therapeutic protocols so that septic dialysis patients can be quickly treated with the most appropriate antibiotic agents.

**V. Buddharaju, MD**

*References*

1. Sarnak MJ, Jaber BL. Mortality caused by sepsis in patients with end stage renal disease compared with the general population. *Kidney Int.* 2000;58:1758-1764.
2. Powe NR, Jaar B, Furth SL, Hermann J, Briggs W. Septicemia in dialysis patients: incidence, risk factors, and prognosis. *Kidney Int.* 1999;55:1081-1090.
3. Kumar ARD, Wood KE, Light RB, et al. Duration of hypotension prior to initiation of effective antimicrobial therapy is a critical determinant of survival in human septic shock. *Crit Care Med.* 2006;34:1589-1596.

---

**Dental Health and Mortality in People With End-Stage Kidney Disease Treated With Hemodialysis: A Multinational Cohort Study**

Palmer SC, on behalf of the ORAL-D Study Investigators (Univ of Otago, Christchurch, New Zealand; et al)
*Am J Kidney Dis* 66:666-676, 2015

---

*Background.*—Dental disease is more extensive in adults with chronic kidney disease, but whether dental health and behaviors are associated with survival in the setting of hemodialysis is unknown.

*Study Design.*—Prospective multinational cohort.

*Setting & Participants.*—4,205 adults treated with long-term hemodialysis, 2010 to 2012 (Oral Diseases in Hemodialysis [ORAL-D] Study).

*Predictors.*—Dental health as assessed by a standardized dental examination using World Health Organization guidelines and personal oral care, including edentulousness; decayed, missing, and filled teeth index; teeth brushing and flossing; and dental health consultation.

*Outcomes.*—All-cause and cardiovascular mortality at 12 months after dental assessment.

*Measurements.*—Multivariable-adjusted Cox proportional hazards regression models fitted with shared frailty to account for clustering of mortality risk within countries.

*Results.*—During a mean follow-up of 22.1 months, 942 deaths occurred, including 477 cardiovascular deaths. Edentulousness (adjusted HR, 1.29; 95% CI, 1.10-1.51) and decayed, missing, or filled teeth score ≥14 (adjusted HR, 1.70; 95% CI, 1.33-2.17) were associated with early all-cause mortality, while dental flossing, using mouthwash, brushing teeth daily, spending at least 2 minutes on oral hygiene daily, changing a toothbrush at least every 3 months, and visiting a dentist within the past

6 months (adjusted HRs of 0.52 [95% CI, 0.32-0.85], 0.79 [95% CI, 0.64-0.97], 0.76 [95% CI, 0.58-0.99], 0.84 [95% CI, 0.71-0.99], 0.79 [95% CI, 0.65-0.95], and 0.79 [95% CI, 0.65-0.96], respectively) were associated with better survival. Results for cardiovascular mortality were similar.

*Limitations.*—Convenience sample of clinics.

*Conclusions.*—In adults treated with hemodialysis, poorer dental health was associated with early death, whereas preventive dental health practices were associated with longer survival (Fig 3, Table 4).

▶ Nephrologists and other health care providers continue to seek ways to improve the health and longevity of patients with chronic kidney disease and renal failure requiring dialysis. Prior research has suggested that poor oral health and chronic inflammation related to periodontal disease can adversely affect the quality of life, nutritional status, and potentially the long-term outcome of

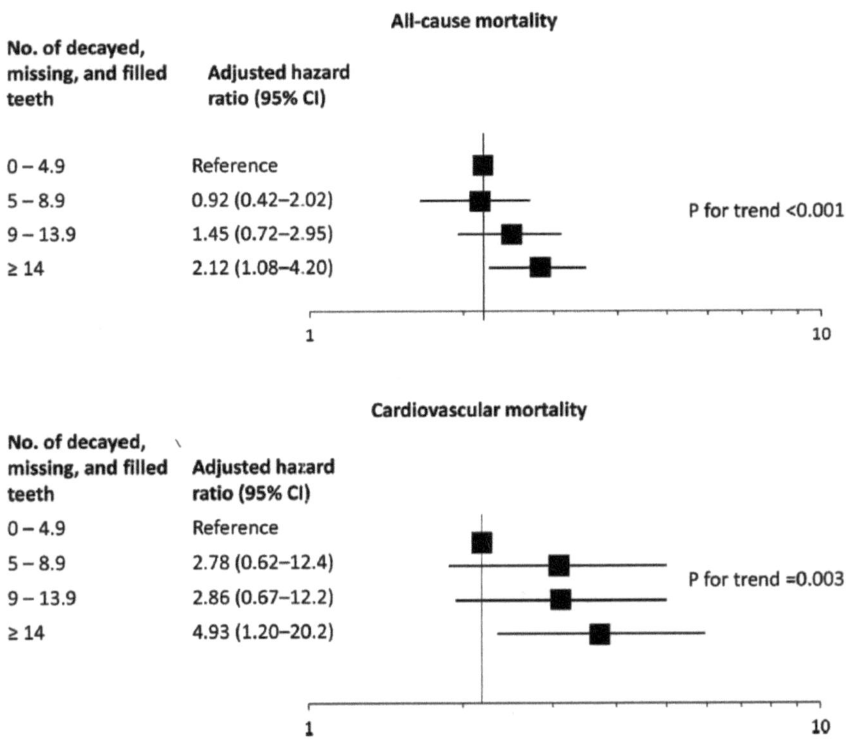


FIGURE 3.—Multivariable adjusted hazard ratios for cardiovascular mortality for World Health Organization categories of decayed, missing, and filled teeth index. The maximum number of decayed missing and filled teeth was 32, including the third molars. The decayed, missing, and filled teeth index is dichotomized according to World Health Organization criteria as very low to moderate, <14, and high, ≥14.[27] A larger number of affected teeth indicates more extensive dental disease. Abbreviation: CI, confidence interval. *Editor's Note*: Please refer to original journal article for full references. (Reprinted from Palmer SC, on behalf of the ORAL-D Study Investigators. Dental health and mortality in people with end-stage kidney disease treated with hemodialysis: a multinational cohort study. *Am J Kidney Dis.* 2015;66:666-676, with permission from The Authors.)

TABLE 4.—Dental Health, Oral Hygiene Habits, and Dental Care Practice Variables Associated With All-Cause and Cardiovascular Mortality in Adults With End-Stage Kidney Disease

| | Death From Any Cause | Death From Cardiovascular Event |
|---|---|---|
| Edentulousness | 1.29 (1.10-1.51) | 1.28 (1.02-1.60) |
| Decayed, missing, filled teeth index ≥ 14[a] | 1.70 (1.33-2.17) | 1.81 (1.26-2.59) |
| Use of dental floss | 0.52 (0.32-0.85) | 0.25 (0.09-0.68) |
| Use of mouthwash | 0.79 (0.64-0.97) | 0.60 (0.44-0.82) |
| Brushing teeth daily | 0.76 (0.58-0.99) | 0.74 (0.52-1.07) |
| Oral hygiene ≥ 2 min daily | 0.84 (0.71-0.99) | 0.72 (0.57-0.92) |
| Change toothbrush every 3 mo or less | 0.79 (0.65-0.95) | 0.73 (0.56-0.95) |
| Age of first dental visit < 30 y | 0.95 (0.79-1.15) | 1.00 (0.77-1.30) |
| Last dental visit within 6 mo | 0.79 (0.65-0.96) | 0.73 (0.55-0.97) |

*Note:* Values are given as adjusted hazard ratio (95% confidence interval). The analyses were stratified by country and adjusted for age, sex, race (European vs non-European), smoking history (ever smoker vs nonsmoker), income (above average vs below average), medical history (diabetes, myocardial infarction), dialysis vintage, and mean arterial blood pressure, serum phosphorus, and hemoglobin values. All participants with recorded data for all exposure variables (n = 4,054/4,205) were included in the survival analyses for edentulousness and the decayed, missing, and filled teeth index and all dentate participants with complete exposure data (n = 3,243/3,338) were included in survival analyses for oral hygiene and dental care practices.

*Editor's Note*: Please refer to original journal article for full references.

[a]The decayed, missing, and filled teeth index is dichotomized according to World Health Organization criteria as very low to moderate, <14, and high, ≥14.[27]

Reprinted from Palmer SC, on behalf of the ORAL-D Study Investigators. Dental health and mortality in people with end-stage kidney disease treated with hemodialysis: a multinational cohort study. *Am J Kidney Dis.* 2015;66:666-676, with permission from The Authors.

patients with advanced renal disease.[1,2] As the authors note, the Oral Disease in Hemodialysis (ORAL-D study) is the first cohort study to investigate how, and whether, oral disease and preventative dental practices affect the outcome of these patients independent of socioeconomic factors and preexisting underlying cardiovascular disease.[3] The authors evaluated the oral health of dialysis patients throughout Europe. Demographic, clinical, laboratory, and dialysis-related data were available. All participants received a standardized oral and periodontal examination and completed an extensive anonymous questionnaire regarding their self-reported dental hygiene practices. Specific and total all-cause mortality data were available from a centralized mandatory dialysis database data. The clinicians who determined the cause of death and related comorbidities were not aware of the patients' dental status or data. After exclusion for incomplete data or cognitive dysfunction, data were available from more than 4200 participants with a mean follow-up of 22 months.

It has been suggested that the periodontal inflammation associated with dental disease may adversely affect cardiovascular health.[4] Therefore, this outcome and its related comorbidities were separately evaluated, and careful statistical evaluation was performed to adjust for the heterogeneity in risks of survival observed across the various participating countries. In addition, multivariate adjusted models were used to control for a wide array of clinical and epidemiological factors, including age, sex, smoking history, presence of diabetes, dialysis vintage, hypertension, anemia, and serum phosphate levels.

Overall, about 20% of the patients were edentulous, two-thirds demonstrated extensive oral disease (14 or more decayed missing or filled teeth), about a third had seen a dentist within the previous 6 months, used use mouthwash, and changed their toothbrush at least every 3 months. About two-thirds spent 2 minutes or more a day on oral hygiene, and about 10% used dental floss. As shown in Fig 3, dental fitness had a clear relationship to all-cause and cardiovascular mortality. Table 4 demonstrates the association between oral hygiene habits and mortality.

Even with the limitations inherent in a longitudinal observational study, the data are significant and clinically immediately applicable. Poor oral health is associated with a worse outcome in this population that is already overly burdened with health risks. Moreover, "best practice" oral hygiene habits were associated with improved survival.

Of course, these types of observational data cannot prove causality, but if we think about the major clinical factors that have been undertaken to improve clinical outcomes in patients with advanced kidney disease (ie, improved diabetes control, blood pressure control, statin use, nocturnal dialysis, daily dialysis, ultrapure water treatment, to name a few), the potential impact of improved oral hygiene seems remarkably straightforward and eminently appealing. It seems likely that to have the greatest impact on overall health, these good oral habits should be started as early as possible. Thus, the Oral-D study suggests that what we all learned as children should now be shared with our patients: Brush your teeth and go to the dentist.

**V. Buddharaju, MD**

*References*

1. Ruospo M, Palmer SC, Craig JC, et al. Prevalence and severity of oral disease in adults with chronic kidney disease: a systematic review of observational studies. *Nephrol Dial Transplant.* 2014;29:364-375.
2. Grubbs V, Plantinga LC, Tuot DS, Powe NR. Chronic kidney disease and use of dental services in a United States public healthcare system: a retrospective cohort study. *BMC Nephrol.* 2012;13:16.
3. Strippoli GF, Palmer SC, Ruospo M, et al. Oral disease in adults treated with hemodialysis: prevalence, predictors, and association with mortality and adverse cardiovascular events: the rationale and design of the Oral Diseases in Hemodialysis (ORAL-D) study, a prospective, multinational, longitudinal, observational, cohort study. *BMC Nephrol.* 2013;14:90.
4. Beck JD, Slade G, Offenbacher S. Oral disease, cardiovascular disease and systemic inflammation. *Periodontol 2000.* 2000;23:110-120.

## Frailty and Cognitive Function in Incident Hemodialysis Patients

McAdams-DeMarco MA, Tan J, Salter ML, et al (Johns Hopkins Bloomberg School of Public Health, Baltimore, MD; et al)
*Clin J Am Soc Nephrol* 10:2181-2189, 2015

*Background and Objectives.*—Patients of all ages undergoing hemodialysis (HD) have a high prevalence of cognitive impairment and worse cognitive function than healthy controls, and those with dementia are at high risk of death. Frailty has been associated with poor cognitive function in older adults without kidney disease. We hypothesized that frailty might also be associated with poor cognitive function in adults of all ages undergoing HD.

*Design, Setting, Participants, & Measurements.*—At HD initiation, 324 adults enrolled (November 2008 to July 2012) in a longitudinal cohort study (Predictors of Arrhythmic and Cardiovascular Risk in ESRD) were classified into three groups (frail, intermediately frail, and nonfrail) based on the Fried frailty phenotype. Global cognitive function (3MS) and speed/attention (Trail Making Tests A and B [TMTA and TMTB, respectively]) were assessed at cohort entry and 1-year follow-up. Associations between frailty and cognitive function (at cohort entry and 1-year follow-up) were evaluated in adjusted (for sex, age, race, body mass index, education, depression and comorbidity at baseline) linear (3MS, TMTA) and Tobit (TMTB) regression models.

*Results.*—At cohort entry, the mean age was 54.8 years (SD 13.3), 56.5% were men, and 72.8% were black. The prevalence of frailty and intermediate frailty were 34.0% and 37.7%, respectively. The mean 3MS was 89.8 (SD 7.6), TMTA was 55.4 (SD 29), and TMTB was 161 (SD 83). Frailty was independently associated with lower cognitive function at cohort entry for all three measures (3MS: −2.4 points; 95% confidence interval [95% CI], −4.2 to −0.5; $P = 0.01$; TMTA: 12.1 seconds; 95% CI, 4.7 to 19.4; $P < 0.001$; and TMTB: 33.2 seconds; 95% CI, 9.9 to 56.4; $P = 0.01$; all tests for trend, $P < 0.001$) and with worse 3MS at 1-year follow-up (−2.8 points; 95% CI, −5.4 to −0.2; $P = 0.03$).

*Conclusions.*—In adult incident HD patients, frailty is associated with worse cognitive function, particularly global cognitive function (3MS).

▶ Cognitive impairment is common in all adults of all ages undergoing hemodialysis. A second demographic indicator is frailty, which has been defined as a measure of measure of physiologic reserve.[1] Frailty has been associated with an increased risk for hospitalization, falls, and increased mortality[1-3] and has recently been thought to be important risk factor in ESRD patients of all ages. Both frailty and cognitive dementia are associated with a higher risk of mortality. The authors suggest that frail adults initiating hemodialysis may have a greater likelihood of cognitive function, and that poor cognitive function may link frailty to adverse outcomes.

To test their hypothesis the authors utilized a longitudinal cohort study of 324 adults undergoing hemodialysis. Patients were classified into 3 groups based on the Fried frailty phenotype (frail, intermediate frail, and nonfrail). Global cognitive function and speed/attention were assessed at cohort entry and 1-year follow-up. Data were evaluated and adjusted for sex, age, race, body mass index, education, depression and comorbidity at baseline and follow-up. Comorbidities assessed included cardiovascular disease (coronary artery disease, MI, angina), congestive heart failure, rheumatoid arthritis (only by self-report), cancer (only by chart abstraction), diabetes, hypertension, or chronic obstructive pulmonary disease.

The prevalence of frailty and intermediate frailty were 34.0% and 37.7%, respectively, and frailty was independently associated with lower cognitive function at cohort entry for all 3 measures and with worsening global cognitive function at 1-year follow-up (22.8 points; 95% confidence interval, 25.4–20.2; $P = .03$).

The frailty risks among dialysis patients was 4 times that found in community-dwelling older adults, and the authors noted that frailty is a risk factor that is distinct from, but related to, cognitive impairments and comorbidity.

How do these findings help us? We have all seen frail patients, and although their phenotype causes us to consider, almost reflexively, the risks associated with frailty, cognitive limitations are not necessarily part of that immediate calculus. Recent data have demonstrated that marked changes in cerebral perfusion can occur during the hemodialysis treatment. Whether these changes are in any way linked to the alterations in global cognitive function that were present at baseline and worsened over follow-up will require further study. The researchers demonstrated that the influence of frailty on cognitive function persisted even after adjustment for a variety of key predictors of cognitive function including age, race, and education.

Their findings suggest that evaluation for both frailty and cognitive dysfunction should be part of an initial assessment in individuals with advanced kidney disease, and, where possible, steps should be taken to identify interventions that may help improve cognitive function among these frail patients. Such steps may both improve their quality of life and reduce mortality.

**R. Ledesma, MD**

*References*


1. Fried LP, Tangen CM, Walston J, et al. Cardiovascular Health Study Collaborative Research Group. Frailty in older adults: evidence for a phenotype. *J Gerontol A Biol Sci Med Sci.* 2001;6:M146-M156.
2. Robertson DA, Savva GM, Kenny RA. Frailty and cognitive impairment—a review of the evidence and causal mechanisms. *Ageing Res Rev.* 2013;12:840-851.
3. McAdams-DeMarco MA, Law A, Salter ML, et al. Frailty as a novel predictor of mortality and hospitalization in individuals of all ages undergoing hemodialysis. *J Am Geriatr Soc.* 2013;61:896-901.

**PART FOUR**

# PULMONARY DISEASE

JANET R. MAURER, MD, MBA

# Introduction

The Pulmonary Disease section of the 2016 YEAR BOOK of Medicine includes abstract selections concerning asthma, cystic fibrosis, chronic obstructive disease, lung cancer, pleural disease, interstitial disease, community-acquired pneumonia and lung transplantation. In addition, several abstracts are included from the areas of sleep and critical care medicine. While a variety of topics are addressed in these different areas, there are some recurrent themes to point out. First, there is an ongoing interest in epidemiology of disease. This data typically comes from large cross-sectional studies or may be derived as secondary data from clinical trials. Second, there is continued interest in the long-term outcomes of diseases. Large registries now collect data on almost all common diseases and many less common diseases. There are several studies in this section that inform us about the natural history of disease—community-acquired pneumonia, pulmonary arterial hypertension, pulmonary embolism, lung cancer screening results. These data can help us better design appropriate follow-up for these diseases. Third, there are important new therapies and refinements of older treatments that provide better quality of life and sometimes longer life or even potential cures for some pulmonary diseases. Patients with cystic fibrosis, idiopathic pulmonary fibrosis, chronic obstructive lung disease, lung cancer and acute respiratory distress syndrome have been among the beneficiaries of these treatment advances.

**Janet R. Maurer, MD, MBA**

# 29 Asthma, Allergy, and Cystic Fibrosis

**Evolving Concepts of Asthma**

Gauthier M, Ray A, Wenzel SE (Univ of Pittsburgh, PA)

*Am J Respir Crit Care Med* 192:660-668, 2015

Our understanding of asthma has evolved over time from a singular disease to a complex of various phenotypes, with varied natural histories, physiologies, and responses to treatment. Early therapies treated most patients with asthma similarly, with bronchodilators and corticosteroids, but these therapies had varying degrees of success. Similarly, despite initial studies that identified an underlying type 2 inflammation in the airways of patients with asthma, biologic therapies targeted toward these type 2 pathways were unsuccessful in all patients. These observations led to increased interest in phenotyping asthma. Clinical approaches, both biased and later unbiased/statistical approaches to large asthma patient cohorts, identified a variety of patient characteristics, but they also consistently identified the importance of age of onset of disease and the presence of eosinophils in determining clinically relevant phenotypes. These paralleled molecular approaches to phenotyping that developed an understanding that not all patients share a type 2 inflammatory pattern. Using biomarkers to select patients with type 2 inflammation, repeated trials of biologics directed toward type 2 cytokine pathways saw newfound success, confirming the importance of phenotyping in asthma. Further research is needed to clarify additional clinical and molecular phenotypes, validate predictive biomarkers, and identify new areas for possible interventions.

▶ This outstanding review from the ATS Discovery Series details the history (Fig 1 in the original article) of consecutive important discoveries in asthma beginning in the late 17th century. This figure takes us all the way through to the present and the sophisticated immunotherapies in use today. In the fast-paced world of sophisticated pharmacotherapies discovery, what was lost on the majority of providers not engaged in research was the innate variability of asthmatics and phenotypes they represented. The fact that one type of therapy does not fit all was learned through trial and error, but the ability to judge this pretherapy trial was missing. Science and research has led us to a better understanding of the cellularity of inflammation and cytokines involved in variable forms of asthma. Table 1 in the original article details the currently available immunotherapies and the biomarkers utilized to monitor efficacy. Fig 2 in the original article differentiates known asthmatic phenotypes (eg, Type 2 High and Type 2 Low asthma, Type I high) based on cellularity-prominent inflammation, and ties in such factors as ages of development of asthma (young vs older), corticosteroid responsiveness vs less or nonresponsive, and so on. Although this figure and the accompanying text can guide the reader through this sophisticated yet easy to understand synopsis, it is clear that abundant opportunities for research exist. The summary of this "discovery" piece is that one day we'll be able to design patient-specific, targeted therapies based on the patient's asthma phenotype, rather than the current trial-and-error method that the majority of us use in clinical practice.

**S. K. Willsie, DO, MA**

---

**Therapeutic approaches to asthma–chronic obstructive pulmonary disease overlap syndromes**

Barnes PJ (Natl Heart and Lung Inst, London, United Kingdom)

*J Allergy Clin Immunol* 136:531-545, 2015

---

The recognition that there are some patients with features of asthma and chronic obstructive pulmonary disease (COPD) has highlighted the need to develop more specific treatments for these clinical phenotypes. Some patients with COPD have predominantly eosinophilic inflammation and might respond to high doses of inhaled corticosteroids and newly developed specific antieosinophil therapies, including blocking antibodies against IL-5, IL-13, IL-33, and thymic stromal lymphopoietin, as well as oral chemoattractant receptor-homologous molecule expressed on $T_H2$ cells antagonists. Other patients have severe asthma or are asthmatic patients who smoke with features of COPD-induced inflammation and might benefit from treatments targeting neutrophils, including macrolides, CXCR2 antagonists, phosphodiesterase 4 inhibitors, p38 mitogen-activating protein kinase inhibitors, and antibodies against IL-1 and IL-17. Other patients appear to have largely fixed obstruction with little inflammation and might respond to long-acting bronchodilators, including long-acting muscarinic antagonists, to reduce hyperinflation. Highly selected patients with severe asthma might benefit from bronchial thermoplasty. Some patients with overlap syndromes can be conveniently treated with triple fixed-dose combination inhaler therapy with an inhaled corticosteroid, long-acting $\beta_2$-agonist, and long-acting muscarinic antagonist, several of which are now in development. Corticosteroid resistance is a feature of asthma-COPD overlap syndrome, and understanding the various molecular mechanisms of this resistance has identified novel therapeutic targets and presented the prospect of therapies that can restore corticosteroid responsiveness (Fig 1, Table 1).

▶ This publication, penned by Peter J. Barnes, agrees that the asthma–chronic obstructive pulmonary disease (COPD) overlap syndrome (ACOS) consists of

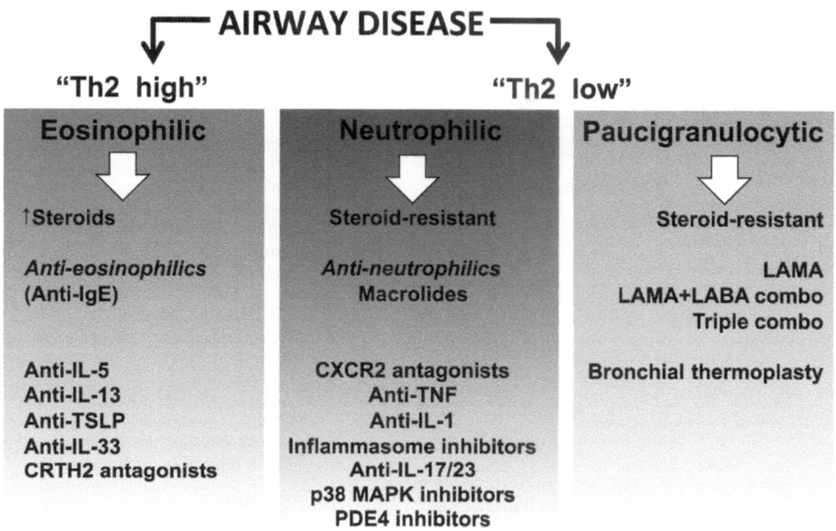


**FIGURE 1.**—Airway diseases can show different patterns of inflammation in sputum and can be classified as "$T_H2$ high" or "$T_H2$ low." $T_H2$-high disease is associated with eosinophilic inflammation and usually indicates steroid responsiveness. If there is a poor response to steroids, there might be an indication for antieosinophilic therapies, including mAbs to block IgE, IL-5, IL-13, TSLP, and IL-33 or oral CRTH2 (DP2) antagonists. $T_H2$-low or non-$T_H2$ disease can be neutrophilic and targeted by macrolides; CXCR2 antagonists; antibodies to block IL-1, TNF, IL-17, or IL-23; inflammasome inhibitors; p38 MAPK; or PDE4 inhibitors. Paucigranulocytic disease results in no increase in inflammatory cell counts and might respond to long-acting bronchodilators, which reduce hyperinflation, including LABAs, LAMAs, or their combination or triple combination with an ICS. Selected asthmatic patients might respond to bronchial thermoplasty. (Reprinted from Barnes PJ. Therapeutic approaches to asthma–chronic obstructive pulmonary disease overlap syndromes. *J Allergy Clin Immunol.* 2015;136:531-545, with permission from American Academy of Allergy, Asthma & Immunology.)

features of both asthma and COPD,[1,2] specifically different phenotypes that require specific therapeutic approaches. Barnes suggests that the phenotypes be divided into 3 major types based on sputum cellularity. These 3 phenotypes are delineated in Fig 1 and Table 1 and include (1) COPD patients who have increased sputum eosinophil counts that may respond to corticosteroids or specific anti-eosinophil therapy ("Th2 high"), (2) severe asthmatics who are current smokers who have predominantly neutrophilic inflammation in their sputum ("Th2 low"), and (3) asthmatic patients who have largely irreversible airflow obstruction and might or might not have increased inflammation: these are divided into eosinophil-predominant, neutrophil-predominant, mixed pattern, and no inflammation (paucigranulocytic; "Th2 low").[3] Existing therapies are listed in Fig 1, and new therapies in development are listed by type of cellular inflammation in Table 1. Th2 high or Eosinophilic ACOS is currently treated by inhaled corticosteroids, and anti-immunoglobulin E, in severe or unresponsive cases. New therapies in development include the anti-interleukin (IL)-5, anti-IL-13, anti-TSLP, anti-IL-33 and CRTH2 antagonists. The Th2 low or neutrophilic ACOS/steroid-resistant phenotype is currently treated with macrolides; in addition, future therapies being explored include

TABLE 1.—Targeting Different Inflammatory Phenotypes of ACOS

| Inflammatory Phenotype | Current Therapies | New Therapies in Development |
|---|---|---|
| Eosinophilic | ICSs | Anti–IL-5/IL-5Rα (mepolizumab, reslizumab, benralizumab) |
| | Anti-IgE (omalizumab) | Anti–IL-13/IL-4Rα (lebrikizumab, tralokinumab, dupilumab) |
| | | GATA3 inhibitors (SB010) |
| | | Anti–IL-33/ST2 |
| | | Anti–IL-25 |
| | | Anti-TSLP |
| | | CRTH2 antagonists |
| Neutrophilic | Macrolides | Anti–IL-1, inflammasome inhibitors |
| | | Anti–IL-17/IL-17Rα (ixekizumab, brodalumab) |
| | | Anti–IL-23, anti-p40 (guselkumab) |
| | | CXCR2 antagonists |
| | | p38 MAPK inhibitors/JAK inhibitors |
| | | PDE4 inhibitors (roflumilast) |
| Paucigranulocytic | LAMA (tiotropium) | |
| | LAMA + LABA (indacaterol/ glycopyrronium, vilanterol/ umeclidinium) | Triple inhalers (corticosteroid/LABA/ LAMA) |
| | Bronchial thermoplasty | |

IL-4Ra, IL-4 receptor a; IL-5Ra, IL-5 receptor a; IL-17Ra, IL-17 receptor a.
Reprinted from Barnes PJ. Therapeutic approaches to asthma–chronic obstructive pulmonary disease overlap syndromes. *J Allergy Clin Immunol.* 2015;136:531-545, with permission from American Academy of Allergy, Asthma & Immunology.

anti-TNF, anti-IL-1, inflammasone inhibitors, anti-IL-17/23, p38 MAPK inhibitors, and PDE4 inhibitors. The Th2 low, paucigranulocytic phenotype (also considered granulocyte resistant), is currently treated with long-acting muscarinic antagonists (LAMA), LAMA-long acting beta agonist (LABA) combination, or triple combination (LAMA + LABA + ICS). Future therapies include potentially bronchial thermoplasty. This is a fascinating "must read" for those who may be frustrated with how to treat the patient with ACOS. Barnes's easy-to-understand phenotypes greatly assist in the therapeutic possibilities currently available.

**S. K. Willsie, DO, MA**

## *References*

1. Gibson PG, Simpson JL. The overlap syndrome of asthma and COPD: what are its features and how important is it? *Thorax.* 2009;64:728-735.
2. Barrecheguren M, Esquinas C, Miravitlles M. The asthma-chronic obstructive pulmonary disease overlap syndrome (ACOS): opportunities and challenges. *Curr Opin Pulm Med.* 2015;21:74-79.
3. Simpson JL, Scott R, Boyle MJ, Gibson PG. Inflammatory subtypes in asthma: assessment and identification using induced sputum. *Respirology.* 2006;11: 54-61.

**Anticholinergic vs Long-Acting β-Agonist in Combination With Inhaled Corticosteroids in Black Adults With Asthma: The BELT Randomized Clinical Trial**

Wechsler ME, for the BELT Investigators (Brigham and Women's Hosp, Boston, MA; et al)

*JAMA* 314:1720-1730, 2015

*Importance.*—The efficacy and safety of long-acting β-agonists (LABAs) have been questioned. Black populations may be disproportionately affected by LABA risks.

*Objective.*—To compare the effectiveness and safety of tiotropium vs LABAs, when used with inhaled corticosteroids (ICS) in black adults with asthma and to determine whether allelic variation at the Arg16Gly locus of the $\beta_2$-adrenergic receptor (*ADRB2*) gene is associated with treatment response.

*Design, Setting, and Participants.*—A multisite (n = 20), open-label, parallel-group, pragmatic randomized clinical trial conducted from March 2011 through July 2013, enrolling black adults with moderate to severe asthma in the United States.

*Interventions.*—Patients eligible for, or receiving, step 3 or step 4 combination therapy per National Heart, Lung, and Blood Institute guidelines, received ICS plus either once-daily tiotropium (n = 532) or twice-daily LABAs (n = 538,) and were followed up for up to 18 months. Patients underwent genotyping, attended study visits at baseline, 1, 6, 12, and 18 months, and completed monthly questionnaires.

*Main Outcomes and Measures.*—The primary outcome was time to asthma exacerbation, defined as a worsening asthma event requiring oral or parenteral corticosteroids. Secondary outcomes included patient-reported outcomes (Asthma Quality of Life Questionnaire, Asthma Control Questionnaire [ACQ], Asthma Symptom Utility Index, and Asthma Symptom-Free Days questionnaire), spirometry ($FEV_1$), rescue medication use, asthma deteriorations, and adverse events.

*Results.*—There was no difference between LABA + ICS vs tiotropium + ICS in time to first exacerbation (mean No. of exacerbations/person-year, 0.42 vs 0.37 (rate ratio, 0.90 [95% CI, 0.73 to 1.11], log-rank $P = .31$). There was no difference in change in $FEV_1$ at 12 months (0.003 L for LABA + ICS vs −0.018 L for tiotropium + ICS; between-group difference, 0.020 [95% CI, −0.021 to 0.061], $P = .33$) and at 18 months (−0.053 L vs −0.078 L; between-group difference, 0.025 [95% CI, −0.045 to 0.095], $P = .49$). There were no differences in ACQ score at 18 months (change in score from baseline, −0.68 for LABA + ICS vs −0.72 for tiotropium + ICS; between-group difference, 0.04 [95% CI, −0.18 to 0.27], $P = .70$). There were no differences in other patient-reported outcomes. Arg16Gly *ADRB2* alleles were not associated with differences in the effects of tiotropium + ICS vs LABA + ICS (hazard ratio for time to first exacerbation, 0.84 [95% CI, 0.47 to 1.51] for Arg/Arg vs 0.85 [95% CI, 0.63 to 1.15] for Arg/Gly or Gly/Gly, $P = .97$).

*Conclusions/Relevance.*—Among black adults with asthma treated with ICS, adding a LABA did not improve time to asthma exacerbation compared with adding tiotropium. These findings were not affected by polymorphisms at the Arg16Gly locus of *ADRB2*. These findings do not support the superiority of LABA + ICS compared with tiotropium + ICS for black patients with asthma.

*Trial Registration.*—ClinicalTrials.gov identifier: NCT01290874

▶ Previous studies[1-4] have suggested that African Americans may be disproportionately and adversely affected by long-acting beta-agonists (LABA), particularly when administered without inhaled corticosteroids (ICS). This study aimed to evaluate the efficacy and safety in black subjects of long-acting ICS twice daily (bid) + either LABA bid or once daily anticholinergic therapy in the form of 2.5 or 5 µg of inhaled tiotropium (T) in black adults with asthma. In addition, determination was made as to whether the Arg16Gly locus of the adrenergic receptor (*ADRB2*) gene was associated with treatment response. This practice-based effectiveness, prospective, open-label trial enrolled subjects from 20 sites, and > 1000 subjects participated for up to 18 months with 10 963 patient-months of follow-up. Fig 3 in the original article demonstrates outcomes between the treatment groups over time. No superiority was seen between the ICS + LABA vs ICS + T. No difference in response was noted between treatments due to the *ADRB2* Arg16Gly polymorphism. High rates of exacerbations were seen in all treatment groups and the study was underpowered to evaluate for differences in hospitalization or death. Despite the nonadherence to both treatment regimens, this study provides a basis for further study, including longer term, additional therapeutic interventions, and larger subject numbers to evaluate for safety and efficacy.

**S. K. Willsie, DO, MA**

*References*


1. Drazen JM, O'Byrne PM. Risks of long-acting β-agonists in achieving asthma control. *N Engl J Med.* 2009;360:1671-1672.
2. Peters J. ACP Journal Club: β-agonists increase asthma-related intubations and deaths in patients with asthma. *Ann Intern Med.* 2010;153:JC3-JC5.
3. Nelson HS, Weiss ST, Bleecker ER, Yancey SW, Dorinsky PM, SMART Study Group. The Salmeterol Multicenter Asthma Research Trial: a comparison of usual pharmacotherapy for asthma or usual pharmacotherapy plus salmeterol. *Chest.* 2006;129:15-26.
4. Bailey W, Castro M, Matz J, et al. Asthma exacerbations in African Americans treated for 1 year with combination fluticasone propionate and salmeterol or fluticasone propionate alone. *Curr Med Res Opin.* 2008;24:1669-1682.


## New and Emerging Treatments for Cystic Fibrosis

Barry PJ, Jones AM (Univ Hosp South Manchester NHS Trust, United Kingdom)

*Drugs* 75:1165-1175, 2015

Recently, a significant number of additional key medications have become licensed in Europe for the treatment of patients with cystic fibrosis

(CF), including a number of inhaled antibiotics, such as nebulised aztreonam and dry powder versions of colistin and tobramycin for inhalation; dry powder inhaled mannitol, an agent to improve airway hydration and aid airway clearance; and ivacaftor, an oral therapy that directly acts on dysfunctional CFTR to correct the basic defect encountered in CF patients with the *G551D* CF gene mutation. The marked success of ivacaftor both in clinical trials and in postlicensing evaluation studies in treating patients with G551D and other gating mutations has greatly encouraged the ongoing development of similar therapies that can directly

**TABLE 1.**—New Therapeutic Agents Under Investigation for the Treatment of Cystic Fibrosis

| Therapy | Mechanism of Action | Phase of Development |
|---|---|---|
| Therapies targeted at the basic defect | | |
| Gene therapy | Restore wild-type CFTR into airway cells | Phase II trial completed |
| PTC 124 | Makes ribosomes less sensitive to premature stop codons in mRNA | Phase III trial completed; further trial in development |
| Ivacaftor | CFTR potentiator | Available to patients |
| Lumacaftor | CFTR corrector | Phase III trials completed |
| VX-661 | CFTR corrector | Phase III trials enrolling |
| Anti-infectives | | |
| Aztreonam lysine | Nebulised anti-pseudomonas agent | Available to patients |
| Liposomal amikacin | Nebulised anti-pseudomonas agent | Phase II trials completed |
| Fosfomycin/ tobramycin | Nebulised anti-pseudomonal agent | Phase II trials completed |
| Aerosolised levofloxacin | Nebulised anti-pseudomonal agent | Phase III trial completed |
| Dry-powder ciprofloxacin | Inhaled anti-pseudomonal agent | Phase I trial completed |
| KB001 | Recombinant mAb against pseudomonas | Phase I study completed |
| Dry powder vancomycin | Inhaled anti-MRSA agent | Phase II trial completed |
| OligoG | Disrupts bacterial biofilms | Phase IIa study completed |
| Anti-inflammatory therapies | | |
| Sildenafil | Phosphodiesterase inhibitor | Phase IIa trial completed |
| Inhaled glutathione | Restore depleted anti-oxidant levels | Two recent trials completed; both failed to achieve primary outcome |
| N6022 | Intravenous inhibitor of *s*-nitrogluthathione reductase | Phase I trial completed |
| N91115 | Oral inhibitor of *s*-nitrogluthathione reductase | Human studies planned |
| CTX-4430 | Leukotriene A4 inhibitor | Phase I trial completed |
| Agents to improve mucociliary clearance | | |
| Dry-powder mannitol | Inhaled osmotic agent | Available to patients |
| Pancreatic enzymes | | |
| Liprotamase | Pancreatic enzyme replacement | One phase III trial completed and further planned |
| Burlulipase | Pancreatic enzyme replacement | Phase II study completed |

mRNA, messenger RNA; MRSA, methicillin-resistant Staphylococcus aureus.

Reprinted from Barry PJ, Jones AM. New and emerging treatments for cystic fibrosis. *Drugs*. 2015;75:1165-1175, with permission from Springer International Publishing Switzerland.

target the underlying cause of CF. Other therapies, including a number of anti-infectives, anti-inflammatories and replacement pancreatic enzymes, are currently undergoing clinical studies. This article reviews those treatments that have been recently licensed for CF and highlights some of the exciting emerging therapies presently under evaluation in clinical trials. In addition, it discusses some of the potential challenges being encountered by research and clinical teams in developing and delivering treatments for this condition (Table 1).

▶ This excellent review article is worthy of a read so that physicians and other health care providers can retain an awareness of new therapeutics in the pipeline for cystic fibrosis. Table 1 is helpful because it details drugs currently under study, lists in which phase of study they are currently or have completed, and highlights the mechanisms of action for the various drugs.

**S. K. Willsie, DO, MA**

---

**Lumacaftor–Ivacaftor in Patients with Cystic Fibrosis Homozygous for Phe508del *CFTR***

Wainwright CE, for the TRAFFIC and TRANSPORT Study Groups (Univ of Queensland School of Medicine, Brisbane, Australia; et al)

*N Engl J Med* 373:220-231, 2015

---

*Background.*—Cystic fibrosis is a life-limiting disease that is caused by defective or deficient cystic fibrosis transmembrane conductance regulator (CFTR) protein activity. Phe508del is the most common *CFTR* mutation.

*Methods.*—We conducted two phase 3, randomized, double-blind, placebo-controlled studies that were designed to assess the effects of lumacaftor (VX-809), a CFTR corrector, in combination with ivacaftor (VX-770), a CFTR potentiator, in patients 12 years of age or older who had cystic fibrosis and were homozygous for the Phe508del *CFTR* mutation. In both studies, patients were randomly assigned to receive either lumacaftor (600 mg once daily or 400 mg every 12 hours) in combination with ivacaftor (250 mg every 12 hours) or matched placebo for 24 weeks. The primary end point was the absolute change from baseline in the percentage of predicted forced expiratory volume in 1 second ($FEV_1$) at week 24.

*Results.*—A total of 1108 patients underwent randomization and received study drug. The mean baseline $FEV_1$ was 61% of the predicted value. In both studies, there were significant improvements in the primary end point in both lumacaftor–ivacaftor dose groups; the difference between active treatment and placebo with respect to the mean absolute improvement in the percentage of predicted $FEV_1$ ranged from 2.6 to 4.0 percentage points ($P < 0.001$), which corresponded to a mean relative treatment difference of 4.3 to 6.7% ($P < 0.001$). Pooled analyses showed that the rate of pulmonary exacerbations was 30 to 39% lower in the lumacaftor–ivacaftor groups than in the placebo group; the rate of events leading to hospitalization or the use of intravenous antibiotics was lower in the lumacaftor–ivacaftor groups as well. The incidence of adverse events was generally similar in the lumacaftor–ivacaftor and placebo groups. The rate of discontinuation due to an adverse event was 4.2% among patients who received lumacaftor–ivacaftor versus 1.6% among those who received placebo.

*Conclusions.*—These data show that lumacaftor in combination with ivacaftor provided a benefit for patients with cystic fibrosis homozygous for the Phe508del *CFTR* mutation. (Funded by Vertex Pharmaceuticals and others; TRAFFIC and TRANSPORT ClinicalTrials.gov numbers, NCT01807923 and NCT01807949.)

▶ Cystic fibrosis (CF) is caused by genetic mutations, resulting in either deficient or dysfunctional CF transmembrane conductance regulator (CFTR) protein. The most common CFTR mutation, present in approximately 45% of CF patients (who are homozygotes), is the Phe508del mutation.[1] Lumacaftor (LU) is an investigational CFTR corrector that has been shown in vitro to correct the Phe508del and increase the amount of cell surface-localized protein.[2] Ivacaftor (IV) is a CFTR potentiator that increases the open probability of CFTR channels in vitro and improves clinical outcomes in patients who have CF and at lease 1 copy of most class III mutations.[3-6] Neither LU or IV alone have been shown to be efficacious in treating homozygotes for the Phe508del mutation; however, a Phase II trial showed that, given together, LU and IV were beneficial in this population.[7] The present investigation reports on 2 Phase III trials of 2 doses of LU given with IV in patients with CF who are homozygotes for the PHe508del mutation. Table 1 in the original article displays the baseline data for the 2 test groups (LU 600 mg daily and IV 250 mg every 12 h; LU 400 mg every 12 h and IV 250 mg every 12 h); and the placebo group. Fig 1 in the original article displays the change in forced expiratory volume in 1 second by group over 24 weeks' time (A) and the differences between characteristics between posttreatment and baseline data (B). Fig 2 in the original article shows a Kaplan-Meier curve depicting time to first exacerbation (A) and time to exacerbation through week 24. Both treatment groups showed superiority to placebo ($P < 0.001$, events leading to hospitalization; $P < 0.003$ for events leading to hospitalization for LU 600 mg daily group and $P < 0.001$ for LU 400 mg every 12 h group). Ninety-three percent of treatment groups finished the study and the LU and IV combination therapy had an overall acceptable safety profile. Pulmonary function was improved on this combination therapy in the homozygote population of Phe508del CF patients.

**S. K. Willsie, DO, MA**

*References*


1. US CF Foundation, Johns Hopkins University, the Hospital for Sick Children. The clinical and functional translation of CFTR (CFTR2). 2011. http://cftr2.org.
2. Van Goor F, Hadida S, Grootenhuis PD, et al. Correction of the F508del-CFTR protein processing defect in vitro by the investigational drug VX-809. *Proc Natl Acad Sci U S A*. 2011;108:18843-18848.

3. Ramsey BW, Davies J, McElvaney NG, et al. A CFTR potentiator in patients with cystic fibrosis and the G551D mutation. *N Engl J Med.* 2011;365:1663-1672.
4. Davies JC, Wainwright CE, Canny GJ, et al. Efficacy and safety of ivacaftor in patients aged 6 to 11 years with cystic fibrosis with a G551D mutation. *Am J Respir Crit Care Med.* 2013;187:1219-1225.
5. McKone EF, Borowitz D, Drevinek P, et al. Long-term safety and efficacy of ivacaftor in patients with cystic fibrosis who have the Gly551Asp-CFTR mutation: a phase 3, open-label extension study (PERSIST). *Lancet Respir Med.* 2014;2:902-910.
6. Rowe SM, Heltshe SL, Gonska T, et al. Clinical mechanism of the cystic fibrosis transmembrane conductance regulator potentiator ivacaftor in G551D-mediated cystic fibrosis. *Am J Respir Crit Care Med.* 2014;190:175-184.
7. Boyle MP, Bell SC, Konstan MW, et al. A CFTR corrector (lumacaftor) and a CFTR potentiator (ivacaftor) for treatment of patients with cystic fibrosis who have a phe508del CFTR mutation: a phase 2 randomised controlled trial. *Lancet Respir Med.* 2014;2:527-538.

# 30 Chronic Obstructive Pulmonary Disease

---

**Economic Burden of COPD in the Presence of Comorbidities**

Mannino DM, Higuchi K, Yu T-C, et al (Univ of Kentucky College of Public Health, Lexington; Novartis Pharmaceuticals Corporation, East Hanover, NJ; et al)

*Chest* 148:138-150, 2015

---

*Background.*—The morbidity and mortality associated with COPD exacts a considerable economic burden. Comorbidities in COPD are associated with poor health outcomes and increased costs. Our objective was to assess the impact of comorbidities on COPD-associated costs in a large administrative claims dataset.

*Methods.*—This was a retrospective observational study of data from the Truven Health MarketScan Commercial Claims and Encounters and the MarketScan Medicare Supplemental Databases from January 1, 2009, to September 30, 2012. Resource consumption was measured from the index date (date of first occurrence of non-rule-out COPD diagnosis) to 360 days after the index date. Resource use (all-cause and disease-specific [ie, COPD- or asthma-related] ED visits, hospitalizations, office visits, other outpatient visits, and total length of hospital stay) and health-care costs (all-cause and disease-specific costs for ED visits, hospitalizations, office visits, and other outpatient visits and medical, prescription, and total health-care costs) were assessed. Generalized linear models were used to evaluate the impact of comorbidities on total health-care costs, adjusting for age, sex, geographic location, baseline health-care use, employment status, and index COPD medication.

*Results.*—Among 183,681 patients with COPD, the most common comorbidities were cardiovascular disease (34.8%), diabetes (22.8%), asthma (14.7%), and anemia (14.2%). Most patients (52.8%) had one or two comorbidities of interest. The average all-cause total healthcare costs from the index date to 360 days after the index date were highest for patients with chronic kidney disease ($41,288) and anemia ($38,870). The impact on total health-care costs was greatest for anemia ($10,762 more, on average, than a patient with COPD without anemia).

*Conclusions.*—Our analysis demonstrated that high resource use and costs were associated with COPD and multiple comorbidities.

▶ COPD is a huge disease burden in the United States and is estimated to cost more than $50 billion a year in direct medical costs and indirect costs such as loss of productivity. With the increasing knowledge that COPD is a systemic inflammatory disease, a great focus has been placed on the many medical comorbidities that complicate its management. Common comorbidities, such as cardiovascular disease, gastroesophageal reflux disease, an increase in various neoplasms, and mood disorders, are now well described and known to increase management costs while reducing health status, quality of life, and prognosis. Unfortunately, in patients with a COPD diagnosis, optimal management of comorbidities by physicians and others can suffer because of fear that more aggressive management will worsen the COPD symptoms or just a feeling that the COPD is the worst problem and that should be the primary focus of care. Either approach is less than ideal for the COPD patient. In this study by Mannino et al, which includes a claims analysis from 2 very large databases, we can get a better idea of the presence of comorbidities in a large population of COPD patients as well as the increased cost of managing patients with these comorbidities. Identifying and managing comorbidities early may help contain these costs especially while health care costs are continuing to increase. A recent study from British Columbia using the provincial health plan's services database and the vital statistics database documented an increase in the excess cost of care of COPD patients over a matched cohort of non-COPD patients between 2001 and 2010. The excess costs in this government-sponsored health system were more than $5400 compared to the matched cohort. Care providers need to pay as much attention to the comorbidities of COPD patients as they do to the lung disease to help contain these costs.

**J. R. Maurer, MD, MBA**

---

**Lung-Function Trajectories Leading to Chronic Obstructive Pulmonary Disease**

Lange P, Celli B, Agustí A, et al (Copenhagen Univ, Denmark; Harvard Med School, Boston, MA; Univ of Barcelona, Spain; et al)

*N Engl J Med* 373:111-122, 2015

---

*Background.*—Chronic obstructive pulmonary disease (COPD) is thought to result from an accelerated decline in forced expiratory volume in 1 second ($FEV_1$) over time. Yet it is possible that a normal decline in $FEV_1$ could also lead to COPD in persons whose maximally attained $FEV_1$ is less than population norms.

*Methods.*—We stratified participants in three independent cohorts (the Framingham Offspring Cohort, the Copenhagen City Heart Study, and the Lovelace Smokers Cohort) according to lung function ($FEV_1$ $\geq$80% or <80% of the predicted value) at cohort inception (mean age of patients, approximately 40 years) and the presence or absence of COPD at the last study visit. We then determined the rate of decline in $FEV_1$ over time among the participants according to their $FEV_1$ at cohort inception and COPD status at study end.

*Results.*—Among 657 persons who had an $FEV_1$ of less than 80% of the predicted value before 40 years of age, 174 (26%) had COPD after 22 years of observation, whereas among 2207 persons who had a baseline $FEV_1$ of at least 80% of the predicted value before 40 years of age, 158 (7%) had COPD after 22 years of observation ($P < 0.001$). Approximately half the 332 persons with COPD at the end of the observation period had had a normal $FEV_1$ before 40 years of age and had a rapid decline in $FEV_1$ thereafter, with a mean (±SD) decline of 53 ± 21 ml per year. The remaining half had had a low $FEV_1$ in early adulthood and a subsequent mean decline in $FEV_1$ of 27 ± 18 ml per year ($P < 0.001$), despite similar smoking exposure.

*Conclusions.*—Our study suggests that low $FEV_1$ in early adulthood is important in the genesis of COPD and that accelerated decline in $FEV_1$ is not an obligate feature of COPD. (Funded by an unrestricted grant from GlaxoSmithKline and others.)

▶ Chronic obstructive pulmonary disease (COPD) is a common illness and recently was noted to be the third most common cause of death in the world.[1] COPD is generally considered to come from inhaled exposure to a variety of substances primarily the components of cigarette smoking, biomass smoke, and some components of modern air pollution. Generally, the lung function in susceptible persons has been has been significantly accelerated beyond expected age-related declines, and this results in typical obstructive spirometry findings. However, it has also been noted both that lung function declines in exposed and susceptible patients do not follow a common pathway in lung function decline and that as many as 10% to 15% of patients with obstructive findings on spirometry in adulthood do not have any known identifiable exposure that would predispose them to this disease. In this study, the authors used 3 large longitudinal population cohorts to follow lung function over time. The novel finding in this study is that a subgroup of the population without an exposure or genetics predisposing to COPD will never reach normal adult lung function and, as they normally age, their lung function will decline spirometrically into the definition of obstructive disease. Are these the children living in households of parents who smoke, or did they have respiratory disease as children, or is their level of lung function genetically determined? And what predisposes someone to more rapid or less rapid decline in lung function? These are all incompletely answered questions and the subject of future investigation—investigation that is necessary not only to understand this population but to provide for early intervention and management.

**J. R. Maurer, MD, MBA**

*Reference*

1. Lozano R, Naghavi M, Foreman K, et al. Global and regional mortality from 235 causes of death for 20 age groups in 1990 and 2010: a systematic analysis for the Global Burden of Disease Study 2010. *Lancet.* 2012;380:2095-2128.

# 31 Lung Cancer

**Current Cigarette Smoking Among Adults — United States, 2005–2014**

Jamal A, Homa DM, O'Connor E, et al (Natl Ctr for Chronic Disease Prevention and Health Promotion)

*MMWR Morb Mortal Wkly Rep* 64:1233-1240, 2015

*Background.*—In the United States, smoking tobacco is the leading cause of preventable disease and death. More than 480,000 premature deaths and over $300 billion in direct health-related expenditures and lost productivity are linked to cigarette smoking. A survey by the Centers for Disease Control and Prevention (CDC) sought to assess the progress that has been made in the United States toward the goal set in *Healthy People 2020* of reducing the percentage of US adults who smoke cigarettes to 12% or less.

*Outcome.*—Between 2005 and 2014 smoking declined among US adults from 20.9% to 16.8%, a fall of 19.8%. The difference between smoking percentages from 2013 (17.8%) to 2014 (16.8%) was significant. However, there was no significant change between the percentage of adults who were former smokers between 2005 and 2014 (21.9% versus 21.5%).

A comparison of gender and age differences noted the prevalence of cigarette smoking was higher in male subjects than female subjects (18.8% versus 14.8%) and highest among adults age 25 to 44 years (20.0%). The lowest level was noted among those age 65 years or older (8.5%).

Analyzing ethnic and racial factors, smoking prevalence was highest in American Indian/Alaska Natives (29.2%) and multiracial adults (27.9%). It was lowest among Asian Americans (9.5%).

The highest prevalence of smoking among those age 25 years or older was noted in those with a General Education Development certificate (43.0%); the lowest was in those with a graduate degree (5.4%). Higher smoking prevalence was noted among those living below poverty level (26.3%) compared to those at or above this level (15.2%). Those in the Midwest smoked considerably more than those in the West (20.7% versus 13.1%). Higher smoking prevalences were also noted for those with a disability or limitation (21.9%) rather than those not disabled (16.1%). In addition, lesbian, gay, or bisexual adults (23.9%) smoked more than straight adults (16.6%).

Persons insured by Medicaid only in 2014 (29.1%) and those who were uninsured (27.9%) reported a higher smoking prevalence than those with private health insurance (12.9%) or Medicare only (12.5%). Among those covered only by Medicaid, the youngest age group (18- to 24-year-olds)

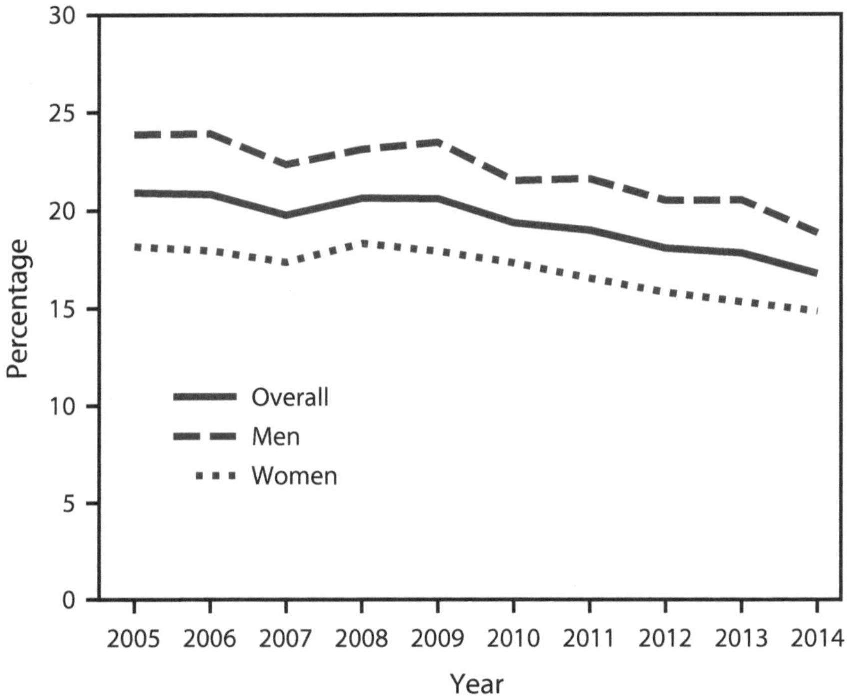


FIGURE 1.—Percentage of adults who were current cigarette smokers,* overall and by sex — National Health Interview Survey, United States, 2005–2014. *Persons who reported smoking ≥100 cigarettes during their lifetime and who, at the time of interview, reported smoking every day or some days.(Reprinted from Jamal A, Homa DM, O'Connor E, et al. Current cigarette smoking among adults – United States, 2005-2014. *MMWR Morb Mortal Wkly Rep*. 2015;64:1233-1240.)

had a smoking prevalence of 18.2%, whereas those age 25 to 44 years and those age 45 to 64 years had prevalences of 35.6% and 29.7%, respectively.

The number of daily smokers fell from 36.4 million to 30.7 million between 2005 and 2014. "Sometimes" smokers increased from 8.7 to 9.3 million over that time period. Mean number of cigarettes smoked per day fell from 16.7 to 13.8 for daily smokers. Declines were noted for the number of those who smoked 20 to 29 cigarettes per day and those smoking 30 or more per day.

*Implications.*—Cigarette smoking and smoking-related disease and death for US adults can be reduced, as illustrated by the fall between 2005 and 2014 in these areas. Ongoing changes in the US health care system may provide opportunities to improve the use of clinical preventive services that can reduce smoking and its hazards among adults (Fig 1).

▶ This report from the Centers for Disease Control and Prevention (CDC) summarizes smoking prevalence data obtained from the 2014 National Health Interview Survey, which included 36 697 adult respondents aged >18 years. Current smoking was defined as smoking every day or some days, former smoking was defined as smoking >100 cigarettes over a lifetime but not currently smoking, and never smoking was defined as total smoking of <100 cigarettes over a lifetime. Fig 1 demonstrates that cigarette smoking among US adults is declining. Smoking prevalence is higher among adult men (18.8%) than women (14.8%), and highest among adults aged 25 to 44 years (20%). Forty million Americans are current smokers, 5 million fewer than in 2005.

The great news is that smoking prevalence is steadily, albeit slowly, declining. The sobering details are that, as has been consistently observed over time, health disparities in cigarette use are clear. Smoking prevalence is higher in Native Americans than whites, in persons with lower education levels, and in persons living below the poverty level. The detrimental effect of smoking in these populations already at higher medical risk is substantial. Smoking prevalence may also reflect different types of health insurance. As challenging as it has been and will be to tackle tobacco cessation, the 480 000 cigarette-related premature deaths that occur in the United States each year[1] and the reinforcement of this report that efforts to facilitate smoking cessation can be successful, demand that we continue to do so, patient by patient.

**L. T. Tanoue, MD**

*Reference*

1. US Department of Health and Human Services. *The Health Consequences of Smoking—50 Years of Progress: A Report of the Surgeon General.* Atlanta, GA: Centers for Disease Control and Prevention, US Department of Health and Human Services; 2014.

---

**An Official American Thoracic Society/American College of Chest Physicians Policy Statement: Implementation of Low-Dose Computed Tomography Lung Cancer Screening Programs in Clinical Practice**

Wiener RS, Gould MK, Arenberg DA, et al; on behalf of the ATS/CHEST Committee on Low-Dose CT Lung Cancer Screening in Clinical Practice
*Am J Respir Crit Care Med* 192:881-891, 2015

---

*Rationale.*—Annual low-radiation-dose computed tomography (LDCT) screening for lung cancer has been shown to reduce lung cancer mortality among high-risk individuals and is now recommended by multiple organizations. However, LDCT screening is complex, and implementation requires careful planning to ensure benefits outweigh harms. Little guidance has been provided for sites wishing to develop and implement lung cancer screening programs.

*Objectives.*—To promote successful implementation of comprehensive LDCT screening programs that are safe, effective, and sustainable.

*Methods.*—The American Thoracic Society (ATS) and American College of Chest Physicians (CHEST) convened a committee with expertise in lung cancer screening, pulmonary nodule evaluation, and implementation science. The committee reviewed the evidence from systematic reviews, clinical practice guidelines, surveys, and the experience of early-adopting LDCT screening programs and summarized potential strategies to implement LDCT screening programs successfully.

*Measurements and Main Results.*—We address steps that sites should consider during the main three phases of developing an LDCT screening program: planning, implementation, and maintenance. We present multiple strategies to implement the nine core elements of comprehensive lung cancer screening programs enumerated in a recent CHEST/ATS statement, which will allow sites to select the strategy that best fits with their local context and workflow patterns. Although we do not comment on cost-effectiveness of LDCT screening, we outline the necessary costs associated with starting and sustaining a high-quality LDCT screening program.

*Conclusions.*—Following the strategies delineated in this policy statement may help sites to develop comprehensive LDCT screening programs that are safe and effective.

▶ With the recommendation of the US Preventive Services Task Force (USPSTF) for lung cancer screening in late 2013 and the endorsement of screening by the Centers for Medicare and Medicaid Services (CMS) earlier this year, implementation of lung cancer screening with low-dose chest CT (LDCT) scanning will be occurring broadly across the country.[1,2] It is important to recognize that lung cancer screening involves much more than the ordering of a LDCT; the necessary components of high-quality screening essentially mandate a programmatic approach.[3] This statement from the American Thoracic Society and the American College of Chest Physicians does not seek to recapitulate extensive discussions of the balance of benefit and risk related to screening, which are available elsewhere but provides a superb structure for planning, implementing, and maintaining a comprehensive screening program. The statement outlines practical suggestions for planning, including for example the involvement of a multidisciplinary steering committee as well as engagement of local hospital or health care system leadership. Recommendations for implementation take into consideration the policy requirements stated by CMS and USPSTF, as well as the costs related to the many components of screening, including personnel, equipment, smoking cessation, information technology, for example. The statement provides the website for the American Thoracic Society patient decision aid (http://www.thoracic.org/patient/patient-resources/resources/decision-aid-lcs.pdf) and discusses the use of other publicly available decision tools, the use of which is a CMS requirement for screening. Maintenance of screening programs is the least well-defined domain because processes for data collection in regional or national registries have as yet not been fully identified. For individuals or institutions seeking guidance for the development of lung cancer screening programs, the roadmap provided by this statement is well worth considering.

**L. T. Tanoue, MD**

*References*

1. U.S. Preventive Services Task Force. *Final Recommendation Statement: Lung Cancer: Screening*. October 2014. Available at: http://www.uspreventiveservicestaskforce.

org/Page/Document/RecommendationStatementFinal/lung-cancer-screening. Accessed January 8, 2016.
2. Centers for Medicare & Medicaid Services. *Decision Memo for Screening for Lung Cancer with Low Dose Computed Tomography (LDCT) (CAG-00439N)*. Available at: https://www.cms.gov/medicare-coverage-database/details/nca-decision-memo.aspx?NCAId=274. Accessed January 8, 2016.
3. Mazzone P, Powell CA, Arenberg D, et al. Components necessary for high-quality lung cancer screening: American college of chest physicians and American thoracic society policy statement. *Chest*. 2015;147:295-303.

**Long-Term Follow-up Results of the DANTE Trial, a Randomized Study of Lung Cancer Screening with Spiral Computed Tomography**

Infante M, Cavuto S, Lutman FR, et al (Humanitas Res Hosp, Rozzano (Milan), Italy; IRCCS-Arcispedale Santa Maria Nuova, Reggio Emilia, Italy; et al)
*Am J Respir Crit Care Med* 191:1166-1175, 2015

*Rationale.*—Screening for lung cancer with low-dose spiral computed tomography (LDCT) has been shown to reduce lung cancer mortality by 20% compared with screening with chest X-ray (CXR) in the National Lung Screening Trial, but uncertainty remains concerning the efficacy of LDCT screening in a community setting.

*Objectives.*—To explore the effect of LDCT screening on lung cancer mortality compared with no screening. Secondary endpoints included incidence, stage, and resectability rates.

*Methods.*—Male smokers of 20+ pack-years, aged 60 to 74 years, underwent a baseline CXR and sputum cytology examination and received five screening rounds with LDCT or a yearly clinical review only in a randomized fashion.

*Measurements and Main Results.*—A total of 1,264 subjects were enrolled in the LDCT arm and 1,186 in the control arm. Their median age was 64.0 years (interquartile range, 5), and median smoking exposure was 45.0 pack-years. The median follow-up was 8.35 years. One hundred four patients (8.23%) were diagnosed with lung cancer in the screening arm (66 by CT), 47 of whom (3.71%) had stage I disease; 72 control patients (6.07%) were diagnosed with lung cancer, with 16 (1.35%) being stage I cases. Lung cancer mortality was 543 per 100,000 person years (95% confidence interval, 413—700) in the LDCT arm versus 544 per 100,000 person-years (95% CI, 410—709) in the control arm (hazard ratio, 0.993; 95% confidence interval, 0.688—1.433).

*Conclusions.*—Because of its limited statistical power, the results of the DANTE (Detection And screening of early lung cancer with Novel imaging TEchnology) trial do not allow us to make a definitive statement about the efficacy of LDCT screening. However, they underline the importance of obtaining additional data from randomized trials with intervention-free reference arms before the implementation of population screening (Table 4).

▶ The DANTE study (Detection and Screening of Early Lung Cancer With Novel Imaging Technology and Molecular Assays) is a randomized trial that

TABLE 4.—Lung Cancer–Specific and All-Cause Mortality Rates (per 100,000 Person-Years

| | LDCT | Control | All |
|---|---|---|---|
| Study subjects, n (%) | 1,264 (51.59) | 1,186 (49.41) | 2,450 (100) |
| FU, person-years | 10,875 | 10,104 | 20,979 |
| Cause of death, n (%) | | | |
| Cancer of the lung | 59 (4.66) | 55 (4.64) | 114 (4.65) |
| Cancer of other organs | 54 | 59 | |
| Nonneoplastic disease | 65 | 62 | |
| Unknown* | 2 | — | |
| Total deaths | 180 (14.24) | 176 (14.84) | 356 (14.53) |
| Lung cancer mortality (95% CI) | 543 (413–700) | 544 (410–709) | 543 (448–653) |
| All-cause mortality (95% CI) | 1,655 (1,422–1,916) | 1,742 (1,494–2,019) | 1,697 (1,525–1,883) |

*Definition of abbreviations*: CI = confidence interval; FU = follow-up; LDCT = low-dose spiral computed tomography.
*One patient died of disseminated cancer of unknown origin, and one patient died of unknown causes in a foreign country.
Reprinted from Infante M, Cavuto S, Lutman FR, et al. Long-term follow-up results of the DANTE Trial, a randomized study of lung cancer screening with spiral computed tomography. *Am J Respir Crit Care Med*. 2015;191:1166-1175, with permission from American Thoracic Society.

evaluated the effect on lung cancer mortality of screening low-dose chest computed tomography (LDCT) versus clinical review annually for 5 years. Study subjects were men aged 60 to 75 years with a 20 pack-year history of smoking who were currently smoking or had quit within 10 years of enrollment, had a life expectancy of at least the duration of the trial, and had no history of previous malignancy within 10 years. DANTE was carried out at 2 hospitals in Milan, Italy. Although a shift toward earlier stage disease was observed in the LDCT arm, at the end of the study, there was no difference in lung cancer–specific or all-cause mortality rates between the 2 arms of the study (Table 4).

Before drawing conclusions about the negative results of the DANTE trial, it is important to recognize the limitations of its design. Two thousand four hundred subjects were recruited for this study; the relatively small sample size achieved a power that could demonstrate a 50% mortality reduction in the LDCT arm. Stated in another way, DANTE lacks sufficient power to demonstrate a more reasonable mortality reduction goal. By comparison, the National Lung Screening Trial (NLST) enrolled more than 50 000 subjects to demonstrate a 20% reduction in lung cancer mortality in the LDCT-screened arm.[1] DANTE set a lower smoking pack-year history threshold than the NLST, in which the smoking requirement for entry was > 30 pack-years. Further, the exclusion of women from the DANTE study population may have had an effect because female subjects in the NLST had a greater mortality benefit compared with male subjects.

A point worth noting in the DANTE results is that the surgical mortality was 3.3%, several-fold higher than the 1% surgical mortality in the NLST, and procedure rates for benign disease were also higher. DANTE was performed in 2 community hospitals, whereas the NLST predominantly took place in tertiary academic medical centers. These observations raise the concern that generalization of screening to the broader community may not occur with the same low rates of surgical complications as were seen in the NLST.

There is 1 other large European lung cancer screening study that has as yet to release its results. The Dutch-Belgian randomized lung cancer multislice computed tomography screening trial (NELSON) randomized 15 000 subjects to annual screening with LDCT versus no screening.[2,3] Although it remains to be seen whether NELSON is adequately powered to give us more information about mortality benefit, all of these studies inform the discussion about the balance between benefits and harms related to LDCT screening for lung cancer.

**L. T. Tanoue, MD**

*References*

1. Aberle DR, Adams AM, Berg CD, et al. Reduced lung-cancer mortality with low-dose computed tomographic screening. *N Engl J Med.* 2011;365:395-409.
2. Baecke E, de Koning HJ, Otto SJ, van Iersel CA, van Klaveren RJ. Limited contamination in the Dutch-Belgian randomized lung cancer screening trial (NELSON). *Lung Cancer.* 2010;69:66-70.
3. van Iersel CA, de Koning HJ, Draisma G, et al. Risk-based selection from the general population in a screening trial: selection criteria, recruitment and power for the Dutch-Belgian randomised lung cancer multi-slice CT screening trial (NELSON). *Int J Cancer.* 2007;120:868-874.

**Racial Differences in Outcomes within the National Lung Screening Trial: Implications for Widespread Implementation**

Tanner NT, Gebregziabher M, Hughes Halbert C, et al (Ralph H. Johnson Veterans Affairs Hosp, Charleston, SC; et al)

*Am J Respir Crit Care Med* 192:200-208, 2015

*Rationale.*—Black individuals with lung cancer (LC) experience higher mortality because they present with more advanced disease and are less likely to undergo curative resection for early-stage disease. The National Lung Screening Trial (NLST) demonstrated improved LC mortality by screening high-risk patients with low-dose computed tomography (LDCT). The benefit of LDCT screening in black individuals is unknown.

*Objectives.*—Examine results of the NLST by race.

*Methods.*—This was a secondary analysis of a randomized trial (NCT00047385) performed in 33 U.S. centers.

*Measurements and Main Results.*—Overall and lung cancer-specific mortality were measured. Screening with LDCT reduced LC mortality in all racial groups but more so in black individuals (hazard ratio [HR], 0.61 vs. 0.86). Smoking increased the likelihood of death from LC, and when stratified by race black smokers were twice as likely to die as white smokers (HR, 4.10 vs. 2.25). Adjusting for sociodemographic and behavioral characteristics, black individuals experienced higher all-cause mortality than white individuals (HR, 1.35; 95% confidence interval, 1.22–1.49); however, black individuals screened with LDCT had a reduction in all-cause mortality. Black individuals were younger, were more likely to be current smokers, had more comorbidities, and had fewer years of formal education than white individuals ($P < 0.05$).

*Conclusions.*—Black individuals screened with LDCT had decreased mortality from lung cancer. However, the demographics associated with improved LC survival were less commonly found in black individuals. The overall mortality in the NLST was higher for black individuals than white individuals, but improved in black individuals screened, suggesting that this subgroup may have had improved access to care. To realize the reductions in mortality from LC screening, dissemination efforts need to be tailored to meet the needs of this community.

▶ It is well known that the National Lung Screening Trial (NLST) demonstrated the efficacy of low-dose computed tomography (LDCT) for the early detection of lung cancer.[1] The NLST study population included persons aged 55 to 74, who were currently smoking or had quit within the previous 15 years and had accumulated at least 30 pack-years of smoking. Since NLST was published, a number of secondary analyses have demonstrated that the benefit of screening is not evenly distributed in the study population.[2,3] Assessment of lung cancer risk, and the potential benefit as well as harm of screening related to that risk, is an important part of the discussion with individual patients as to whether to screen or not.

This study by Tanner and colleagues adds the consideration of race to this discussion. Compared with whites, black participants in NLST were younger and had fewer years of education, more comorbidities, and lower overall cigarette consumption, although they were more likely to be current smokers. All racial groups demonstrated a reduction in lung cancer mortality with screening with LDCT, but blacks who were screened with LDCT also had a statistically significant reduction in all-cause mortality that was not observed in whites. The authors speculate that screening might have improved access to primary medical care, with benefit realized in the management of comorbid disease or abnormalities identified on the screening studies themselves.

Race-related health disparities in lung cancer outcomes have long been observed.[4,5] Besides the benefit in all-cause mortality related to LDCT screening, another striking difference noted in NLST was that black current smokers were 4 times more likely to die from lung cancer than black former smokers, and twice as likely to die from lung cancer as white smokers. Understanding these disparities and addressing them deliberately will be important to achieving the goals of saving lives by lung cancer screening.

**L. T. Tanoue, MD**

*References*

1. Aberle DR, Adams AM, Berg CD, et al. Reduced lung-cancer mortality with low-dose computed tomographic screening. *N Engl J Med.* 2011;365:395-409.
2. Bach PB, Gould MK. When the average applies to no one: personalized decision making about potential benefits of lung cancer screening. *Ann Intern Med.* 2012;157:571-573.
3. Kovalchik SA, Tammemagi M, Berg CD, et al. Targeting of low-dose CT screening according to the risk of lung-cancer death. *N Engl J Med.* 2013;369:245-254.
4. Bach PB, Cramer LD, Warren JL, Begg CB. Racial differences in the treatment of early-stage lung cancer. *N Engl J Med.* 1999;341:1198-1205.
5. Siegel R, Ward E, Brawley O, Jemal A. Cancer statistics, 2011: the impact of eliminating socioeconomic and racial disparities on premature cancer deaths. *CA Cancer J Clin.* 2011;61:212-236.

**Recent Trends in the Identification of Incidental Pulmonary Nodules**

Gould MK, Tang T, Liu I-LA, et al (Kaiser Permanente Southern California, Pasadena; et al)
*Am J Respir Crit Care Med* 192:1208-1214, 2015

*Rationale.*—Pulmonary nodules are common incidental findings, but information about their incidence in the era of computed tomography (CT) is lacking.

*Objectives.*—To examine recent trends in pulmonary nodule identification.

*Methods.*—We used electronic health records and natural language processing to identify members of an integrated health system who had nodules measuring 4 to 30 mm. We calculated rates of chest CT imaging, nodule identification, and receipt of a new lung cancer diagnosis within 2 years of nodule identification, and standardized rates by age and sex to estimate the frequency of nodule identification in the U.S. population in 2010.

*Measurements and Main Results.*—Between 2006 and 2012, more than 200,000 adult members underwent 415,581 chest CT examinations. The annual frequency of chest CT imaging increased from 1.3 to 1.9% for all adult members, whereas the frequency of nodule identification increased from 24 to 31% for all scans performed. The annual rate of chest CT increased from 15.4 to 20.7 per 1,000 person-years, and the rate of nodule identification increased from 3.9 to 6.6 per 1,000 person-years, whereas the rate of a new lung cancer diagnosis remained stable. By extrapolation, more than 4.8 million Americans underwent at least one chest CT scan and 1.57 million had a nodule identified, including 63,000 who received a new lung cancer diagnosis within 2 years.

*Conclusions.*—Incidental pulmonary nodules are an increasingly common consequence of routine medical care, with an incidence that is much greater than recognized previously. More frequent nodule identification has not been accompanied by increases in the diagnosis of cancerous nodules (Table 2).

▶ This population study provides us with an appreciation that the number of pulmonary nodules identified in the course of general medical evaluation has logarithmically increased. It has been widely cited that approximately 150 000 pulmonary nodules are identified in the United States annually, but this estimate dates back to the 1950s.[1] Extrapolating from a robust data set collected from Kaiser Permanente Southern California (KPSC), Gould and colleagues now estimate that, at present, approximately 1 500 000 nodules are identified in the country each year.

Pulmonary nodules are commonly identified as incidental findings on chest computed tomography (CT) scans. Table 2 demonstrates the increase in the utilization of chest CT scanning in KPSC from 2006 to 2012. Approximately 25% to 30% of those scans identified new nodules. Of note, the rate of a positive CT scan per 1000 person years increased from 3.9 in 2006 to 6.6 in 2012. By contrast, over the same period of time, the incidence of lung cancer

TABLE 2.—Frequency of Chest CT Imaging and Positive Chest CT Scans, Adult Member–Level Data 2006 to 2012

| Year | Total Members (*N*) | Members with ≥1 Chest CT Scan [*n* (*% of Members*)] | Members with ≥1 Positive Chest CT Scan [*n* (*% of Members Scanned*)] | Time at Risk for Scanning* (*Person-Years*) | Time at Risk for Having Positive Scan† (*Person-Years*) | ≥1 Chest CT Scan Performed‡ [*Rate per 1,000 Person-Years (95% CI)*] | ≥1 Positive CT Scan‡ [*Rate per 1,000 Person-Years (95% CI)*] |
|---|---|---|---|---|---|---|---|
| 2006 | 2,623,719 | 34,915 (1.3) | 8,973 (25.7) | 2,270,315 | 2,283,728 | 15.4 (15.2–15.5) | 3.9 (3.8–4.0) |
| 2007 | 2,673,078 | 37,294 (1.4) | 10,860 (29.1) | 2,323,514 | 2,336,821 | 16.1 (15.9–16.2) | 4.6 (4.6–4.7) |
| 2008 | 2,672,351 | 41,073 (1.5) | 12,132 (29.5) | 2,349,300 | 2,363,762 | 17.5 (17.3–17.7) | 5.1 (5.0–5.2) |
| 2009 | 2,663,055 | 45,411 (1.7) | 13,794 (30.4) | 2,352,838 | 2,368,731 | 19.3 (19.1–19.5) | 5.8 (5.7–5.9) |
| 2010 | 2,698,679 | 47,773 (1.8) | 15,592 (32.6) | 2,388,202 | 2,404,342 | 20.0 (19.8–20.2) | 6.5 (6.4–6.6) |
| 2011 | 2,822,145 | 51,499 (1.8) | 16,289 (31.6) | 2,514,851 | 2,532,401 | 20.5 (20.3–20.7) | 6.4 (6.3–6.5) |
| 2012 | 2,916,094 | 53,949 (1.9) | 17,368 (32.2) | 2,607,705 | 2,626,455 | 20.7 (20.5–20.9) | 6.6 (6.5–6.7) |
| 2006–2012 Total | 19,069,121 | 311,914 (1.6) | 95,008 (30.5) | 16,806,725 | 16,916,239 | 18.6 (18.5–18.6) | 5.6 (5.6–5.7) |
| 2006–2012 Unique members§ | 4,613,081 | 218,079 (4.7) | 68,998 (31.6) | | | | |

*Definition of abbreviations*: CI = confidence interval; CT = computed tomography.
*Follow-up endpoints were defined as yearly first chest CT scan, disenrollment, death, or the end of each year, whichever occurred first.
†Follow-up endpoints were defined as yearly first positive chest CT scan, disenrollment, death, or the end of each year, whichever occurred first.
‡Ninety-five percent CIs were determined based on a Poisson model for a rare event.
§Members with more than 1 year of membership were counted once.

Reprinted from Gould MK, Tang T, Liu I-LA, et al. Recent trends in the identification of incidental pulmonary nodules. *Am J Respir Crit Care Med*. 2015;192:1208-1214, with permission from American Thoracic Society.

diagnosis after a positive CT scan did not increase, holding steady at approximately 2.9 lung cancers per 10 000 person-years. This suggests that increased rates of CT imaging and the consequent increased rates of nodule identification did not identify more lung cancer cases but did produce many more false-positive findings.

The explosion in nodule identification with CT scanning should not be surprising. Utilization of CT imaging continues to accelerate as CT has become a routine tool in even simple diagnostic evaluations.[2] Image quality has improved with technologic advances, allowing the identification of nodules as small as 1 to 2 mm. Cost and radiation exposure have both diminished. We can expect even higher numbers of nodules to be identified in the future, particularly as lung cancer screening is implemented.

The realization that most incidental nodules identified on CT are not cancers highlights the value of standardizing the approach to their evaluation. Evidence-based guidelines for nodule evaluation are widely available though not widely applied in practice.[3,4] For now, broader dissemination and application of these guidelines should be encouraged to minimize unwarranted testing, both invasive and noninvasive, and to maximize the identification of those nodules that actually are cancers.

**L. T. Tanoue, MD**

*References*

1. Ost D, Fein AM, Feinsilver SH. Clinical practice. The solitary pulmonary nodule. *N Engl J Med.* 2003;348:2535-2542.
2. Brenner DJ, Hall EJ. Computed tomography—an increasing source of radiation exposure. *N Engl J Med.* 2007;357:2277-2284.
3. Gould MK, Fletcher J, Iannettoni MD, et al. Evaluation of patients with pulmonary nodules: when is it lung cancer?: ACCP evidence-based clinical practice guidelines (2nd edition). *Chest.* 2007;132:108S-130S.
4. Tanner NT, Aggarwal J, Gould MK, et al. Management of pulmonary nodules by community pulmonologists: a Multicenter Observational Study. *Chest.* 2015;148: 1405-1414.

## Close Surveillance with Long-Term Follow-up of Subjects with Preinvasive Endobronchial Lesions

van Boerdonk RAA, Smesseim I, Heideman DAM, et al (VU Univ Med Ctr, Amsterdam, the Netherlands; et al)
*Am J Respir Crit Care Med* 192:1483-1489, 2015

*Rationale.*—Autofluorescence bronchoscopy (AFB) and computed tomography (CT) enable lung cancer (LC) detection at the early (pre-)invasive stage. However, LC risk in patients with preinvasive endobronchial lesions is unclear.

*Objectives.*—To assess LC incidence and identify potential risk determinants in patients with preinvasive lesions.

*Methods.*—In our tertiary care referral center, 164 subjects with preinvasive lesions were monitored up to 12.5 years by repeated AFB and CT.

Occurrence of LC was monitored. Clinical management depended on histological grade, with cancer patients receiving standard care. Potential risk determinants (smoking status, baseline histology, cancer history, and chronic obstructive pulmonary disease [COPD] status) were evaluated in relation to cancer occurrence, event-free survival (EFS), and overall survival (OS).

*Measurements and Main Results.*—During surveillance (median of 30 mo, range 4–152) of 164 subjects with preinvasive lesions (80 high grade and 84 low grade at inclusion), 61 LCs were detected in 55 subjects (median time to event 16.5 mo). Twenty-three LCs (38%) were detected by CT, and 38 (62%) were detected by AFB. More cancers (36 of 61; 59%) developed from separate, rather than initial lesional sites. Subjects with high-grade lesions were more likely to be diagnosed with LC at the same or another site in the lungs than those with low-grade lesions ($P = 0.03$). Independent risk determinants for OS were previous curatively treated cancer and COPD ($P \leq 0.05$).

*Conclusions.*—Presence of preinvasive lesions, especially high-grade lesions, may serve as LC risk markers. LCs occur both at preinvasive lesion sites and elsewhere in the bronchial epithelium or lung parenchyma. Prospective validation of biomarkers and randomized intervention studies are needed to determine optimal management strategies.

▶ Autofluorescence bronchoscopy (AFB) is an endoscopic technique that takes advantage of the endogenous fluorescent and spectral properties of the bronchial mucosa and can distinguish between normal and dysplastic bronchial epithelium.[1,2] AFB has been used primarily for surveillance in populations deemed at very high risk of lung cancer. It has not been readily adopted into clinical practice because of the impracticality of bronchoscopy as a repeated surveillance intervention in asymptomatic patients and because of the lack of evidence that airway hyperplasia or dysplasia consistently progress to invasive malignancy.

In this study by van Boerdonk and colleagues, AFB was used in the surveillance of patients referred to a tertiary center because of a high risk of lung cancer recurrence or the development of a second prior lung cancer. The study population consisted of 164 patients who on baseline AFB had 1 or more preinvasive squamous endobronchial lesions (hyperplasia, squamous metaplasia, carcinoma in situ). Follow-up with surveillance AFB included a median of 5 AFB/subject (range 2-27 AFB/subject), over a median of 30 months (range 4-152 months). The rate of development of lung cancer over the follow-up was high, with 61 cancers developing in 55 individuals, the majority of which occurred within 5 years. As shown in Fig 2 in the original article, patients with high-grade endobronchial lesions were more likely to develop invasive cancer than those with low-grade lesions, although the rate of cancer was high in the latter group as well. Interestingly, of the 35 lung cancers identified by AFB, 10 developed at sites separate from the abnormal lesion(s) that had been identified at the baseline AFB. AFB did not identify lung cancers in 26 patients whose tumors were detected by interval (nonscreening) CT.

There are several points worth noting. First, the presence of preinvasive endobronchial squamous lesions appears to be a marker of lung cancer risk. Second, the finding that cancers did not necessarily occur in the site of identified airway lesions supports the concept of "field cancerization," where all cells are exposed to a carcinogen (such as tobacco smoke), many may develop genetic changes that increase cancer risk, and some may have sufficient cumulative injury to become malignant. Dysplasia and/or hyperplasia may be useful as biomarkers for higher cancer risk elsewhere in the lung. Third, both high-grade and low-grade lesions were associated with elevated lung cancer risk. Finally, in this study, AFB and chest CT were complementary techniques, evaluating predominantly the airway and the parenchyma, respectively. This raises the intriguing consideration that bimodal surveillance combining an airway examination with parenchymal imaging might be beneficial in a population identified at high risk for lung cancer because of the presence of preinvasive endobronchial lesions.

**L. T. Tanoue, MD**

*References*

1. Edell E, Lam S, Pass H, et al. Detection and localization of intraepithelial neoplasia and invasive carcinoma using fluorescence-reflectance bronchoscopy: an international, multicenter clinical trial. *J Thorac Oncol*. 2009;4:49-54.
2. Chiyo M, Shibuya K, Hoshino H, et al. Effective detection of bronchial preinvasive lesions by a new autofluorescence imaging bronchovideoscope system. *Lung Cancer*. 2005;48:307-313.

**Stereotactic Body Radiation Therapy Versus No Treatment for Early Stage Non-Small Cell Lung Cancer in Medically Inoperable Elderly Patients: A National Cancer Data Base Analysis**

Nanda RH, Liu Y, Gillespie TW, et al (Emory Univ, Atlanta, GA; et al)
*Cancer* 121:4222-4230, 2015

*Background.*—Stereotactic body radiation therapy (SBRT) has demonstrated high rates of local control with low morbidity and has now emerged as the standard of care for medically inoperable, early stage non–small cell lung cancer (NSCLC). However, the impact of lung SBRT on survival in the elderly population is less clear given competing comorbid conditions. An analysis of the National Cancer Data Base (NCDB) was undertaken to determine whether definitive SBRT improves survival relative to observation alone patients ages 70 years and older.

*Methods.*—The NCDB, a retrospective national database that captures approximately 70% of all patients treated for cancer, was queried for patients aged 70 years or older with early stage (T1-T3N0M0) NSCLC from 2003 to 2006. Overall survival was compared between patients who received stereotactic body radiotherapy alone and those who received no treatment. An extended Cox proportional hazards model was applied to estimate the treatment effect of SBRT.

*Results.*—In total, 3147 patients met the selection criteria for this analysis. SBRT was delivered to 258 patients (8.2%), and 2889 patients (91.8%) received no treatment. There was no significant difference in the distribution of Charlson/Deyo comorbidity index scores between the 2 groups ($P = .076$). Multivariable analysis revealed improved overall survival with SBRT compared with observation for the entire cohort (hazard ratio, 0.64; $P < .001$).

*Conclusions.*—SBRT is associated with improved survival in elderly patients with early stage NSCLC who have concurrent comorbid conditions compared with observation alone. The current data support the use of SBRT for the treatment of elderly patients with early stage NSCLC who have limiting comorbid conditions (Fig 3, Table 3).

▶ Stereotactic body radiation therapy (SBRT) is usually the treatment of choice for patients with early-stage non–small cell lung cancer (NSCLC) who are deemed medically inoperable because of concerns for surgery-related morbidity

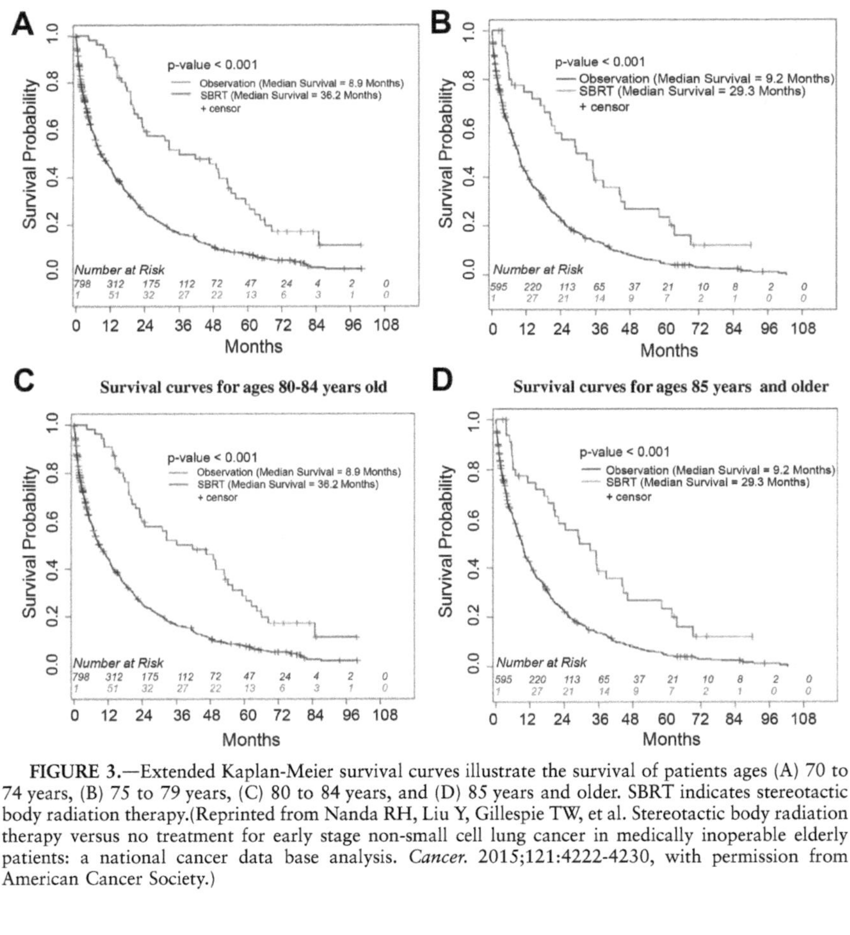


FIGURE 3.—Extended Kaplan-Meier survival curves illustrate the survival of patients ages (A) 70 to 74 years, (B) 75 to 79 years, (C) 80 to 84 years, and (D) 85 years and older. SBRT indicates stereotactic body radiation therapy.(Reprinted from Nanda RH, Liu Y, Gillespie TW, et al. Stereotactic body radiation therapy versus no treatment for early stage non-small cell lung cancer in medically inoperable elderly patients: a national cancer data base analysis. *Cancer.* 2015;121:4222-4230, with permission from American Cancer Society.)

TABLE 3.—Multivariable Interaction Model for Treatment Effect by Age or Charlson/Deyo Score

| Strata | Treatment | HR (95% CI) | HR *P* |
|---|---|---|---|
| Age, y | | | |
| 70-74 | SBRT vs observation | 0.72 (0.53-0.97) | .028[a] |
| 75-79 | SBRT vs observation | 0.66 (0.49-0.88) | .004[a] |
| 80-84 | SBRT vs observation | 0.59 (0.42-0.83) | .003[a] |
| ≥85 | SBRT vs observation | 0.56 (0.37-0.85) | .006[a] |
| Charlson/Deyo score | | | |
| 0 | SBRT vs observation | 0.64 (0.52-0.78) | <.001[a] |
| 1 | SBRT vs observation | 0.79 (0.56-1.11) | .173 |
| ≥2 | SBRT vs observation | 0.51 (0.33-0.77) | .002[a] |

Abbreviations: CI, confidence interval; HR, hazard ratio; SBRT, stereotactic body radiation therapy.
[a]These *P* values indicate a statistically significant difference.
Reprinted from Nanda RH, Liu Y, Gillespie TW, et al. Stereotactic body radiation therapy versus no treatment for early stage non-small cell lung cancer in medically inoperable elderly patients: a national cancer data base analysis. *Cancer.* 2015;121:4222-4230, with permission from American Cancer Society.

and mortality related to pulmonary physiologic limitations or medical comorbidities.[1] Age is also a factor in the decision about surgery. Although many studies have demonstrated that fit older persons tolerate surgery for early-stage NSCLC with good results, it is consistently observed that older patients undergo surgery for early-stage NSCLC at a lower rate than younger patients.[2] This may reflect a perception that survival benefit is less clear, particularly if there are concomitant comorbidities. SBRT may be better tolerated in older patients because of the ease of dose delivery in only a few fractions and high-precision treatment, minimizing the volume of normal tissues irradiated.

This study used data from the National Cancer Data Base to evaluate the difference in survival between elderly patients (age >70 years; median age 79 years) with early-stage NSCLC (T1-3 N0 M0) who received SBRT compared with those who received no treatment. Median survival for the SBRT-treated group was 29 months vs 10.1 months in the group that was observed without cancer-specific treatment, with a statistically significant increase in survival observed even in patients >85 years (Fig 3). Further, SBRT resulted in significant survival improvement regardless of the presence of comorbidities, even in patients with a Charlson/Deyo comorbidity score of >2 (Table 3).

SBRT is rapidly becoming a widely available treatment for patients with early-stage NSCLC. Although surgery remains the treatment of choice for patients who can physiologically tolerate resection, SBRT is increasingly a reasonable alternative. Direct head-to-head trials comparing the outcomes of lobectomy vs SBRT have been few and with relatively small numbers of patients,[3,4] but factors beyond technical issues, including the presence of medical comorbidities, age, and patient preference, should be considered in the choice of treatment for individual cases.

**L. T. Tanoue, MD**

*References*

1. Timmerman R, Paulus R, Galvin J, et al. Stereotactic body radiation therapy for inoperable early stage lung cancer. *JAMA*. 2010;303:1070-1076.
2. Detterbeck FC, Postmus PE, Tanoue LT. The stage classification of lung cancer: diagnosis and management of lung cancer, 3rd ed: American College of Chest Physicians evidence-based clinical practice guidelines. *Chest*. 2013;143: e191S-e210S.
3. Chang JY, Senan S, Paul MA, et al. Stereotactic ablative radiotherapy versus lobectomy for operable stage I non-small-cell lung cancer: a pooled analysis of two randomised trials. *Lancet Oncol*. 2015;16:630-637.
4. Palma D, Visser O, Lagerwaard FJ, Belderbos J, Slotman B, Senan S. Treatment of stage I NSCLC in elderly patients: a population-based matched-pair comparison of stereotactic radiotherapy versus surgery. *Radiother Oncol*. 2011;101:240-244.

# 32 Pleural, Interstitial Lung, and Pulmonary Vascular Disease

**Comorbidities in idiopathic pulmonary fibrosis patients: a systematic literature review**

Raghu G, Amatto VC, Behr J, et al (Univ of Washington, Seattle; Boehringer Ingelheim Pharma GmbH & Co. KG, Ingelheim am Rhein, Germany; Comprehensive Pneumology Ctr, Munich, Germany)

*Eur Respir J* 46:1113-1130, 2015

Idiopathic pulmonary fibrosis (IPF) is associated with a fatal prognosis and manifests in patients over 60 years old who may have comorbidities. The prevalence and impact of comorbidities on the clinical course of IPF is unclear.

This systematic literature review examined the prevalence of comorbidities and mortality associated with comorbidities in IPF patients. Relevant observational studies published in English from January 1990 to January 2015 identified *via* MEDLINE and EMBASE were included; bibliographies of articles were also searched.

Among the 126 studies included, prevalence of pulmonary hypertension (PH) was 3–86%, 6–91% for obstructive sleep apnoea, 3–48% for lung cancer and 6–67% for chronic obstructive pulmonary disease (COPD). Nonrespiratory comorbidities included ischaemic heart disease (IHD) (3–68%) and gastro-oesophageal reflux (GER) (0–94%). Mortality was highest among patients with IPF and lung cancer. Most studies assessed relatively small samples of patients with IPF.

PH, COPD, lung cancer, GER and IHD are significant comorbidities; differences in IPF severity, case definitions and patient characteristics limited the comparability of findings. The identification and prompt treatment of comorbidities may have a clinically significant impact on overall outcome that is meaningful for patients with IPF.

► Chronic illness such as idiopathic pulmonary fibrosis (IPF), which occur primarily in older patients, nearly always occur in patients with 1 or more comorbidities. This article is intended to be a comprehensive review of the comorbidities in IPF. Comorbidities are more than just coincidental. For example, gastroesophageal reflux disease has been described in nearly all IPF patients, and aspiration into the lung is associated with progression of disease.[1] Ischemic heart disease may be the ultimate cause of death, rather than the IPF. The authors found it difficult to do a comprehensive assessment of the comorbidities of IPF because studies were small and limited in scope. That is probably because IPF is such a rapidly progressive disease, resulting in death in less than 5 years, that little attention has been paid to the other illnesses patients might have. In an era in which new drugs may well extend the life of many of these patients, it is important to look for and manage more aggressively comorbidities that may significantly affect quality of life or longevity (such as gastroesophageal reflux or ischemic heart disease). Now that many of these patients are treated in centers specializing in the management of IPF, that should be easy to do. We should also be able to collect better data on the prevalence and impact of the various comorbidities. For example, Oldham et al have recently identified hypothyroidism as an important and common comorbidity that appears to be predictive of worse survival in this disease.[2]

**J. R. Maurer, MD, MBA**

*References*

1. Lee JS, Collard HR, Anstrom KJ, et al. Anti-acid treatment and disease progression in idiopathic pulmonary fibrosis: an analysis of data from three randomised controlled trials. *Lancet Respir Med.* 2013;1:369-376.
2. Oldham JM, Kumar D, Lee C, et al. Thyroid disease is prevalent and predicts survival in patients with idiopathic pulmonary fibrosis. *Chest.* 2015;148:692-700.

---

**Global incidence and mortality of idiopathic pulmonary fibrosis: a systematic review**

Hutchinson J, Fogarty A, Hubbard R, et al (Univ of Nottingham, United Kingdom)

*Eur Respir J* 46:795-806, 2015

---

As idiopathic pulmonary fibrosis emerges as an important public health problem, there is a need to coordinate data on incidence and mortality globally. This study aims to systematically assess all available studies to investigate the global burden of disease.

Medline and Embase databases were searched systematically for all population-based studies of incidence or mortality of idiopathic pulmonary fibrosis. Clinical case series and prevalence studies were excluded. The search was supplemented using the Google search engine, hand-searching of references and conference abstracts. Data were extracted independently by two authors using a pre-specified proforma, with assessment of methodological quality.

34 studies were identified, providing data from 21 countries from 1968–2012. 28 studies reported incidence data and eight reported mortality data. In studies from the year 2000 onwards, we estimated a conservative incidence range of 3–9 cases per 100000 per year for Europe and North America. Incidence was lower in East Asia and South America. The majority of studies showed an increase in incidence over time.

The incidence of idiopathic pulmonary fibrosis is increasing worldwide and rates are coming together across countries. Current data suggest incidence is similar to that of conditions such as stomach, liver, testicular and cervical cancers.

▶ The global incidence and mortality of idiopathic pulmonary fibrosis is unclear. Studies in recent years seem to suggest that the disease is increasing in incidence, but because of the variability in the methodologies used to define cases and the disease itself, it is difficult to compare different studies. In addition, several country-specific studies looking at incidence and prevalence have been published, but, again, because of the small size of populations and differing methodologies, it is difficult to derive a global picture of the disease. Unlike obstructive lung disease, which is a highly studied pulmonary disease, idiopathic pulmonary fibrosis has much less global literature. There are several reasons for this. It is much less common than obstructive disease; it is rapidly progressive and therefore difficult to study over time; and until recently it had really no effective treatment, so all care was basically supportive. Now, with the emergence of some therapies that may increase the life span of these patients, it has become a disease that can be studied over time and that might place greater demands on health care systems, and thus it is a focus of increased research. To better understand the epidemiology of this disease and its impact, the authors here have endeavored to describe the global burden of this disease with the limited literature available. In the available data, the incidence does appear to be increasing across much of the world; however, more consistent global disease definitions and research methodology will help to better understand why this is true.

**J. R. Maurer, MD, MBA**

---

**The Use of Indwelling Tunneled Pleural Catheters for Recurrent Pleural Effusions in Patients With Hematologic Malignancies: A Multicenter Study**

Gilbert CR, Lee HJ, Skalski JH, et al (Milton S. Hershey Med Ctr, PA; Johns Hopkins Univ, Baltimore, MA; Mayo Clinic, Rochester, MN; et al)
*Chest* 148:752-758, 2015

---

*Background.*—Malignant pleural effusion is a common complication of advanced malignancies. Indwelling tunneled pleural catheter (IPC) placement provides effective palliation but can be associated with complications, including infection. In particular, hematologic malignancy and the associated immunosuppressive treatment regimens may increase infectious complications. This study aimed to review outcomes in patients with hematologic malignancy undergoing IPC placement.

*Methods.*—A retrospective multicenter study of IPCs placed in patients with hematologic malignancy from January 2009 to December 2013 was performed. Inclusion criteria were recurrent, symptomatic pleural effusion and an underlying diagnosis of hematologic malignancy. Records were reviewed for patient demographics, operative reports, and pathology, cytology, and microbiology reports.

*Results.*—Ninety-one patients (mean ± SD age, 65.4 ± 15.4 years) were identified from eight institutions. The mean ± SD in situ dwell time of all catheters was 89.9 ± 127.1 days (total, 8,160 catheter-days). Seven infectious complications were identified, all of the pleural space. All patients were admitted to the hospital for treatment, with four requiring additional pleural procedures. Two patients died of septic shock related to pleural infection.

*Conclusions.*—We present, to our knowledge, the largest study examining clinical outcomes related to IPC placement in patients with hematologic malignancy. An overall 7.7% infection risk and 2.2% mortality were identified, similar to previously reported studies, despite the significant immunosuppression and pancytopenia often present in this population. IPC placement appears to remain a reasonable clinical option for patients with recurrent pleural effusions related to hematologic malignancy.

▶ Malignant pleural effusions are common in adults and can present difficult management challenges. Traditionally drainage followed by talc pleurodesis was commonly used; however, morbidity and sometimes failure from these procedures has led to widespread adoption of the use of tunneled indwelling pleural catheters. This approach has been recommended by British Thoracic Guidelines that state tunneled catheters can be "effective in controlling recurrent and symptomatic malignant effusions in select patients."[1] In 2012, Davies et al published a randomized controlled trial evaluating tunneled catheters versus tube drainage with talc pleurodesis in terms of dyspnea relief and found that dyspnea relief was not significantly different at 6 weeks.[2] Of concern, however, was the infectious complication rate which was much higher in the tunneled catheter group (25%) than in the talc slurry group. Other studies have also documented significant complication rates with this management approach. Of particular interest to the authors of this study was the infectious complication rate of hematologic malignancies because these patients tend to be at increased risk for infections related to the tumor biology and their chemotherapeutic regimens. The authors identified an infection rate in line with that of studies involving a more heterogeneous group of malignancies, but there were also 2 deaths due to sepsis from the indwelling catheters. At the time of this report, only 7 catheters remained in place; the mean dwell time for catheters was about 3 months, and the most common reason for removal was patient death (in more than half of the patients in the study). In this very ill population, it appears tunneled catheters have an acceptable infectious complication rate and are a reasonable option in the setting of very limited life spans.

**J. R. Maurer, MD, MBA**

*References*

1. Roberts ME, Neville E, Berrisford RG, Antunes G, Ali NJ, BTS Pleural Disease Guideline Group. Management of a malignant pleural effusion: British Thoracic Society pleural disease guideline 2010. *Thorax.* 2010;65:ii32-ii40.

2. Davies HE, Mishra EK, Kahan BC, et al. Effect of an indwelling pleural catheter vs chest tube and talc pleurodesis for relieving dyspnea in patients with malignant pleural effusion: the TIME2 randomized controlled trial. *JAMA*. 2012;307: 2383-2389.

**Five-Year Outcomes of Patients Enrolled in the REVEAL Registry**

Farber HW, Miller DP, Poms AD, et al (Boston Univ School of Medicine, MA; ICON Clinical Res, San Francisco, CA; Duke Univ Med Ctr, Durham, NC)
*Chest* 148:1043-1054, 2015

*Background.*—Pulmonary arterial hypertension (PAH) is a rare, severe disease characterized by worsening right-sided heart failure, decreasing functional status, and poor survival. The present study characterizes the 5-year survival in the United States of a new and previous diagnosis of PAH in patients stratified by baseline functional class (FC). The Registry to Evaluate Early and Long-term PAH Disease Management (REVEAL Registry) is a 55-center observational US registry of the demographics, disease course, and management of patients with World Health Organization (WHO) group 1 PAH.

*Methods.*—The REVEAL Registry enrolled newly and previously diagnosed patients aged ≥ 3 months with WHO group 1 PAH consecutively from March 2006 to December 2009. Demographics, disease characteristics, and hemodynamic data were collected at enrollment. Survival analysis was conducted by FC and other subgroups in patients aged ≥ 18 years.

*Results.*—Survival differences between previously diagnosed and newly diagnosed patients at 1 year (90.4% vs 86.3%) were maintained to 5 years; 5-year survival for previously diagnosed patients was 65.4% compared with 61.2% for newly diagnosed patients. Previously diagnosed patients in FC I, II, III, and IV had an estimated 5-year survival rate of 88.0%, 75.6%, 57.0%, and 27.2%, respectively, compared with 72.2%, 71.7%, 60.0%, and 43.8% for newly diagnosed patients in FC I, II, III, and IV, respectively.

*Conclusions.*—Patient survival of advanced PAH remains poor at 5 years despite treatment advances. New York Heart Association FC remains one of the most important predictors of future survival. These observations reinforce the importance of continuous monitoring of FC in patients with PAH.

*Trial Registry.*—ClinicalTrials.gov; No.: NCT00370214; URL: www.clinicaltrials.gov (Figs 3 and 4).

▶ The Registry to Evaluate Early and Long-term PAH (REVEAL) provides data on World Health Organization group 1 pulmonary arterial hypertension patients in the era in which there has been a variety of treatments available for the disease. These data can be compared with historical data when no effective treatment existed.[1] In those data, the median survival for patients with pulmonary hypertension was 2.8 years (not differentiated by functional class). Previously published subgroup analysis from REVEAL has shown that the ability to improve with treatment or failure to improve predicts better or worse survival. The present report looks at survival in both newly diagnosed and previously diagnosed patients registered between 2006 and 2009 and followed for 5 years. It is stratified by initial functional class. This is important because the survival curves show that a better functional class is associated with better survival. Whether this is because the patient has a different phenotype of disease or is earlier in the disease and will progress or gets treatment earlier and that improves outcome is not known. However, it is also clear that newly registered patients with worse function continue to have poor outcomes. In fact, the median survival of those patients appears to be similar to the historical premodern treatment survivals. Previously diagnosed patients entering the registry with better function (Class I and II) interestingly had better survivals than newly diagnosed patients (Figs 3 and 4). This probably reflects survivor bias of previously diagnosed patients. The data produced by registries such as REVEAL are useful in creating survival prediction models.[2] Data from these models can help guide management of the disease as well as appropriate timing for referral for transplant when treatments are failing.

**J. R. Maurer, MD, MBA**

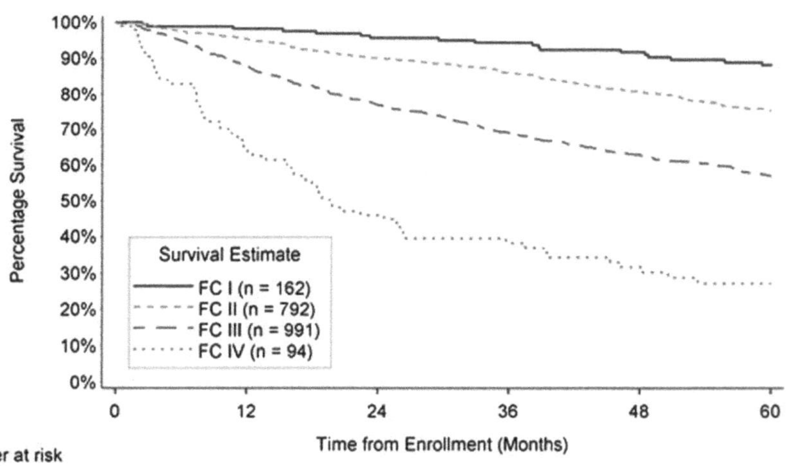


| Number at risk | | | | | | |
|---|---|---|---|---|---|---|
| FC I | 162 | 158 | 149 | 142 | 133 | 122 |
| FC II | 792 | 748 | 694 | 638 | 568 | 514 |
| FC III | 991 | 860 | 731 | 621 | 537 | 467 |
| FC IV | 94 | 60 | 42 | 29 | 24 | 17 |

**FIGURE 3.**—Kaplan-Meier estimates of 5-y survival for the subgroup of previously diagnosed patients, by FC at enrollment. FC I: Patients with pulmonary hypertension but without resulting limitation of physical activity. Ordinary physical activity does not cause undue dyspnea or fatigue, chest pain, or near syncope. FC II: Patients with pulmonary hypertension resulting in slight limitation of physical activity. They are comfortable at rest. Ordinary physical activity causes undue dyspnea or fatigue, chest pain, or near syncope. FC III: Patients with pulmonary hypertension resulting in marked limitation of physical activity. They are comfortable at rest. Less than ordinary activity causes undue dyspnea or fatigue, chest pain, or near syncope. FC IV: Patients with pulmonary hypertension with inability to carry out any physical activity without symptoms. These patients manifest signs of right-sided heart failure. Dyspnea, fatigue, or both may even be present at rest. Discomfort is increased by any physical activity. FC = functional class.(Reprinted from Farber HW, Miller DP, Poms AD, et al. Five year outcomes of patients enrolled in the REVEAL REgistry. *Chest*. 2015;148:1043-1054, with permission.)

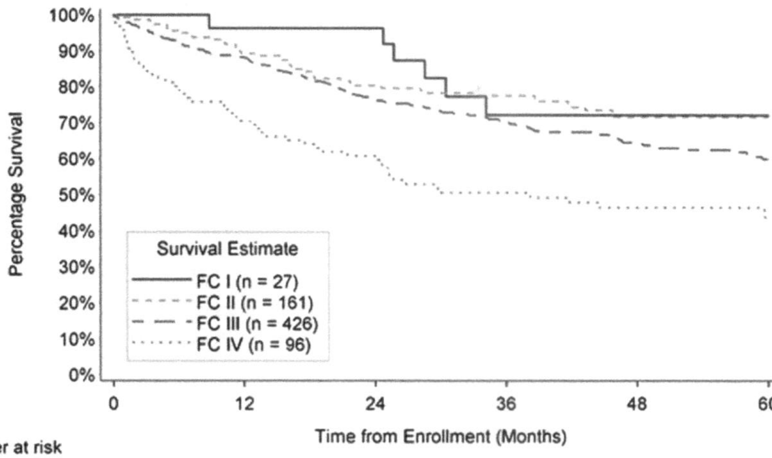


| Number at risk | | | | | | |
|---|---|---|---|---|---|---|
| FC I | 27 | 26 | 23 | 14 | 11 | 9 |
| FC II | 161 | 140 | 123 | 109 | 75 | 54 |
| FC III | 426 | 372 | 309 | 269 | 171 | 96 |
| FC IV | 96 | 66 | 55 | 41 | 31 | 16 |

FIGURE 4.—Kaplan-Meier estimates of 5-y survival for the subgroup of newly diagnosed patients, by FC at enrollment. FC I: Patients with pulmonary hypertension but without resulting limitation of physical activity. Ordinary physical activity does not cause undue dyspnea or fatigue, chest pain, or near syncope. FC II: Patients with pulmonary hypertension resulting in slight limitation of physical activity. They are comfortable at rest. Ordinary physical activity causes undue dyspnea or fatigue, chest pain, or near syncope. FC III: Patients with pulmonary hypertension resulting in marked limitation of physical activity. They are comfortable at rest. Less than ordinary activity causes undue dyspnea or fatigue, chest pain, or near syncope. FC IV: Patients with pulmonary hypertension with inability to carry out any physical activity without symptoms. These patients manifest signs of right-sided heart failure. Dyspnea, fatigue, or both may even be present at rest. Discomfort is increased by any physical activity. See Fig 3 legend for expansion of abbreviation.(Reprinted from Farber HW, Miller DP, Poms AD, et al. Five year outcomes of patients enrolled in the REVEAL REgistry. *Chest.* 2015;148:1043-1054, with permission.)

## *References*

1. D'Alonzo GE, Barst RJ, Ayres SM, et al. Survival in patients with primary pulmonary hypertension. Results from a national prospective registry. *Ann Intern Med.* 1991;115:343-349.
2. Sitbon O, Benza RL, Badesch DB, et al. Validation of two predictive models for survival in pulmonary arterial hypertension. *Eur Respir J.* 2015;46:152-164.

## Six Months vs Extended Oral Anticoagulation After a First Episode of Pulmonary Embolism: The PADIS-PE Randomized Clinical Trial

Couturaud F, for the PADIS-PE Investigators (Universite de Bretagne Occidentale, Brest, France; et al)
*JAMA* 314:31-40, 2015

*Importance.*—The optimal duration of anticoagulation after a first episode of unprovoked pulmonary embolism is uncertain.

*Objectives.*—To determine the benefits and harms of an additional 18-month treatment with warfarin vs placebo, after an initial 6-month nonrandomized treatment period on a vitamin K antagonist.

*Design, Setting, and Participants.*—Randomized, double-blind trial (treatment period, 18 months; median follow-up, 24 months); 371 adult patients who had experienced a first episode of symptomatic unprovoked pulmonary embolism (ie, with no major risk factor for thrombosis) and had been treated initially for 6 uninterrupted months with a vitamin K antagonist were randomized and followed up between July 2007 and September 2014 in 14 French centers.

*Interventions.*—Warfarin or placebo for 18 months.

*Main Outcomes and Measures.*—The primary outcome was the composite of recurrent venous thromboembolism or major bleeding at 18 months after randomization. Secondary outcomes were the composite at 42 months (treatment period plus 24-month follow-up), as well as each component of the composite, and death unrelated to pulmonary embolism or major bleeding, at 18 and 42 months.

*Results.*—After randomization, 4 patients were lost to follow-up, all after month 18, and 1 withdrew due to an adverse event. During the 18-month treatment period, the primary outcome occurred in 6 of 184 patients (3.3%) in the warfarin group and in 25 of 187 (13.5%) in the placebo group (hazard ratio [HR], 0.22; 95%CI, 0.09-0.55; *P* =.001). Recurrent venous thromboembolism occurred in 3 patients in the warfarin group and 25 patients in the placebo group (HR, 0.15; 95%CI, 0.05-0.43); major bleeding occurred in 4 patients in the warfarin group and in 1 patient in the placebo group (HR, 3.96; 95%CI, 0.44 to 35.89). During the 42-month entire study period (including the study treatment and follow-up periods), the composite outcome occurred in 33 patients (20.8%) in the warfarin group and in 42 (24.0%) in the placebo group (HR, 0.75; 95%CI, 0.47-1.18). Rates of recurrent venous thromboembolism, major bleeding, and unrelated death did not differ between groups.

*Conclusions and Relevance.*—Among patients with a first episode of unprovoked pulmonary embolism who received 6 months of anticoagulant treatment, an additional 18 months of treatment with warfarin reduced the composite outcome of recurrent venous thrombosis and major bleeding compared with placebo. However, benefit was not maintained after discontinuation of anticoagulation therapy.

*Trial Registration.*—Clinicaltrials.gov Identifier: NCT00740883 (Fig 2).

▶ Patients who have an unprovoked pulmonary embolus have a high risk of recurrent emboli when their anticoagulation is discontinued at 3 to 6 months. In this prospective, randomized, double-blinded trial, the question addressed was whether continuing anticoagulation for an extended time would prevent recurrent events. Patients who had standard-of-care 6 months of anticoagulant therapy with warfarin were randomized to have an additional 18 months of treatment or placebo. All were then followed for an additional 18 months (total 42 months from initial embolus) to determine whether any benefit of the additional anticoagulation was durable. The end point of this study was a composite of recurrent events and major bleeding, illustrated in the accompanying

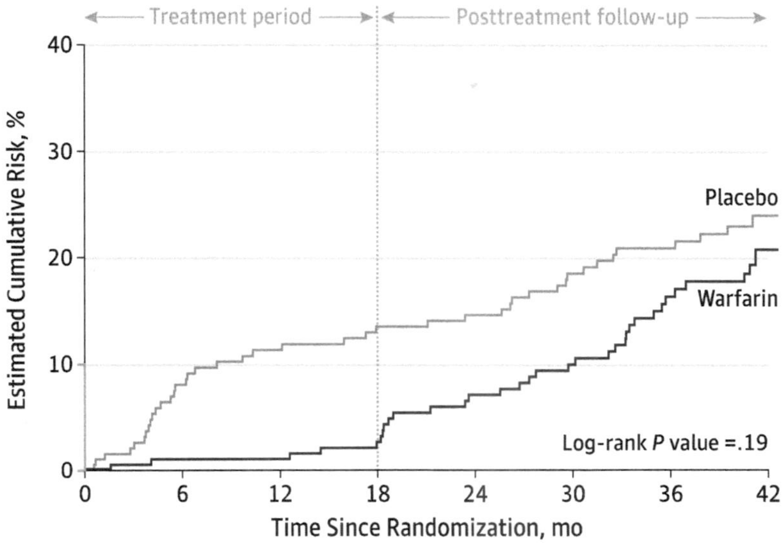


No. at risk

| | | | | | | | | |
|---|---|---|---|---|---|---|---|---|
| Placebo | 187 | 170 | 162 | 158 | 155 | 140 | 117 | 104 |
| Warfarin | 184 | 182 | 180 | 174 | 168 | 150 | 120 | 110 |

FIGURE 2.—Probability of the composite outcome of recurrent venous thromboembolism and major bleeding throughout the study period. The unadjusted hazard ratios for warfarin-placebo were 0.23 (95% CI, 0.09-0.55) during the treatment period and 0.74 (95% CI, 0.47-1.17) for the entire study period. The y axis that is shown in blue indicates the range of estimated cumulative risk from 0%to 10%. For Interpretation of the references to color in this figure legend, the reader is referred to web version of this article.(Reprinted from Couturaud F, for the PADIS-PE Investigators. Six months vs extended oral anticoagulation after a first episode of pulmonary embolism: The PADIS-PE randomized clinical trial. *JAMA*. 2015;314:31-40, with permission from American Medical Association.)

figure (Fig 2). During the 18 months of additional therapy in the intervention group, there was a reduction in recurrent events with minimal increased bleeding risk; however, in the last 18 months of follow-up the risk of recurrent embolism returned. Recurrent episodes of emboli tended to mirror the initial presentation; however, 4 of 52 episodes of recurrent events were fatal. This raises the question—especially with newer types of oral anticoagulation that do not require close monitoring—of whether patients with unprovoked pulmonary emboli should have indefinite anticoagulation.

**J. R. Maurer, MD, MBA**

---

**National Trends in Pulmonary Embolism Hospitalization Rates and Outcomes for Adults Aged ≥65 Years in the United States (1999 to 2010)**

Minges KE, Bikdeli B, Wang Y, et al (Yale-New Haven Hosp, New Haven, CT; Yale School of Medicine, New Haven, CT; et al)

*Am J Cardiol* 116:1436-1442, 2015

---

Little is known about national trends of pulmonary embolism (PE) hospitalizations and outcomes in older adults in the context of recent diagnostic and therapeutic advances. Therefore, we conducted a retrospective cohort study of 100% Medicare fee-for-service beneficiaries hospitalized from 1999 to 2010 with a principal discharge diagnosis code for PE. The adjusted PE hospitalization rate increased from 129/100,000 person-years in 1999 to 302/100,000 person-years in 2010, a relative increase of 134% ($p < 0.001$). Black patients had the highest rate of increase (174 to 548/100,000 person-years) among all age, gender, and race categories. The mean (standard deviation) length of hospital stay decreased from 7.6 (5.7) days in 1999 to 5.8 (4.4) days in 2010, and the proportion of patients discharged to home decreased from 51.1% (95% confidence interval [CI] 50.5 to 51.6) to 44.1% (95% CI 43.7 to 44.6), whereas more patients were discharged with home health care and to skilled nursing facilities. The in-hospital mortality rate decreased from 8.3% (95% CI 8.0 to 8.6) in 1999 to 4.4% (95% CI 4.2 to 4.5) in 2010, as did adjusted 30-day (from 12.3% [95% CI 11.9 to 12.6] to 9.1% [95% CI 8.5 to 9.7]) and 6-month mortality rates (from 23.0% [95% CI 22.5 to 23.4] to 19.6% [95% CI 18.8 to 20.5]). There were no significant racial differences in mortality rates by 2010. There was no change in the adjusted 30-day all-cause readmission rate from 1999 to 2010. In conclusion, PE hospitalization rates increased substantially from 1999 to 2010, with a higher rate for black patients. All mortality rates decreased but remained high. The increase in hospitalization rates and continued high mortality and readmission rates confirm the significant burden of PE for older adults.

▶ Pulmonary embolism is a common, potentially lethal disease. One of the largest risk factors, aside from coagulation abnormalities, is advancing age. The United States and many other industrialized countries have a rapidly increasing population over age of 65 putting them into a high-risk group for pulmonary emboli. In this setting, the authors chose to review Medicare fee-for-service claims data to determine trends in pulmonary emboli hospitalizations in the first decade of the 21st century. That the rates of hospitalization have increased is not surprising because not only is there a much larger population older than 65, but there are also many more people in their 80s and 90s. Despite the more than 100% rise is hospitalization rate, however, the in-hospital, 30-day, and 6-month mortality rates all fell, and 30-day readmissions did not change. Length of stay also shortened. These changes are probably due in part to cost pressures on hospitals but may also be a result of healthier patients in the "younger" Medicare age groups. This could be true even though the percent of patients discharged to home decreased from around 51% to 44%, likely because of the increasing population of the very old. This increasing rate of hospitalization will increase the financial burden of this disease on the Medicare system as the population continues to age. Given the shorter length of stays and decreasing early mortalities, it is conceivable that a low-risk subgroup of these patients could be identified through sophisticated scoring systems—some already exist—and could be treated as outpatients based on careful selection criteria.

**J. R. Maurer, MD, MBA**

# 33 Community-Acquired Pneumonia

## Ten-Year Mortality after Community-acquired Pneumonia: A Prospective Cohort

Eurich DT, Marrie TJ, Minhas-Sandhu JK, et al (Univ of Alberta, Edmonton, Canada; Dalhousie Univ, Halifax, Nova Scotia, Canada)
*Am J Respir Crit Care Med* 192:597-604, 2015

*Rationale.*—Information on the long-term prognosis after community-acquired pneumonia (CAP) is limited.

*Objectives.*—To determine if CAP increases adverse long-term outcomes relative to a control population.

*Methods.*—Between 2000 and 2002, 6,078 adults with CAP from six hospitals and seven emergency departments in Edmonton (AB, Canada) were prospectively recruited and matched on age, sex, and site of treatment with five control subjects without pneumonia (n = 29,402). Mortality, hospitalizations, and emergency department admissions through 2012 were evaluated using multivariable Cox proportional hazards analyses adjusted for socioeconomic status and comorbidities.

*Measurements and Main Results.*—Average age was 59 years (2,682 [44%] ≥65 yr), 3,214 (53%) were men, and 3,425 (56%) were managed as outpatients. Over a median of 9.8 years, 2,858 patients with CAP died compared with 9,399 control subjects (absolute risk difference, 30 per 1,000 patient years [py]; adjusted hazard ratio [aHR], 1.65; 95% confidence interval, 1.57–1.73; $P < 0.001$). Patients with CAP who were younger than 25 years old had the lowest absolute rate difference for mortality (4 per 1,000 py; aHR, 2.40), and patients older than 80 years old had the highest absolute rate difference (92 per 1,000 py; aHR, 1.42). Absolute rates of all-cause hospitalization, emergency department visits, and CAP-related visits were all significantly higher in patients with CAP compared with control subjects ($P < 0.001$ for all comparisons).

*Conclusions.*—Our results indicate that an episode of CAP confers a high risk of long-term adverse events compared with the general population who have not experienced CAP, and this is irrespective of age.

▶ Many studies have focused on hospitalizations for community-acquired pneumonia (CAP) and the huge costs to the health care system. We also know a lot about early mortality rates and increasing mortality rates with age as well as the high propensity for discharged patients to be readmitted shortly after discharge (20%). The long-term survival rates have been less studied. This Canadian study followed all patients presenting to emergency departments or hospitals in Edmonton, Alberta, who had documented evidence of pneumonia and followed them as well as matched controls with no pneumonia for 10 years. It may be intuitive that the older age groups had a higher mortality rate than those under 25, but even in that young group, the death rate was significantly higher than controls. CAP patients died of similar causes as control subjects—primarily cardiovascular and neoplasms—except for respiratory disease, which was more than twice as common in the CAP group. Over the entire population, there were 30 excess deaths per 1000 patient years of follow-up (50% relative increased rate of mortality) compared with non-CAP patients. Of course, most of the absolute increase in deaths occurred in the older age groups, but middle-aged cohorts suffered significant increases and increases in morbidity as well. This study provides a better understanding of the burden placed on the health care system by a problem not previously considered a "chronic disease" and should stimulate more investigation into the pathogenesis and mechanisms that contribute to the ongoing morbidity of these infections.

**J. R. Maurer, MD, MBA**

---

**Association Between Hospitalization for Pneumonia and Subsequent Risk of Cardiovascular Disease**

Corrales-Medina VF, Alvarez KN, Weissfeld LA, et al (Univ of Ottawa, Ontario, Canada; Univ of Pittsburgh, PA; et al)

*JAMA* 313:264-274, 2015

---

*Importance.*—The risk of cardiovascular disease (CVD) after infection is poorly understood.

*Objective.*—To determine whether hospitalization for pneumonia is associated with an increased short-term and long-term risk of CVD.

*Design, Settings, and Participants.*—We examined 2 community-based cohorts: the Cardiovascular Health Study (CHS, n = 5888; enrollment age, ≥65 years; enrollment period, 1989–1994) and the Atherosclerosis Risk in Communities study (ARIC, n = 15 792; enrollment age, 45-64 years; enrollment period, 1987–1989). Participants were followed up through December 31, 2010. We matched each participant hospitalized with pneumonia to 2 controls. Pneumonia cases and controls were followed for occurrence of CVD over 10 years after matching. We estimated hazard ratios (HRs) for CVD at different time intervals, adjusting for demographics, CVD risk factors, subclinical CVD, comorbidities, and functional status.

*Exposures.*—Hospitalization for pneumonia.

*Main Outcomes and Measures.*—Incident CVD (myocardial infarction, stroke, and fatal coronary heart disease).

*Results.*—Of 591 pneumonia cases in CHS, 206 had CVD events over 10 years after pneumonia hospitalization. Compared with controls,

CVD risk among pneumonia cases was highest during the first year after hospitalization and remained significantly higher than among controls through 10 years. In ARIC, of 680 pneumonia cases, 112 had CVD events over 10 years after hospitalization. After the second year, CVD risk among pneumonia cases was not significantly higher than among controls.

| | Pneumonia Cases | Controls | HR (95% CI) |
|---|---|---|---|
| CHS | | | |
| No. of participants | 591 | 1182 | |
| CVD events | | | |
| 0-30 d | 54 | 6 | 4.07 (2.86-5.27) |
| 31-90 d | 11 | 9 | 2.94 (2.18-3.70) |
| 91 d-1 y | 22 | 55 | 2.10 (1.59-2.60) |
| 9-10 y | 4 | 12 | 1.86 (1.18-2.55) |
| ARIC | | | |
| No. of participants | 680 | 1360 | |
| CVD events | | | |
| 0-30 d | 4 | 3 | 2.38 (1.12-3.63) |
| 31-90 d | 4 | 0 | 2.40 (1.23-3.47) |
| 91 d-1 y | 11 | 8 | 2.19 (1.20-3.19) |
| 1-2 y | 8 | 7 | 1.88 (1.10-2.66) |

*Conclusions and Relevance.*—Hospitalization for pneumonia was associated with increased short-term and long-term risk of CVD, suggesting that pneumonia may be a risk factor for CVD.

▶ Several studies published in 2015 placed a sharp focus on cardiac complications of community-acquired pneumonia (CAP). The Corrales-Medina et al study used 2 large databases, 1 with patients 65 or older and 1 with patients younger than 65, and compared cardiovascular events in each group to controls without a pneumonia episode. The impact on cardiovascular risk in both groups, but particularly in the older group, over a long period is striking. In a prospectively designed Italian study, Cangemi et al found that 18% of 301 patients admitted for CAP experienced a cardiac event ranging from acute myocardial infarction to atrial fibrillation. Most of the patients experiencing these events were at least 70 years old. By a year and a half after the hospitalization, 89 patients had died. This included 51% of those who had an in-hospital cardiac event and 26% of those who did not. After discharge, 73 experienced cardiac events; this included 47% of those who had had an in hospital event and 19% of those who had not.[1] Other studies have identified a high risk of new-onset heart failure in older patients after hospitalization for pneumonia.[2] Research is ongoing into the mechanism of how these events are precipitated in at risk patients. New data suggest that the intense inflammation that accompanies pneumonia, particularly severe pneumonia, may be a major culprit. Platelet activation is probably part of that inflammatory milieu, and platelet activation plays a key role in acute coronary ischemia events.[3] If this is found to be a primary cause of the coronary events, a variety of "interruptive" or therapeutic interventions (such as short steroid courses described elsewhere in this Year Book section) might be potentially valuable in ameliorating the risk.

**J. R. Maurer, MD, MBA**

*References*


1. Cangemi R, Calvieri C, Falcone M, et al. SIXTUS Study Group. Relation of cardiac complications in the early phase of community-acquired pneumonia to long-term mortality and cardiovascular events. *Am J Cardiol.* 2015;116:647-651.
2. Corrales-Medina VF, Taljaard M, Yende S, et al. Intermediate and long-term risk of new-onset heart failure after hospitalization for pneumonia in elderly adults. *Am Heart J.* 2015;170:306-312.
3. Feldman C, Anderson R. Community-acquired pneumonia: pathogenesis of acute cardiac events and potential adjunctive therapies. *Chest.* 2015;148:523-532.


---

**Sensitivity, Specificity, and Positivity Predictors of the Pneumococcal Urinary Antigen Test in Community-Acquired Pneumonia**

Molinos L, Zalacain R, Menéndez R, et al (Hosp Universitario Central Asturias, Oviedo, Spain; Hosp de Cruces, Baracaldo (Bizkaia), Spain; Hosp Universitario La Fe, Valencia, Spain; et al)

*Ann Am Thorac Soc* 12:1482-1489, 2015

---


*Rationale.*—Detection of the C-polysaccharide of *Streptococcus pneumoniae* in urine by an immune-chromatographic test is increasingly used to evaluate patients with community-acquired pneumonia.

*Objectives.*—We assessed the sensitivity and specificity of this test in the largest series of cases to date and used logistic regression models to determine predictors of positivity in patients hospitalized with community-acquired pneumonia.

*Methods.*—We performed a multicenter, prospective, observational study of 4,374 patients hospitalized with community-acquired pneumonia.

*Measurements and Main Results.*—The urinary antigen test was done in 3,874 cases. Pneumococcal infection was diagnosed in 916 cases (21%); 653 (71%) of these cases were diagnosed exclusively by the urinary antigen test. Sensitivity and specificity were 60 and 99.7%, respectively. Predictors of urinary antigen positivity were female sex; heart rate $\geq$ 125 bpm, systolic blood pressure < 90 mm Hg, and $SaO_2$ < 90%; absence of antibiotic treatment; pleuritic chest pain; chills; pleural effusion; and blood urea nitrogen $\geq$ 30 mg/dl. With at least six of all these predictors present, the probability of positivity was 52%. With only one factor present, the probability was only 12%.

*Conclusions.*—The urinary antigen test is a method with good sensitivity and excellent specificity in diagnosing pneumococcal pneumonia, and its use greatly increased the recognition of community-acquired pneumonia due to *S. pneumoniae*. With a specificity of 99.7%, this test could be used to direct simplified antibiotic therapy, thereby avoiding excess costs and risk for bacterial resistance that result from broad-spectrum antibiotics. We also identified predictors of positivity that could increase suspicion

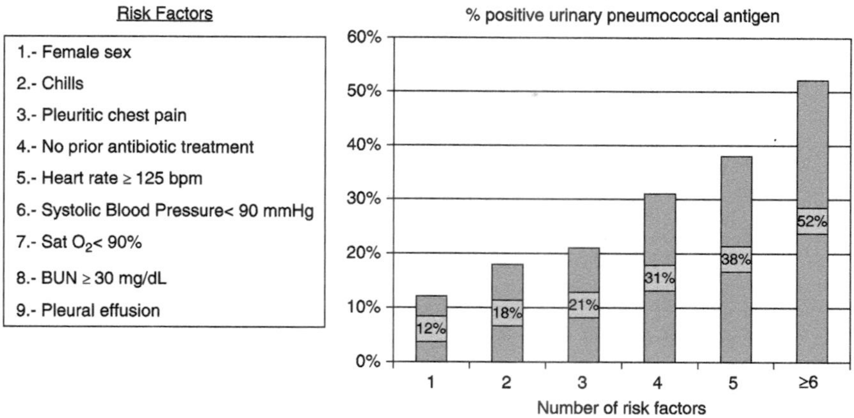


FIGURE 2.—Risk of positive pneumococcal urinary antigen testing in patients with community-acquired pneumonia according to the number of predictors present. BUN = blood urea nitrogen. (Reprinted from Molinos L, Zalacain R, Menéndez R, et al. Sensitivity, specificity, and positivity predictors of the pneumococcal urinary antigen test in community-acquired pneumonia. *Ann Am Thorac Soc* 2015;12:1482-1489, with permission from American Thoracic Society.)

for pneumococcal infection or avoid the unnecessary use of this test (Fig 2).

► *Streptococcus pneumoniae* is the most common bacterial cause of community-acquired pneumonia (CAP), but it is often difficult to get a good-quality sputum for Gram stain and culture, and blood cultures are positive in only 20% to 25% of cases.[1] Guidelines recommend the use of urine antigen testing which detects the C-polysaccharide antigen found in all serotypes.[2,3] However, caregivers have been reluctant to rely on this test to make a diagnosis of pneumococcal pneumonia because reliability of the test has not been clear despite a number of small studies. This report is the largest prospective study to date (4374 patients) that has attempted to determine positivity, sensitivity, and specificity of the test. Another aim was to try to identify patients most likely to present with pneumococcal disease so that the urine antigen test can be selectively applied to those most likely to have pneumococcal disease. In this study, urine antigen testing was much more sensitive than other diagnostic techniques because it alone diagnosed 71% of patients with pneumococcal disease, and it was 99.7% specific in detecting *S pneumoniae*. Using the test when several of the risk factors (Fig 2, p. 1847) for pneumococcal disease identified in the study are present can make a quick and noninvasive diagnosis. As the authors note, early diagnosis will help limit the excessive use of antibiotics and unnecessary additional testing. This study should provide physicians with greater confidence in using the *S pneumoniae* urine antigen in diagnosis and management of CAP.

**J. R. Maurer, MD, MBA**

*References*

1. Said MA, Johnson HL, Nonyane BA, et al. AGEDD Adult Pneumococcal Burden Study Team. Estimating the burden of pneumococcal pneumonia among adults: a systematic review and meta-analysis of diagnostic techniques. *PLoS One*. 2013;8: e60273.
2. Mandell LA, Wunderink RG, Anzueto A, et al. Infectious Diseases Society of America, American Thoracic Society. Infectious Diseases Society of America/American Thoracic Society consensus guidelines on the management of community-acquired pneumonia in adults. *Clin Infect Dis*. 2007;44:S27-S72.
3. Woodhead M, Blasi F, Ewig S, et al. Joint Taskforce of the European Respiratory Society and European Society for Clinical Microbiology and Infectious Diseases. Guidelines for the management of adult lower respiratory tract infections: full version. *Clin Microbiol Infect*. 2011;17:E1-E59.

# 34 Lung Transplantation

**Lung transplantation from donation after cardiocirculatory death: a systematic review and meta-analysis**

Krutsinger D, Reed RM, Blevins A, et al (Univ of Iowa; Univ of Maryland, Baltimore; et al)

*J Heart Lung Transplant* 34:675-684, 2015

*Background.*—Lung transplantation (LTx) can extend life expectancy and enhance the quality of life for select patients with end-stage lung disease. In the setting of donor lung shortage and waiting list mortality, the interest in donation after cardiocirculatory death (DCD) is increasing. We performed a systematic review and meta-analysis to compare outcomes between DCD and conventional donation after brain death (DBD).

*Methods.*—PubMed, CINAHL, Cochrane Database of Systematic Reviews, Database of Abstracts of Reviews of Effects, Cochrane Central Register of Controlled Trials, Scopus, Web of Science, and ClinicalTrials.-gov were searched. We identified original research studies with 1-year post-transplant survival data involving >5 DCD transplants. We performed meta-analyses examining 1-year survival, primary graft dysfunction, and acute rejection after LTx.

*Results.*—We identified 519 citations; 11 observational cohort studies met our inclusion criteria for systematic review, and 6 met our inclusion criteria for meta-analysis. There were no differences found in 1-year mortality after LTx between DCD and DBD cohorts in individual studies or in the meta-analysis (DCD [$n = 271$] vs DBD [$n = 2,369$], relative risk [RR] 0.88, 95% confidence interval [CI] 0.59−1.31, $p = 0.52$, $I^2 = 0\%$). There was also no difference between DCD and DBD in a pooled analysis of 5 studies reporting on primary graft dysfunction (RR 1.09, 95% CI 0.68−1.73, $p = 0.7$, $I^2 = 0\%$) and 4 studies reporting on acute rejection (RR 0.72, 95% CI 0.49−1.05, $p = 0.09$, $I^2 = 0\%$).

*Conclusion.*—Survival after LTx from DCD is comparable to survival after LTx from DBD in observational cohort studies. DCD appears to be a safe and effective method to expand the donor pool.

► Organ donation after circulatory death has some historical roots; however, the most common way that organs are procured is from patients who have suffered brain death but are being maintained on life support so that the cardiocirculatory system is functioning until just before organs are harvested. This clearly limits the organ supply because many patients die of cardiocirculatory arrest without prior complete loss of brain function. It has only been in the past decade or so that non—brain-dead patients have been allowed to clinically die and then have donated organs or that patients arriving clinically dead to emergency facilities have donated organs. Unlike the life-supported patient, organs from the patient who experiences cardiocirculatory arrest has a period of no perfusion to the organs. This ischemic period and the inability at times to optimally control fluid and other management before death has led to some concerns about survival of organs harvested from clinically deceased donors and the outcomes of recipients. Some small and single-center studies have reported reasonable survivals, but this is the largest report and meta-analysis to date. These data show comparable 1-year survivals and, although the numbers are fewer, apparently comparable 3- and 5-year survivals. This needs to be confirmed with larger numbers. Overall, these data support the expanded use of organs donated after cardiocirculatory death, a move that could greatly increase the donor pool.

**J. R. Maurer, MD, MBA**

# 35 Sleep Disorders

**Association of incident obstructive sleep apnoea with outcomes in a large cohort of US veterans**

Molnar MZ, Mucsi I, Novak M, et al (Univ of Tennessee Health Science Ctr, Memphis; Univ of Toronto, Canada; Semmelweis Univ, Budapest, Hungary; et al)

*Thorax* 70:888-895, 2015

*Rationale.*—There is a paucity of large cohort studies examining the association of obstructive sleep apnoea (OSA) with clinical outcomes including all-cause mortality, coronary heart disease (CHD), strokes and chronic kidney disease (CKD).

*Objectives.*—We hypothesised that a diagnosis of incident OSA is associated with higher risks of these adverse clinical outcomes.

*Methods, Measurements.*—In a nationally representative cohort of over 3 million (n = 3 079 514) US veterans (93% male) with baseline estimated glomerular filtration rate (eGFR) ≥60 mL/min/1.73 $m^2$, we examined the association between the diagnosis of incident OSA, treated and untreated with CPAP, and: (1) all-cause mortality, (2) incident CHD, (3) incident strokes, (4) incident CKD defined as eGFR<60 mL/min/1.73 $m^2$, and (5) slopes of eGFR.

*Main Results.*—Compared with OSA-negative patients, untreated and treated OSA was associated with 86% higher mortality risk, (adjusted HR and 95% CI 1.86 (1.81 to 1.91) and 35% (1.35 (1.21 to 1.51)), respectively. Similarly, untreated and treated OSA was associated with 3.5 times (3.54 (3.40 to 3.69)) and 3 times (3.06 (2.62 to 3.56)) higher risk of incident CHD; 3.5 times higher risk of incident strokes (3.48 (3.28 to 3.64) and 3.50 (2.92 to 4.19)) for untreated and treated OSA, respectively. The risk of incident CKD was also significantly higher in untreated (2.27 (2.19 to 2.36)) and treated (2.79 (2.48 to 3.13)) patients with OSA. The median (IQR) of the eGFR slope was −0.41 (−2.01 to 0.99), −0.61 (−2.69 to 0.93) and −0.87 (−3.00 to 0.70) mL/min/1.73 $m^2$ in OSA-negative patients, untreated OSA-positive patients and treated OSA-positive patients, respectively.

*Conclusions.*—In this large and contemporary cohort of more than 3 million US veterans, a diagnosis of incident OSA was associated with higher mortality, incident CHD, stroke and CKD and with faster kidney function decline.

▶ This is an important study because it confirms the findings of previous studies showing an association between incident moderate and severe obstructive sleep apnea (OSA) and cardiovascular disease, declining kidney function, stroke, and mortality. The advantage of this study is its large national sample size (approximately 3 million veterans). The limitations are the biases that are often seen in database studies, which rely on diagnostic codes; namely, the study accuracy is only as good as the accuracy of diagnostic codes entered. The sample size was predominately male and white. The OSA-treated group were surprisingly a small portion of the entire OSA group. Therefore, this study does not really tell us whether OSA treatment with continuous positive airway pressure is associated with better outcomes. Nevertheless, this large study highlights the important consequences of OSA.

**S. Shafazand, MD, MS, FRCP(C), FAASM**

---

## Obstructive Sleep Apnea Is Associated with Nonalcoholic Steatohepatitis and Advanced Liver Histology

Corey KE, Misdraji J, Gelrud L, et al (Massachusetts General Hosp, Boston; Bon Secours Richmond Health System, Richmond, VA; et al)
*Dig Dis Sci* 60:2523-2528, 2015

---

*Background and Aims.*—Nonalcoholic fatty liver disease (NAFLD) and obstructive sleep apnea (OSA) are growing in prevalence in the USA. Existing data on the relationship between OSA and NAFLD are conflicting and limited by the use of various histologic definitions of nonalcoholic steatohepatitis (NASH). Using a robust definition of NASH in a large, well-characterized cohort, we sought to evaluate whether OSA was associated with NASH and advanced fibrosis.

*Methods.*—Two hundred and thirteen subjects undergoing weight loss surgery were queried for OSA and then underwent liver biopsy. NASH was defined, as recommended by the American Association for the Study of Liver Disease, by the presence of all of the following: >5% macrovesicular steatosis, lobular inflammation, and hepatocyte ballooning. NAFLD activity score (NAS) was also determined for each subject.

*Results.*—Subjects with OSA had significantly higher alanine and aspartate aminotransferase levels than subjects without OSA (ALT 54.1 vs. 37.7 U/L, $P = 0.0007$; AST 31.7 vs. 20.5 U/L, $P = 0.0007$). OSA was associated with the presence of NASH, and this remained significant after adjusting for age, gender, race, and diabetes mellitus ($P = 0.03$ OR 2.01; 95%, 1.05–3.87). Steatosis grade, lobular inflammation grade, NAS score, and fibrosis stage were all significantly associated with the presence of OSA and remained so after adjustment.

*Conclusions.*—OSA is associated with elevated aminotransferase levels, the presence of NASH, and advanced NASH histology. Further studies are needed to evaluate the impact of OSA treatment on NASH.

▶ Nonalcoholic fatty liver disease (NAFLD) is the most common cause of liver disease in the United States and is growing in prevalence. Nonalcoholic steatohepatitis (NASH), the progressive form of NAFLD, can lead to cirrhosis and eventual need for liver transplantation. Animal studies suggest an association between intermittent hypoxemia (hallmark of obstructive sleep apnea [OSA]) and hepatocellular damage.[1] Human studies are conflicted in whether there is an association between OSA and NASH. In this study, the authors report on a cross-sectional analysis of liver biopsy results from a cohort of predominately women being evaluated for weight loss surgery. The diagnosis of NASH was based on objective criteria noted on liver biopsy. However, OSA diagnosis was based on patient self-report of a previous polysomnography. As a result, there was no information on OSA severity, nor were the investigators able to confirm the diagnosis of OSA in most instances. This is an important limitation of the study. As a cross-sectional study, no conclusions can be made about causation; however, this is an important study of reasonable size showing an association between OSA and liver fibrosis. Additional studies are needed to determine whether severity of OSA (Apnea Hypopnea Index, oxygen desaturation index) is associated with increasing severity of NASH. Additionally, it is not known whether treatment of OSA will play a role on reversing liver injury.

**S. Shafazand, MD, MS, FRCP(C), FAASM**

*Reference*

1. Savransky V, Nanayakkara A, Vivero A, et al. Chronic intermittent hypoxia predisposes to liver injury. *Hepatology.* 2007;45:1007-1013.

---

**Racial/Ethnic Differences in Sleep Disturbances: The Multi-Ethnic Study of Atherosclerosis (MESA)**

Chen X, Wang R, Zee P, et al (Harvard School of Public Health, Boston, MA; Harvard Med School, Boston, MA; Northwestern Univ School of Medicine, Chicago, IL; et al)

*Sleep* 38:877-888, 2015

---

*Objectives.*—There is limited research on racial/ethnic variation in sleep disturbances. This study aimed to quantify the distributions of objectively measured sleep disordered breathing (SDB), short sleep duration, poor sleep quality, and self-reported sleep disturbances (e.g., insomnia) across racial/ethnic groups.

*Design.*—Cross-sectional study.

*Setting.*—Six US communities.

*Participants.*—Racially/ethnically diverse men and women aged 54–93 y in the Multi-Ethnic Study of Atherosclerosis Sleep Cohort (n = 2,230).

*Interventions.*—N/A.

*Measurements and Results.*—Information from polysomnography-measured SDB, actigraphy-measured sleep duration and quality, and self-reported daytime sleepiness were obtained between 2010 and 2013. Overall, 15.0% of individuals had severe SDB (apnea-hypopnea index [AHI] $\geq$ 30); 30.9% short sleep duration (< 6 h); 6.5% poor sleep quality (sleep efficiency < 85%); and 13.9% had daytime sleepiness. Compared with Whites, Blacks had higher odds of sleep apnea syndrome (AHI $\geq$ 5

**TABLE 2.**—Sleep Disturbances of Study Participants Across Racial/Ethnic Groups

| | White | | Black | | Hispanic | | Chinese | | |
|---|---|---|---|---|---|---|---|---|---|
| | n | % or Mean (SD) | n | % or Mean (SD) | n | % or Mean (SD) | n | % or Mean (SD) | *P* Value[a] |
| Diagnosed sleep apnea, % | | | | | | | | | |
| No | 738 | 89.2 | 551 | 90.0 | 485 | 92.0 | 253 | 96.6 | 0.002 |
| Yes | 89 | 10.8 | 61 | 10.0 | 42 | 8.0 | 9 | 3.4 | |
| Total | 827 | | 612 | | 527 | | 262 | | |
| Habitual snoring, % | | | | | | | | | |
| No | 530 | 64.0 | 390 | 63.7 | 267 | 50.6 | 149 | 56.9 | < 0.001 |
| Yes | 298 | 36.0 | 222 | 36.3 | 261 | 49.4 | 113 | 43.1 | |
| Total | 828 | | 612 | | 528 | | 262 | | |
| AHI (events/h), mean (SD) | 734 | 13.3 (15.5) | 572 | 14.9 (17.8) | 487 | 16.6 (17.2) | 241 | 16.0 (16.6) | 0.005 |
| SDB category, % | | | | | | | | | |
| Normal (AHI < 5) | 273 | 37.2 | 209 | 36.5 | 139 | 28.5 | 81 | 33.6 | 0.024 |
| Mild SDB (AHI = 5–14) | 239 | 32.6 | 178 | 31.1 | 162 | 33.3 | 65 | 27.0 | |
| Moderate SDB (AHI = 15–29) | 131 | 17.9 | 100 | 17.5 | 100 | 20.5 | 52 | 21.6 | |
| Severe SDB (AHI ≥ 30) | 91 | 12.4 | 85 | 14.9 | 86 | 17.7 | 43 | 17.8 | |
| Total | 734 | | 572 | | 487 | | 241 | | |
| Sleep apnea syndrome[b], % | | | | | | | | | |
| No | 680 | 92.6 | 499 | 87.2 | 438 | 89.9 | 217 | 90.0 | 0.014 |
| Yes | 54 | 7.4 | 73 | 12.8 | 49 | 10.1 | 24 | 10.0 | |
| Total | 734 | | 572 | | 487 | | 241 | | |
| Sleep duration (h), mean (SD) | 787 | 6.85 (1.22) | 590 | 6.05 (1.41) | 496 | 6.56 (1.37) | 229 | 6.35 (1.34) | < 0.001 |
| Sleep duration category, % | | | | | | | | | |
| < 6 h | 152 | 19.3 | 256 | 43.4 | 156 | 31.5 | 85 | 37.1 | < 0.001 |

| | | | | | | | | | |
|---|---|---|---|---|---|---|---|---|---|
| 6–7 h | 249 | 31.6 | 193 | 32.7 | 150 | 30.2 | 61 | 26.6 | |
| 7–8 h | 271 | 34.4 | 97 | 16.4 | 124 | 25.0 | 64 | 28.0 | |
| ≥ 8 h | 115 | 14.6 | 44 | 7.5 | 66 | 13.3 | 19 | 8.3 | |
| Total | 787 | | 590 | | 496 | | 229 | | |
| Sleep maintenance efficiency (%), mean (SD) | 787 | 91.4 (3.4) | 590 | 90.3 (3.9) | 496 | 90.5 (3.4) | 229 | 90.7 (3.6) | < 0.001 |
| Sleep quality[c], % | | | | | | | | | |
| Good | 748 | 95.0 | 541 | 91.7 | 463 | 93.4 | 214 | 93.5 | 0.098 |
| Poor | 39 | 5.0 | 49 | 8.3 | 33 | 6.7 | 15 | 6.6 | |
| Total | | 787 | | 590 | | 496 | | 229 | |
| Insomnia[d], % | | | | | | | | | |
| No | 642 | 77.5 | 459 | 75.0 | 388 | 73.5 | 220 | 84.0 | 0.007 |
| Yes | 186 | 22.5 | 153 | 25.0 | 140 | 26.5 | 42 | 16.0 | |
| Total | | 828 | | 612 | | 528 | | 262 | |
| Excessive daytime sleepiness[e], % | | | | | | | | | |
| No | 734 | 88.7 | 497 | 81.2 | 456 | 86.4 | 233 | 88.9 | < 0.001 |
| Yes | 94 | 11.4 | 115 | 18.8 | 72 | 13.6 | 29 | 11.1 | |
| Total | | 828 | | 612 | | 528 | | 262 | |

[a]Analysis of variance was conducted for continuous variables and chi-square test was conducted for categorical variables.
[b]Sleep apnea syndrome was defined as having AHI ≥ 5 and the Epworth Sleepiness Scale (ESS) score > 10.
[c]Sleep quality was defined as poor if the actigraphy-measured sleep maintenance efficiency < 85%, whereas sleep quality was defined as good if the sleep maintenance efficiency ≥ 85%.
[d]The 5-item Women's Health Initiative Insomnia Rating Scale (WHIIRS) was used to define insomnia, with the total score of WHIIRS > 10 as having insomnia.
[e]Excessive daytime sleepiness was assessed using the Epworth Sleepiness Scale (ESS) score > 10. AHI, apnea-hypopnea index; SD, standard deviation; SDB, sleep disordered breathing.
Reprinted from Chen X, Wang R, Zee P, et al. Racial/ethnic differences in sleep disturbances: the Multi-Ethnic Study of Atherosclerosis (MESA). *Sleep*. 2015;38:877-888.

plus sleepiness) (sex-, age-, and study site-adjusted odds ratio [OR] = 1.78, 95% confidence interval [CI]: 1.20, 2.63), short sleep (OR = 4.95, 95% CI: 3.56, 6.90), poor sleep quality (OR = 1.57, 95% CI: 1.00, 2.48), and daytime sleepiness (OR = 1.89, 95% CI: 1.38, 2.60). Hispanics and Chinese had higher odds of SDB and short sleep than Whites. Among non-obese individuals, Chinese had the highest odds of SDB compared to Whites. Only 7.4% to 16.2% of individuals with an AHI ≥ 15 reported a prior diagnosis of sleep apnea.

*Conclusions.*—Sleep disturbances are prevalent among middle-aged and older adults, and vary by race/ethnicity, sex, and obesity status. The high prevalence of sleep disturbances and undiagnosed sleep apnea among racial/ethnic minorities may contribute to health disparities (Table 2).

▶ The Multi-Ethnic Study of Atherosclerosis (MESA) is a multicenter prospective study designed to look at subclinical cardiovascular disease in a racially and ethnically diverse population. This article presents the initial findings from the MESA sleep ancillary study; 2230 patients underwent polysomnography and actigraphy and completed validated questionnaires for evaluating insomnia and excessive daytime sleepiness. The study cohort was 37% white, 27% black, 24% Hispanic, and 12% Chinese, with a slight predominance of women. The value of this study is that it is population based, using objective measures of sleep apnea and sleep duration and inclusive of multiple races and ethnicities. Table 2 demonstrates the sleep disturbances across the cohort; blacks had the highest prevalence of symptomatic sleep apnea, whereas Chinese had the lowest prevalence of insomnia. This study highlights the high prevalence of undiagnosed sleep disturbances in middle-aged and older adults and identifies racial/ethnic disparities in sleep.

**S. Shafazand, MD, MS, FRCP(C), FAASM**

# 36 Critical Care Medicine

**Acute respiratory distress syndrome in patients with and without diffuse alveolar damage: an autopsy study**

Lorente JA, Cardinal-Fernández P, Muñoz D, et al (Universidad Europea, Madrid, Spain; Hosp Universitario de Sanchinarro, Madrid, Spain; Universidad CES, Medellín, Colombia; et al)

*Intensive Care Med* 41:1921-1930, 2015

*Objective.*—To demonstrate that among patients with acute respiratory distress syndrome (ARDS), the presence of diffuse alveolar damage (DAD) at histological examination, as compared to its absence, defines a specific subphenotype.

*Methods.*—We studied 149 patients who died in our ICU with the clinical diagnosis of ARDS according to the Berlin Definition (BD) and who had autopsy examination. We compared the change over time of different clinical variables in patients with ($n = 49$) and without ($n = 100$) DAD. A predictive model for the presence of DAD was developed and validated in an independent cohort of 57 patients with ARDS and postmortem examination (21 of them with DAD).

*Results.*—Patients with DAD, as compared to patients without DAD, had a lower $PaO_2/FiO_2$ ratio and dynamic respiratory system compliance, and a higher SOFA score and INR, and were more likely to die of hypoxemia and less likely to die of shock. In multivariate analysis, variables associated with DAD [odds ratio, 95 % confidence interval (CI)] were $PaO_2/FiO_2$ ratio [0.988 (0.981–0.995)], dynamic respiratory system compliance [0.937 (0.892–0.984)] and age [0.972 (0.946–0.999)]. Areas under the ROC curve (95 % CI) for the classification of DAD using the regression model or the BD were, respectively, 0.74 (0.65–0.82) and 0.64 (0.55–0.72) ($p = 0.03$). In the validation cohort, the areas under the ROC curve for the diagnosis of DAD were 0.73 (0.56–0.90) and 0.67 (0.54–0.81) for the regression model and the BD, respectively.

*Conclusions.*—The presence of DAD appears to define a specific subphenotype in patients with ARDS. Targeting patients with DAD within the population of patients with the clinical diagnosis of ARDS might be appropriate to find effective therapies for this condition.

▶ This article demonstrates how clinical suspicion and diagnosis may not match histopathological findings and how a predictive model based on the physiology of acute respiratory distress syndrome (ARDS) could lead to a more accurate diagnosis. The Berlin definition for ARDS provides us with a clinical tool based on patient data. Questions remain was to whether chest imaging, $Pao_2/Fio_2$ ratio and other clinical characteristics are accurate enough to make the diagnosis of ARDS. The histopathological findings in this study with nonsurvivors, who met the Berlin definition of ARDS, show that the presence of diffuse alveolar damage (DAD) was not identified in all of the cases. The 2 groups, ARDS patients who had DAD versus those without DAD, demonstrate a difference clinically and their cause of death. Given the limitations in this study, is difficult to establish whether the variables used in this article are sufficient to create a prediction model of which patient has ARDS with DAD. However, the results bring into the spotlight how patients who meet the Berlin definition of ARDS do not necessarily imply the pathology of DAD. Evaluating other variables and adding it to the present criteria could improve accuracy of diagnosis and potentially change patient management. Future studies with ARDS patients could determine the clinical impact of the proposed prediction model in this disease.

**A. J. Malavé, MD**

---

**Driving Pressure and Survival in the Acute Respiratory Distress Syndrome**

Amato MBP, Meade MO, Slutsky AS, et al (Univ of São Paulo, Brazil; McMaster Univ, Hamilton, Ontario, Canada; St. Michael's Hosp, Ontario, Canada; et al)

*N Engl J Med* 372:747-755, 2015

---

*Background.*—Mechanical-ventilation strategies that use lower end-inspiratory (plateau) airway pressures, lower tidal volumes ($V_T$), and higher positive end-expiratory pressures (PEEPs) can improve survival in patients with the acute respiratory distress syndrome (ARDS), but the relative importance of each of these components is uncertain. Because respiratory-system compliance ($C_{RS}$) is strongly related to the volume of aerated remaining functional lung during disease (termed functional lung size), we hypothesized that driving pressure ($\Delta P = V_T/C_{RS}$), in which $V_T$ is intrinsically normalized to functional lung size (instead of predicted lung size in healthy persons), would be an index more strongly associated with survival than $V_T$ or PEEP in patients who are not actively breathing.

*Methods.*—Using a statistical tool known as multilevel mediation analysis to analyze individual data from 3562 patients with ARDS enrolled in nine previously reported randomized trials, we examined $\Delta P$ as an independent variable associated with survival. In the mediation analysis, we estimated the isolated effects of changes in ΔP resulting from randomized ventilator settings while minimizing confounding due to the baseline severity of lung disease.

*Results.*—Among ventilation variables, ΔP was most strongly associated with survival. A 1-SD increment in ΔP (approximately 7 cm of water) was associated with increased mortality (relative risk, 1.41; 95% confidence interval [CI], 1.31 to 1.51; $P < 0.001$), even in patients receiving "protective" plateau pressures and $V_T$ (relative risk, 1.36; 95% CI, 1.17 to 1.58; $P < 0.001$). Individual changes in $V_T$ or PEEP after randomization were not independently associated with survival; they were associated only if they were among the changes that led to reductions in ΔP (mediation effects of ΔP, $P = 0.004$ and $P = 0.001$, respectively).

*Conclusions.*—We found that ΔP was the ventilation variable that best stratified risk. Decreases in ΔP owing to changes in ventilator settings were strongly associated with increased survival. (Funded by Fundação de Amparo e Pesquisa do Estado de São Paulo and others.)

▶ Acute respiratory distress syndrome (ARDS) continues to have a high mortality despite advances in technology and changes in its management. We continue to search for the "smoking gun" that could improve further patient survival. Since the ARDsNET study, our goals of lung protective strategy with low tidal volumes, monitoring plateau pressures, and determining the effective positive end expiratory pressure (PEEP) have remained our main tools in managing this critically ill patients. This article brings to light perhaps another tool in the armamentarium to treat ARDS. Considering the physiology of this syndrome and the parameters adjusted and monitored in mechanical ventilation, driving pressure presents a promising tool. The improvement in mortality, as seen in the comparisons between PEEP and plateau pressures in Figs 1 and 2 of the original article, demonstrates the potential of using driving pressure in treating ARDS and achieving better outcomes in this lethal disease. This article could lead to future studies that will help determine whether driving pressure can become a new standard in the management of ARDS.

**A. J. Malavé, MD**

---

### Effect of Noninvasive Ventilation vs Oxygen Therapy on Mortality Among Immunocompromised Patients With Acute Respiratory Failure: A Randomized Clinical Trial

Lemiale V, for the Groupe de Recherche en Réanimation Respiratoire du patient d'Onco-Hématologie (GRRR-OH) (Saint-Louis Univ Hosp, Paris, France; et al)
*JAMA* 314:1711-1719, 2015

---

*Importance.*—Noninvasive ventilation has been recommended to decrease mortality among immunocompromised patients with hypoxemic acute respiratory failure. However, its effectiveness for this indication remains unclear.

*Objective.*—To determine whether early noninvasive ventilation improved survival in immunocompromised patients with nonhypercapnic acute hypoxemic respiratory failure.

*Design, Setting, and Participants.*—Multicenter randomized trial conducted among 374 critically ill immunocompromised patients, of whom 317 (84.7%) were receiving treatment for hematologic malignancies or solid tumors, at 28 intensive care units (ICUs) in France and Belgium between August 12, 2013, and January 2, 2015.

*Interventions.*—Patients were randomly assigned to early noninvasive ventilation (n = 191) or oxygen therapy alone (n = 183).

*Main Outcomes and Measures.*—The primary outcome was day-28 mortality. Secondary outcomes were intubation, Sequential Organ Failure Assessment score on day 3, ICU-acquired infections, duration of mechanical ventilation, and ICU length of stay.

*Results.*—At randomization, median oxygen flow was 9 L/min (interquartile range, 5-15) in the noninvasive ventilation group and 9 L/min (interquartile range, 6-15) in the oxygen group. All patients in the noninvasive ventilation group received the first noninvasive ventilation session immediately after randomization. On day 28 after randomization, 46 deaths (24.1%) had occurred in the noninvasive ventilation group vs 50 (27.3%) in the oxygen group (absolute difference, −3.2 [95% CI, −12.1 to 5.6]; $P = .47$). Oxygenation failure occurred in 155 patients overall (41.4%), 73 (38.2%) in the noninvasive ventilation group and 82 (44.8%) in the oxygen group (absolute difference, −6.6 [95% CI, −16.6 to 3.4]; $P = .20$). There were no significant differences in ICU-acquired infections, duration of mechanical ventilation, or lengths of ICU or hospital stays.

*Conclusions and Relevance.*—Among immunocompromised patients admitted to the ICU with hypoxemic acute respiratory failure, early noninvasive ventilation compared with oxygen therapy alone did not reduce 28-day mortality. However, study power was limited.

*Trial Registration.*—clinicaltrials.gov Identifier: NCT01915719

▶ The risks of intubation and mechanical ventilation in the intensive care unit (ICU), and especially for immunocompromised hosts, is well known and ranges from ventilatory-associated pneumonia, lung injury, ICU-acquired myopathy/neuropathy, venous thromboembolism, delirium, and cognitive dysfunction. The use of noninvasive ventilation for the treatment of hypoxic respiratory failure is therefore a welcome alternative. Two previous small randomized clinical trials showed that the use of noninvasive ventilation was associated with decreased intubation, ICU complications, and mortality.[1,2] In the present study, the impact of noninvasive ventilation is once again studied, but now in modern-day ICUs.

The study was well designed with excellent follow-up and objective outcomes that are also clinically relevant. There was no blinding of study assignment; however, given the nature of the outcomes, it is unlikely to have introduced any bias. The mortality rate in both arms was high, and there was no difference between the groups on study outcomes. It may be that the study lacked power to show a difference and therefore whether noninvasive ventilation is still a viable treatment option. It is interesting to note that a portion of the patients on the oxygen-only arm was actually receiving high-flow oxygen. Given the recent findings of improved mortality with high-flow nasal cannula versus noninvasive ventilation,[3] any potential impact of noninvasive ventilation may have been reduced.

More studies are needed to further determine what role, if any, noninvasive ventilation plays in the management of acute respiratory failure in immunocompromised hosts, and especially whether high-flow oxygen is indeed a beneficial option.

**S. Shafazand, MD, MS, FRCP(C), FAASM**

*References*

1. Hilbert G, Gruson D, Vargas F, et al. Noninvasive ventilation in immunosuppressed patients with pulmonary infiltrates, fever, and acute respiratory failure. *N Engl J Med.* 2001;344:481-487.
2. Delclaux C, L'Her E, Alberti C, et al. Treatment of acute hypoxemic nonhypercapnic respiratory insufficiency with continuous positive airway pressure delivered by a face mask: a randomized controlled trial. *JAMA.* 2000;284:2352-2360.
3. Frat JP, Thille AW, Mercat A, et al. FLORALI Study Group, REVA Network. High-flow oxygen through nasal cannula in acute hypoxemic respiratory failure. *N Engl J Med.* 2015;372:2185-2196.

**PART FIVE**

# HEART AND CARDIOVASCULAR DISEASE

MICHAEL R. GOLD, MD, PhD

# Introduction

We have witnessed a dramatic decline in cardiovascular mortality over the past 50 years. In fact, in many countries cancer is a larger cause of mortality than heart disease at present. This has been driven by improvements in all facets of cardiovascular care from prevention to pharmacologic therapy and interventional procedures. The advances in our understanding of cardiovascular disease continued in 2016 and some of the most important studies are highlighted in this edition of the YEAR BOOK of Medicine. Topics include treatment of atrial fibrillation, leadless pacemakers, treatments for heart failure, advances in devices and adjunctive medical therapy for coronary artery disease and optimization of outcomes and patient selection for cardiac surgery. These advances will likely result in further reductions in morbidity and mortality associated with cardiovascular disease.

**Michael R. Gold, MD, PhD**

# 37 Arrhythmias

### **Use of the Wearable Cardioverter Defibrillator in High-Risk Cardiac Patients: Data From the Prospective Registry of Patients Using the Wearable Cardioverter Defibrillator (WEARIT-II Registry)**

Kutyifa V, Moss AJ, Klein H, et al (Univ of Rochester Med Ctr, NY)
*Circulation* 132:1613-1619, 2015

*Background.*—Prospective data on the safety and efficacy of the wearable cardioverter defibrillator (WCD) in a real-world setting are lacking. The Prospective Registry of Patients Using the Wearable Defibrillator (WEARIT-II) Registry was designed to provide real-world data on the WCD as a strategy during a period of risk stratification.

*Methods and Results.*—The WEARIT-II Registry enrolled 2000 patients with ischemic (n = 805, 40%), or nonischemic cardiomyopathy (n=927, 46%), or congenital/inherited heart disease (n = 268) prescribed WCD between August 2011 and February 2014. Clinical data, arrhythmia events, implantable cardioverter defibrillator implantation, and improvement in ejection fraction were captured. The median age was 62 years; the median ejection fraction was 25%. The median WCD wear time was 90 days, with median daily use of 22.5 hours. There was a total of 120 sustained ventricular tachyarrhythmias in 41 patients, of whom 54% received appropriate WCD shock. Only 10 patients (0.5%) received inappropriate WCD therapy. The rate of sustained ventricular tachyarrhythmias by 3 months was 3% among patients with ischemic cardiomyopathy and congenital/inherited heart disease, and 1% among nonischemic patients (P=0.02). At the end of WCD use, 840 patients (42%) were implanted with an implantable cardioverter defibrillator. The most frequent reason not to implant an implantable cardioverter defibrillator following WCD use was improvement in ejection fraction.

*Conclusions.*—The WEARIT-II Registry demonstrates a high rate of sustained ventricular tachyarrhythmias at 3 months in at-risk patients who are not eligible for an implantable cardioverter defibrillator, and suggests that the WCD can be safely used to protect patients during this period of risk assessment (Fig 2).

▶ The implantable cardioverter defibrillator (ICD) has been shown to be effective in treating ventricular tachyarrhythmias and reducing mortality. This has led

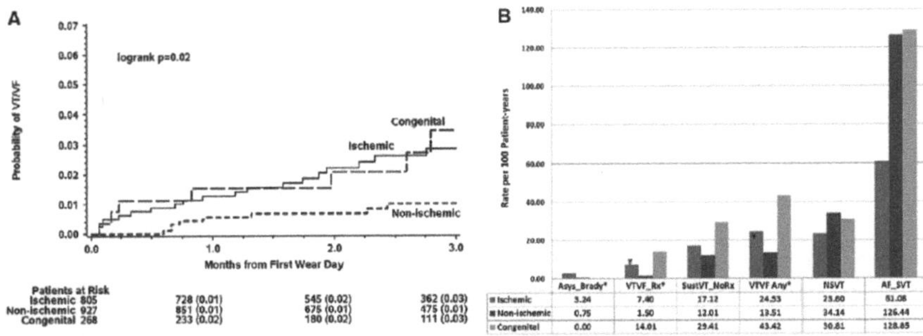


FIGURE 2.—The rate of first arrhythmic events in WCD patients by disease etiology (**A**) and total arrhythmic events in WCD patients by disease etiology (**B**). $^{*}P < 0.05$ for comparison between patients with ischemic, nonischemic, and congenital heart disease. $^{¥}P < 0.05$ for comparison between patients with ischemic and nonischemic heart disease. AF indicates atrial fibrillation; Asys_brady asystole, bradyarrhythmia; NSVT, nonsustained ventricular tachycardia; SustVT_NoRx, sustained VT with no treatment by WCD; SVT, supraventricular tachycardia; VF, ventricular fibrillation; VT, ventricular tachycardia; VTVF_Rx, appropriate therapy; and WCD, wearable cardioverter defibrillator. (Reprinted from Kutyifa V, Moss AJ, Klein H, et al. Use of the wearable cardioverter defibrillator in high-risk cardiac patients: data from the prospective registry of patients using the wearable cardioverter defibrillator (WEARIT-II registry). *Circulation.* 2015;132:1613-1619, with permission from American Heart Association, Inc.)

to guidelines for the use of this device and significant growth in its utilization over the past 2 decades. However, there are many patients who are perceived at risk but may have relative contraindications (eg, recent infection or surgery) or uncertainty regarding the persistence of their risk, most commonly because of new-onset heart failure or cardiomyopathy with short duration of medical therapy. This has led to the development of a wearable defibrillator that can be used as a "bridge" to ICD. WEARIT-II is a large (2000-patient) prospective registry of the use of this device. The important observations from this study are that patients tolerate the wearable device well with good compliance, termination of ventricular arrhythmias was high, and the risk of inappropriate shocks was low. Another important observation was that the risk of ventricular tachycardia or fibrillation was much lower among patients with nonischemic cardiomyopathy (Fig 2). This study provides additional important data on the safety, tolerance, and effectiveness of the wearable defibrillator. However, more information is needed to help optimize patient selection.

**M. Gold, MD, PhD**

---

**Incidence, Cause, and Comparative Frequency of Sudden Cardiac Death in National Collegiate Athletic Association Athletes: A Decade in Review**

Harmon KG, Asif IM, Maleszewski JJ, et al (Univ of Washington, Seattle; Univ of South Carolina Greenville; Mayo Clinic, Rochester, MN; et al)

*Circulation* 132:10-19, 2015

---

*Background.*—The incidence and cause of sudden cardiac death (SCD) in athletes is debated with hypertrophic cardiomyopathy often reported as the most common cause.

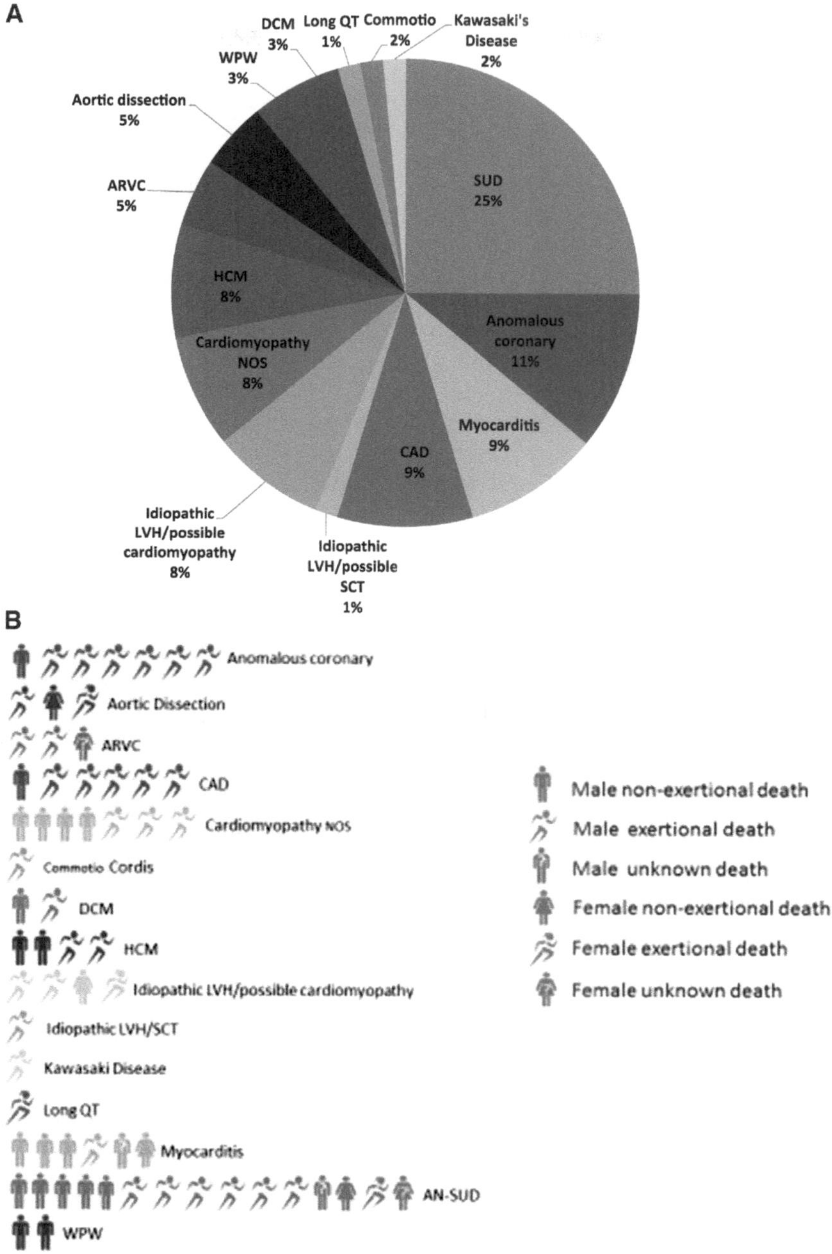


FIGURE 2.—A, Causes of sudden cardiac death in athletes. B, Cause and activity at time of death. One person figure equals 1 death; female figures follow male figures, unless no male deaths were present. AN-SUD indicates autopsy-negative sudden unexplained death; ARVC, arrhythmogenic right ventricular cardiomyopathy; CAD, coronary artery disease; DCM, dilated cardiomyopathy; HCM, hypertrophic cardiomyopathy; LVH, left ventricular hypertrophy; NOS, not otherwise specified; SCT, sickle cell trait; SUD, sudden unexplained death; and WPW, Wolff-Parkinson-White. (Reprinted from Harmon KG, Asif IM, Maleszewski JJ, et al. Incidence, cause, and comparative frequency of sudden cardiac death in national collegiate athletic association athletes: a decade in review. *Circulation*. 2015;132:10-19, with permission from American Heart Association, Inc.)

*Methods and Results.*—A database of all National Collegiate Athletic Association deaths (2003–2013) was developed. Additional information and autopsy reports were obtained when possible. Cause of death was adjudicated by an expert panel. There were 4 242 519 athlete-years (AY) and 514 total student athlete deaths. Accidents were the most common cause of death (257, 50%, 1:16 508 AY) followed by medical causes (147, 29%, 1:28 861 AY). The most common medical cause of death was SCD (79, 15%, 1:53 703 AY). Males were at higher risk than females 1:37 790 AY versus 1:121 593 AY (incidence rate ratio, 3.2; 95% confidence interval, 1.9–5.5; $P < 0.00001$), and black athletes were at higher risk than white athletes 1:21 491 AY versus 1:68 354 AY (incidence rate ratio, 3.2; 95% confidence interval, 1.9–5.2; $P < 0.00001$). The incidence of SCD in Division 1 male basketball athletes was 1:5200 AY. The most common findings at autopsy were autopsy-negative sudden unexplained death in 16 (25%), and definitive evidence for hypertrophic cardiomyopathy was seen in 5 (8%). Media reports identified more deaths in higher divisions (87%, 61%, and 44%), whereas the percentages from the internal database did not vary (87%, 83%, and 89%). Insurance claims identified only 11% of SCDs.

*Conclusions.*—The rate of SCD in National Collegiate Athletic Association athletes is high, with males, black athletes, and basketball players at substantially higher risk. The most common finding at autopsy is autopsy-negative sudden unexplained death. Media reports are more likely to capture high-profile deaths, and insurance claims are not a reliable method for case identification (Fig 2).

▶ Sudden cardiac death (SCD) is a particularly tragic event in the young. SCD in young athletes has been an often-studied problem with much controversy regarding how to screen for such events. It has been often reported that hypertrophic cardiomyopathy is the most common cause among athletes < 40 years old. In the present study, a meticulous analysis of death in college athletes was performed. Accidents are the most common form of death. With regard to SCD, there were significant heterogeneities with regard to the incidence of events. Men and black athletes each have about a 3-fold higher incidence of SCD than women and nonblacks, respectively. The incidence of SCD was highest among basketball players. Importantly, hypertrophic cardiomyopathy was not the leading cause of SCD. Rather, autopsy-negative SCD was reported in 25% of all events (Fig 2). Presumably this included a variety of channelopathies. These findings raise important questions regarding risk stratification for SCD and challenge the potential utility of screening echocardiography.

**M. Gold, MD, PhD**

**Apixaban in Comparison With Warfarin in Patients With Atrial Fibrillation and Valvular Heart Disease: Findings From the Apixaban for Reduction in Stroke and Other Thromboembolic Events in Atrial Fibrillation (ARISTOTLE) Trial**

Avezum A, Lopes RD, Schulte PJ, et al (Dante Pazzanese Inst of Cardiology, São Paulo, Brazil; Duke Clinical Res Inst, Durham, NC; et al)
*Circulation* 132:624-632, 2015

*Background.*—Apixaban is approved for the prevention of stroke and systemic embolism in patients with nonvalvular atrial fibrillation. However, the Apixaban for Reduction in Stroke and Other Thromboembolic Events in Atrial Fibrillation (ARISTOTLE) trial included a substantial number of patients with valvular heart disease and only excluded patients with clinically significant mitral stenosis or mechanical prosthetic heart valves.

*Methods and Results.*—We compared the effect of apixaban and warfarin on rates of stroke or systemic embolism, major bleeding, and death in patients with and without moderate or severe valvular heart disease using Cox proportional hazards modeling. Of the 18 201 patients enrolled in ARISTOTLE, 4808 (26.4%) had a history of moderate or severe valvular heart disease or previous valve surgery. Patients with valvular heart disease had higher rates of stroke or systemic embolism and bleeding than patients without valvular heart disease. There was no evidence of a differential effect of apixaban over warfarin in patients with and without valvular heart disease in reducing stroke and systemic embolism (hazard ratio [HR], 0.70; 95% confidence interval [CI], 0.51–0.97 and HR, 0.84; 95%, CI 0.67–1.04; interaction $P = 0.38$), causing less major bleeding (HR, 0.79; 95% CI, 0.61–1.04 and HR, 0.65; 95% CI, 0.55–0.77; interaction $P = 0.23$), and reducing mortality (HR, 1.01; 95% CI, 0.84–1.22 and HR, 0.84; 95% CI, 0.73–0.96; interaction $P = 0.10$).

*Conclusions.*—More than a quarter of the patients in ARISTOTLE with nonvalvular atrial fibrillation had moderate or severe valvular heart disease. There was no evidence of a differential effect of apixaban over warfarin in reducing stroke or systemic embolism, causing less bleeding, and reducing death in patients with and without valvular heart disease.

*Clinical Trial Registration.*—URL: http://www.clinicaltrials.gov. Unique identifier: NCT00412984 (Fig 2).

► Atrial fibrillation (AF) remains the most common pathologic arrhythmia in clinical practice. The prevention of stroke or systemic embolus is one of the major goals of the treatment of AF. The development of novel oral anticoagulants (NOAC) has markedly simplified the management of "nonvalvular" AF, avoiding the need for dietary restriction and frequent monitoring anticoagulation status. One controversy in the selection of oral anticoagulants in this setting has been the definition nonvalvular AF. The Aristotle study was one of several large

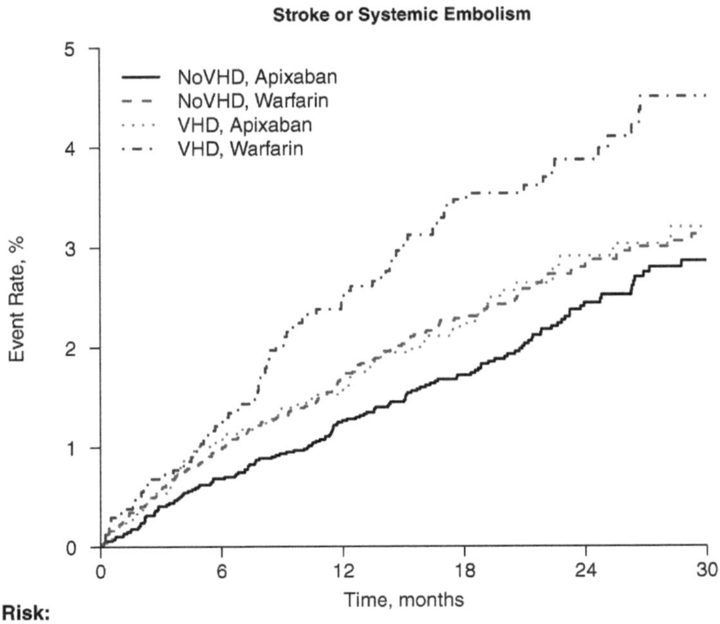


**No. at Risk:**

| | 0 | 6 | 12 | 18 | 24 | 30 |
|---|---|---|---|---|---|---|
| NoVHD, Apixaban | 6681 | 6430 | 6253 | 4534 | 2676 | 1370 |
| NoVHD, Warfarin | 6708 | 6398 | 6207 | 4494 | 2628 | 1375 |
| VHD, Apixaban | 2438 | 2305 | 2222 | 1573 | 919 | 467 |
| VHD, Warfarin | 2370 | 2228 | 2138 | 1547 | 915 | 478 |

FIGURE 2.—Kaplan–Meier estimates. Stroke or systemic embolism in patients with and without valvular heart disease by treatment assignment. VHD indicates valvular heart disease. (Reprinted from Avezum A, Lopes RD, Schulte PJ, et al. Apixaban in comparison with warfarin in patients with atrial fibrillation and valvular heart disease: findings from the apixaban for reduction in stroke and other thromboembolic events in atrial fibrillation (ARISTOTLE) trial. *Circulation.* 2015;132:624-632, with permission from American Heart Association, Inc.)

randomized trials of NOAC. This was a randomized trial of apixaban versus warfarin, showing less bleeding and fewer strokes with the former. In the present analysis, eligible patients without a mechanical prosthetic valve or mitral stenosis were evaluated. Apixaban had similar benefit in this group compared with subjects without any or minimal valvular abnormalities (Fig 2). Importantly, valvular heart disease was a marker of increased risk, regardless of the anticoagulant. These data help clarify and potentially expand the use of NOACs, which should only be avoided in the presence of mechanical heart valves or mitral stenosis. In addition, the presence of valvular abnormalities should lower the threshold for anticoagulation in the presence of AF, as reflected by the CHADSVASC scoring system.

**M. Gold, MD, PhD**

**Ablation Versus Amiodarone for Treatment of Persistent Atrial Fibrillation in Patients With Congestive Heart Failure and an Implanted Device: Results From the AATAC Multicenter Randomized Trial**

Di Biase L, Mohanty P, Mohanty S, et al (Texas Cardiac Arrhythmia Inst at St. David's Med Ctr, Austin; et al)

*Circulation* 133:1637-1644, 2016

*Background.*—Whether catheter ablation (CA) is superior to amiodarone (AMIO) for the treatment of persistent atrial fibrillation (AF) in patients with heart failure is unknown.

*Methods and Results.*—This was an open-label, randomized, parallel-group, multicenter study. Patients with persistent AF, dual-chamber implantable cardioverter defibrillator or cardiac resynchronization therapy defibrillator, New York Heart Association II to III, and left ventricular ejection fraction <40% within the past 6 months were randomly assigned (1:1 ratio) to undergo CA for AF (group 1, n = 102) or receive AMIO (group 2, n = 101). Recurrence of AF was the primary end point. All-cause mortality and unplanned hospitalization were the secondary end points. Patients were followed up for a minimum of 24 months. At the end of follow-up, 71 (70%; 95% confidence interval, 60%–78%) patients in group 1 were recurrence free after an average of 1.4 ± 0.6 procedures in comparison with 34 (34%; 95% confidence interval, 25%–44%) in group 2 (log-rank $P < 0.001$). The success rate of CA in the different centers after a single procedure ranged from 29% to 61%. After adjusting for covariates in the multivariable model, AMIO therapy was found to be significantly more likely to fail (hazard ratio, 2.5; 95% confidence interval, 1.5–4.3; $P < 0.001$) than CA. Over the 2-year follow-up, the unplanned hospitalization rate was (32 [31%] in group 1 and 58 [57%] in group 2; $P < 0.001$), showing 45% relative risk reduction (relative risk, 0.55; 95% confidence interval, 0.39–0.76). A significantly lower mortality was observed in CA (8 [8%] versus AMIO 18 [18%]; $P = 0.037$).

*Conclusions.*—This multicenter randomized study shows that CA of AF is superior to AMIO in achieving freedom from AF at long-term follow-up and reducing unplanned hospitalization and mortality in patients with heart failure and persistent AF.

*Clinical Trial Registration.*—URL: http://www.clinicaltrials.gov. Unique identifier: NCT00729911 (Fig 2).

► Catheter ablation has emerged as an important therapy for the treatment of symptomatic atrial fibrillation (AF). Observational studies suggested that arrhythmia control was better with ablation compared with antiarrhythmic drugs. More recently, a number of small, randomized trials confirmed the superiority of ablation for rhythm control. The Ablation versus Amiodarone for Treatment of Atrial Fibrillation in Patients With Congestive Heart Failure and an Implanted ICD/CRTD (AATAC) trial was designed to evaluate optimal therapy in a particularly high-risk cohort. Patients with cardiomyopathy, heart failure, and implantable cardioverter defibrillator or cardiac resynchronization therapy

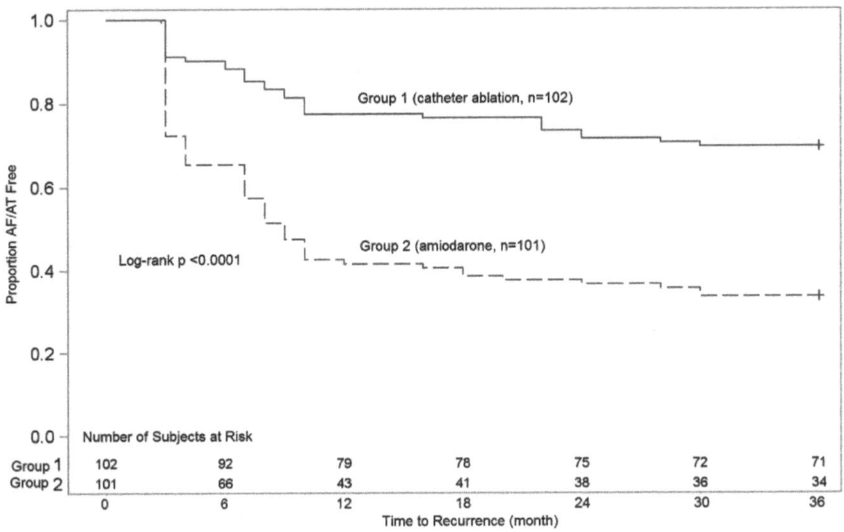


FIGURE 2.—Kaplan–Meier curve comparing AF-free survival between patients undergoing catheter ablation (group 1) and those receiving amiodarone therapy (group 2). At end of the study, 71 (70%; 95% CI, 60%–78%) patients in group 1 were recurrence free in comparison with 34 (34%; 95% CI, 25%–44%) in group 2 (log-rank P<0.001). AF indicates atrial fibrillation; AT, atrial tachycardia; and CI, confidence interval. (Reprinted from Di Biase L, Mohanty P, Mohanty S, et al. Ablation versus amiodarone for treatment of persistent atrial fibrillation in patients with congestive heart failure and an implanted device: results from the AATAC multicenter randomized trial. *Circulation*. 2016;133:1637-1644, with permission from American Heart Association, Inc.)

devices were randomized to full-dose amiodarone therapy or catheter ablation. During the standard 3-month blanking period, cardioversion or repeat ablation could be performed. A strict definition of arrhythmia recurrence ( > 30 seconds) was used because all patients had implanted atrial leads. Recurrence was observed in 70% of the amiodarone group compared with 34% of the ablation group (Fig 2). To achieve this success, ablation patients needed on average 1.4 procedures. Ablation was also associated with reduced hospitalization and mortality, which were predefined secondary end points in this trial. This study provided further support for the efficacy and early adoption of catheter ablation for the treatment of AF. Ongoing pivotal studies such as CABANA will help to define the role of ablation as fist-line therapy for a much broader group of patients.

**M. Gold, MD, PhD**

---

**Ablation of Stable VTs Versus Substrate Ablation in Ischemic Cardiomyopathy: The VISTA Randomized Multicenter Trial**

Di Biase L, Burkhardt JD, Lakkireddy D, et al (Texas Cardiac Arrhythmia Inst at St David's Med Ctr, Austin; Univ of Kansas; et al)

*J Am Coll Cardiol* 66:2872-2882, 2015

---

*Background.*—Catheter ablation reduces ventricular tachycardia (VT) recurrence and implantable cardioverter defibrillator shocks in patients

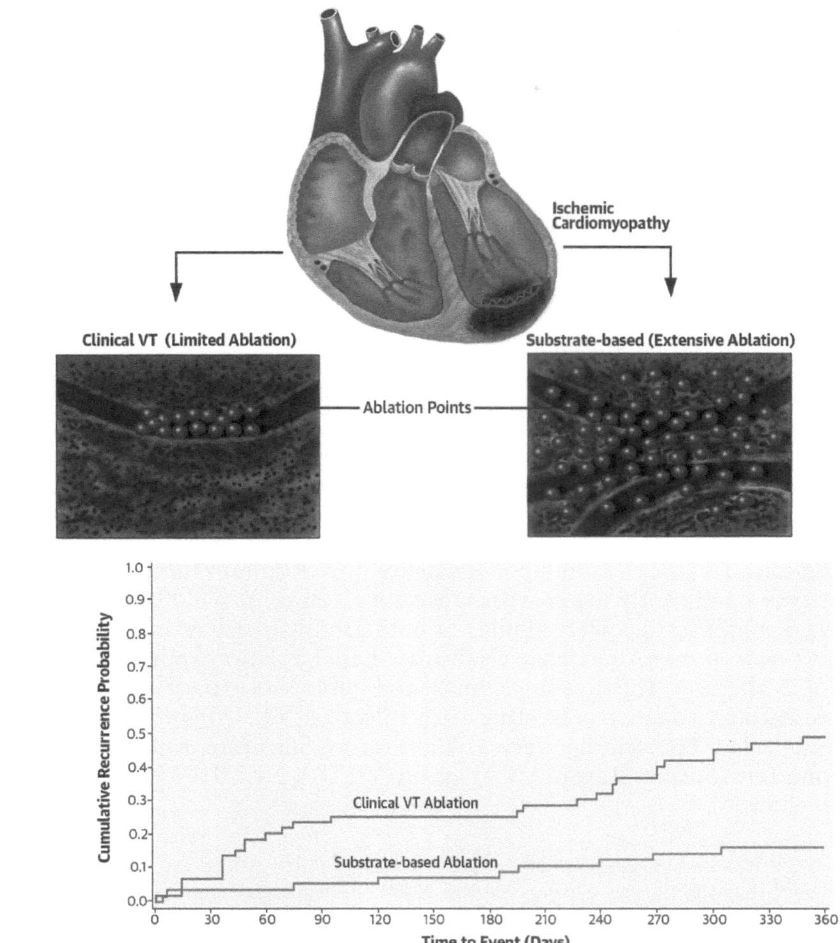


Number at Risk

| Ablation Strategy | | | | | | | | | | | | | |
|---|---|---|---|---|---|---|---|---|---|---|---|---|---|
| Substrate-based | 58 | 56 | 56 | 55 | 55 | 54 | 54 | 52 | 51 | 50 | 50 | 49 | 49 |
| Clinical Stable VT | 60 | 56 | 48 | 46 | 45 | 45 | 45 | 43 | 41 | 38 | 35 | 32 | 31 |

**CENTRAL ILLUSTRATION.—**. VT ablation in patients with ischemia. The curve compares the cumulative probability of VT recurrence (on or off antiarrhythmic drug) between patients undergoing substrate-based ablation and stable clinical ablation. Patients with substrate-based ablation exhibited significantly lower recurrence rate at 12-month follow-up: 9 of 58 (15.5%) compared with 29 of 60 (48.3%) patients in clinical VT ablation (log-rank $p < 0.001$). Median time to recurrence was 7.0 months (interquartile range: 6.3 to 7.8 months) and 2.5 months (interquartile range: 1.2 to 8.6 months), respectively (unadjusted hazard ratio: 0.26 [95% confidence interval: 0.11 to 0.61]). VT = ventricular tachycardia. (Reprinted from Di Biase L, Burkhardt JD, Lakkireddy D, et al. Ablation of stable VTs versus substrate ablation in ischemic cardiomyopathy: the VISTA randomized multicenter trial. *J Am Coll Cardiol.* 2015;66:2872-2882, with permission from the American College of Cardiology Foundation.)

with VT and ischemic cardiomyopathy. The most effective catheter ablation technique is unknown.

*Objectives.*—This study determined rates of VT recurrence in patients undergoing ablation limited to clinical VT along with mappable VTs ("clinical ablation") versus substrate-based ablation.

*Methods.*—Subjects with ischemic cardiomyopathy and hemodynamically tolerated VT were randomized to clinical ablation (n = 60) versus substrate-based ablation that targeted all "abnormal" electrograms in the scar (n = 58). Primary endpoint was recurrence of VT. Secondary endpoints included periprocedural complications, 12-month mortality, and rehospitalizations.

*Results.*—At 12-month follow-up, 9 (15.5%) and 29 (48.3%) patients had VT recurrence in substrate-based and clinical VT ablation groups, respectively (log-rank $p < 0.001$). More patients undergoing clinical VT ablation (58%) were on antiarrhythmic drugs after ablation versus substrate-based ablation (12%; $p < 0.001$). Seven (12%) patients with substrate ablation and 19 (32%) with clinical ablation required rehospitalization ($p = 0.014$). Overall 12-month mortality was 11.9%; 8.6% in substrate ablation and 15.0% in clinical ablation groups, respectively (log-rank $p = 0.21$). Combined incidence of rehospitalization and mortality was significantly lower with substrate ablation ($p = 0.003$). Periprocedural complications were similar in both groups ($p = 0.61$).

*Conclusions.*—An extensive substrate-based ablation approach is superior to ablation targeting only clinical and stable VTs in patients with ischemic cardiomyopathy presenting with tolerated VT. (Ablation of Clinical Ventricular Tachycardia Versus Addition of Substrate Ablation on the Long Term Success Rate of VT Ablation (VISTA); NCT01045668) (Central Illustration).

▶ Ventricular tachycardia and fibrillation (VT/VF) are the most common arrhythmias leading to sudden cardiac death. In high-risk primary or secondary prevention patients, the implantable cardioverter defibrillator (ICD) has been shown to reduce mortality. However, the ICD does not prevent VT/VF but rather effectively treats these arrhythmias. Given the morbidity and mortality associated with ventricular arrhythmias, adjunctive therapy is often used. Several prospective randomized trials have shown that VT ablation is superior to antiarrhythmic drugs among patients with known VT. The VISTA study evaluated 2 ablation strategies in patients with ICDs, coronary artery disease, and known VT. The traditional approach is to ablate the clinical VT, whereas more recently substrate-based ablation has been developed that targets areas within scar. The results were clear (Central Illustration), showing the superiority of substrate ablation. These results have important implications for ablation technique, help redefine success rates in ischemic heart patients, and reinforce the need for ICD back up in patients with sustained VT and structural heart disease.

**M. Gold, MD, PhD**

**Percutaneous Implantation of an Entirely Intracardiac Leadless Pacemaker**

Reddy VY, for the LEADLESS II Study Investigators (Icahn School of Medicine at Mount Sinai, NY; et al)

*N Engl J Med* 373:1125-1135, 2015

*Background.*—Cardiac pacemakers are limited by device-related complications, notably infection and problems related to pacemaker leads. We studied a miniaturized, fully self-contained leadless pacemaker that is nonsurgically implanted in the right ventricle with the use of a catheter.

*Methods.*—In this multicenter study, we implanted an active-fixation leadless cardiac pacemaker in patients who required permanent single-chamber ventricular pacing. The primary efficacy end point was both an acceptable pacing threshold (≤2.0 V at 0.4 msec) and an acceptable sensing amplitude (R wave ≥5.0 mV, or a value equal to or greater than the value at implantation) through 6 months. The primary safety end point was freedom from device-related serious adverse events through 6 months. In this ongoing study, the prespecified analysis of the primary end points was performed on data from the first 300 patients who completed 6 months of follow-up (primary cohort). The rates of the efficacy end point and safety end point were compared with performance goals (based on historical data) of 85% and 86%, respectively. Additional outcomes were assessed in all 526 patients who were enrolled as of June 2015 (the total cohort).

*Results.*—The leadless pacemaker was successfully implanted in 504 of the 526 patients in the total cohort (95.8%). The intention-to-treat primary efficacy end point was met in 270 of the 300 patients in the primary cohort (90.0%; 95% confidence interval [CI], 86.0 to 93.2, $P = 0.007$), and the primary safety end point was met in 280 of the 300 patients (93.3%; 95% CI, 89.9 to 95.9; $P < 0.001$). At 6 months, device-related serious adverse events were observed in 6.7% of the patients; events included device dislodgement with percutaneous retrieval (in 1.7%), cardiac perforation (in 1.3%), and pacing-threshold elevation requiring percutaneous retrieval and device replacement (in 1.3%).

*Conclusions.*—The leadless cardiac pacemaker met prespecified pacing and sensing requirements in the large majority of patients. Device-related serious adverse events occurred in approximately 1 in 15 patients. (Funded by St. Jude Medical; LEADLESS II ClinicalTrials.gov number, NCT02030418.)

▶ Implantable pacemakers have been used for nearly 60 years to treat a variety of bradycardic rhythms, most commonly heart block or sick sinus syndrome. Although pacemaker pulse generators are reliable, the leads remain the weak link of the system. Lead fracture, dislodgment, and infection are important contributors to the comorbidity of permanent pacing. Recently, advances in miniaturization of batteries and electronics has allowed for the development of a leadless pacemaker. The Nanostim used in this study is an active fixation device that is placed in the right ventricle (Fig 1 in the original article). The LEADLESS

II clinical trial was a nonrandomized study of more than 500 subjects. Electrical performance of the device was excellent, and complications rates were surprisingly low given this novel device. One major limitation of this therapy is that it is currently used as only a standalone ventricular pacemaker. Thus, dual-chamber pacer, defibrillator backup, or cardiac resynchronization therapy is not feasible with the Nanostim in its current iteration. Nevertheless, this is breakthrough technology that will likely become the standard for pacing as systems become more sophisticated and multichamber devices are developed.

**M. Gold, MD, PhD**

---

**Association Between Chest Compression Interruptions and Clinical Outcomes of Ventricular Fibrillation Out-of-Hospital Cardiac Arrest**

Brouwer TF, Walker RG, Chapman FW, et al (Academic Med Ctr, Amsterdam, The Netherlands; Physio-Control, Inc, Redmond, WA)
*Circulation* 132:1030-1037, 2015

---

*Background.*—Minimizing pauses in chest compressions during cardiopulmonary resuscitation is a focus of current guidelines. Prior analyses found that prolonged pauses for defibrillation (perishock pauses) are associated with worse survival. We analyzed resuscitations to characterize the association between pauses for all reasons and both ventricular fibrillation termination and patient survival.

*Methods and Results.*—In 319 patients with ventricular tachycardia/fibrillation out-of-hospital cardiac arrest, we analyzed recordings from all defibrillators used during resuscitation and measured durations of all cardiopulmonary resuscitation pauses. Median durations were 32 seconds (25th and 75th percentile, 22 and 52 seconds) for the longest pause for any reason, 23 seconds (25th and 75th percentile, 14 and 34 seconds) for the longest perishock pause, and 24 seconds (25th and 75th percentile, 11 and 38 seconds) for the longest nonshock pause. Multivariable regression models showed lower odds for survival per 5-second increase in the longest overall pause (odds ratio, 0.89; 95% confidence interval, 0.83–0.95), longest perishock pause (odds ratio, 0.85; 95% confidence interval, 0.77–0.93), and longest nonshock pause (odds ratio, 0.83; 95% confidence interval, 0.75–0.91). In 36% of cases, the longest pause was a nonshock pause; this subgroup had lower survival than the group in whom the longest pause was a perishock pause (27% versus 44%, respectively; $P < 0.01$) despite a higher chest compression fraction. Preshock pauses were 8 seconds (25th and 75th percentile, 4 and 17 seconds) for shocks that terminated ventricular fibrillation and 7 seconds (25th and 75th percentile, 4 and 13 seconds) for shocks that did not ($P = 0.18$).

*Conclusions.*—Prolonged pauses have a negative association with survival not explained by chest compression fraction or decreased ventricular fibrillation termination rate. Ventricular fibrillation termination was not

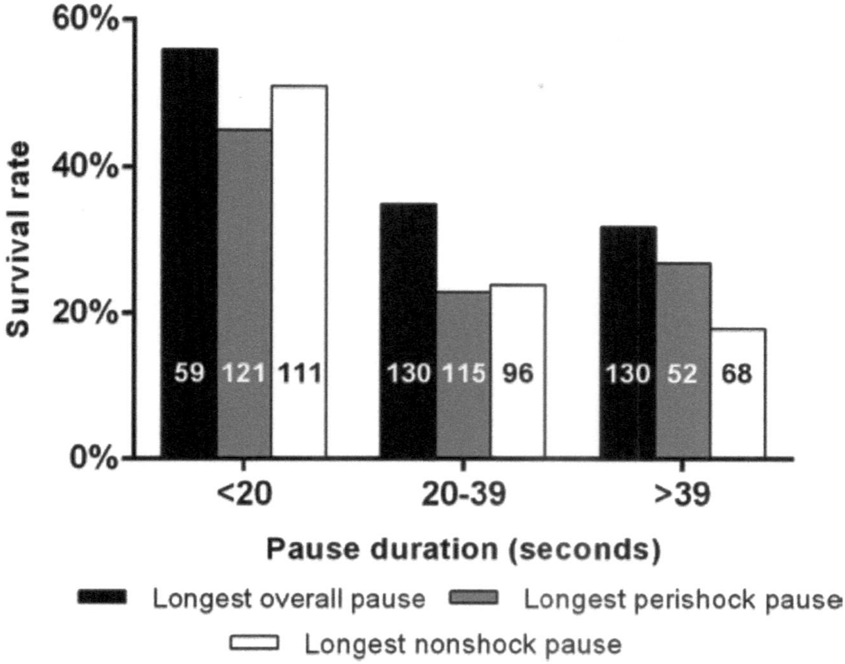


FIGURE 2.—Survival to hospital discharge and duration of longest overall pause (black), longest perishock pause (light gray), and longest nonshock pause (dark gray). Numbers in bars represent the number of patients. $P < 0.01$ for each pause category ($\chi^2$ for trend); see also Table 2 in the original article. (Reprinted from Brouwer TF, Walker RG, Chapman FW, et al. Association between chest compression interruptions and clinical outcomes of ventricular fibrillation out-of-hospital cardiac arrest. *Circulation.* 2015;132:1030-1037, with permission from American Heart Association, Inc.)

the mechanism linking pause duration and survival. Strategies shortening the longest pauses may improve outcome (Fig 2).

▶ Tremendous strides have been made in resuscitation of out-of-hospital cardiac arrests. Studies have shown that ventricular tachycardia and fibrillation (VT/VF) are the most common arrhythmias, although asystole and pulseless electrical activity are increasing in frequency more recently. Two of the most critical components of the resuscitation process are chest compression and electrical defibrillation. Resuscitation science has helped to elucidate the most important strategies to optimize care. In the present observational study, the pauses during chest compression were analyzed in 319 patients with out-of-hospital cardiac arrest secondary to VT/VF. Pauses during compression were noted for the delivery of shocks or for nonshock reasons. The median longest shock was 32 shocks. Multivariate analysis showed that there was a 11% decrease in survival for every 5-second increase in longest pause. This relationship was noted for perishock pauses and non-shock-related pauses as well (Fig 2). Interestingly, this was not related to shock efficacy because the longer pauses were associated with a trend toward higher rather than lower shock efficacy. These data emphasize the importance of minimizing pause duration for any reason during resuscitation and identify a target to improve survival from cardiac arrest due to VT/VF.

**M. Gold, MD, PhD**

# 38 Cardiomyopathy

**Association Between Hypertensive Disorders of Pregnancy and Later Risk of Cardiomyopathy**

Behrens I, Basit S, Lykke JA, et al (Statens Serum Institut, Copenhagen, Denmark; Copenhagen Univ Hosp (Rigshospitalet), Denmark)

*JAMA* 315:1026-1033, 2016

*Importance.*—Women with hypertensive disorders of pregnancy, preeclampsia in particular, have an increased risk of cardiomyopathy during the peripartum period. Whether hypertensive disorders of pregnancy are also associated with cardiomyopathy later in life is unknown.

*Objective.*—To determine whether hypertensive disorders of pregnancy are associated with cardiomyopathy beyond the peripartum period.

*Design, Setting, and Participants.*—Nationwide register–based cohort study using Cox regression to compare rates of cardiomyopathy in women with and without a history of hypertensive disorders of pregnancy in a cohort of 1 075 763 women with at least 1 pregnancy ending in live birth or stillbirth in Denmark, 1978-2012, with follow-up through December 31, 2012.

*Exposures.*—A hypertensive disorder of pregnancy (severe or moderate preeclampsia or gestational hypertension) registered in the National Patient Register.

*Main Outcomes and Measures.*—Cardiomyopathy more than 5 months after delivery (outside the peripartum period) up to 34 years 7 months.

*Result.*—The women in the primary cohort had 2 067 633 eligible pregnancies during the study period, 76 108 of which were complicated by a hypertensive disorder of pregnancy. During follow-up, 1577 women (mean age, 48.5 years at cardiomyopathy diagnosis; 2.6% with multiple pregnancies) developed cardiomyopathy. Compared with women with normotensive pregnancies (18 211 603 person-years of follow-up; n = 1408 cardiomyopathy events, 7.7/100 000 person-years [95% CI, 7.3-8.2]), women with a history of hypertensive disorders of pregnancy had significantly increased rates of cardiomyopathy (in 173 062 person-years of follow-up among women with severe preeclampsia, n = 27 cardiomyopathy events; 15.6/100 000 person-years [95% CI, 10.7-22.7]; adjusted hazard ratio [HR], 2.20 [95% CI, 1.50-3.23]; in 697 447 person-years of follow-up among women with moderate preeclampsia, n = 102 cardiomyopathy events; 14.6/100 000 person-years [95% CI, 12.0-17.8]; adjusted HR, 1.89 [95% CI, 1.55-2.23]; in 213 197 person-years of follow-up among women with gestational hypertension, n = 40 cardiomyopathy events; 17.3/100 000 person-years [95% CI, 12.7-23.6]; adjusted HR, 2.06 [95% CI, 1.50-2.82]). These increases persisted more than 5 years after the latest pregnancy. Mediation analyses suggested that only about 50% of the association was an indirect association through postpregnancy chronic hypertension. In this cohort, 11% of all cardiomyopathy events occurred in women with a history of hypertensive disorders of pregnancy.

*Conclusions and Relevance.*—Women with a history of hypertensive disorders of pregnancy, compared with women without such a history, had a small but statistically significant increased risk of cardiomyopathy more than 5 months after delivery. Further research is necessary to understand whether there is a causal mechanism behind this association.

► Preeclampsia during pregnancy is associated with postpartum cardiomyopathy. However, it is less clear if hypertensive syndromes associated with pregnancy are associated with late cardiomyopathy. To address this issue, this study was performed using the Danish nationwide database. More than 1 million woman with more than 2 million pregnancies were included over a 34-year period. A hypertensive disorder occurred in <4% of pregnancies. The late (>5 months) development of cardiomyopathy occurred about twice as often among women with a hypertensive syndrome during pregnancy (15.6/100 000 person-years) compared with normotensive pregnancies (7.7/100 000 person-years). Adjusting for clinical differences between groups, this difference persisted (hazard ratio 2.2). The authors concluded that this observation was not due solely to chronic hypertension as only about half of the cases occurred in women with a history of chronic hypertension. These interesting observations suggest that the cardiovascular risk of gestational hypertension may be lifelong. If confirmed, this will have important implications for periodic screening and preventative measures in women with hypertensive disorders during pregnancy.

**M. Gold, MD, PhD**

---

**Bariatric Surgery and Emergency Department Visits and Hospitalizations for Heart Failure Exacerbation: Population-Based, Self-Controlled Series**

Shimada YJ, Tsugawa Y, Brown DM, et al (Harvard Med School, Boston, MA; Harvard T.H. Chan School of Public Health, Boston, MA; et al)

*J Am Coll Cardiol* 67:895-903, 2016

---

*Background.*—The United States is battling obesity and heart failure (HF) epidemics. Although studies have suggested relationships between obesity and HF morbidity, little is known regarding the effects of substantial weight reduction in obese patients with HF.

*Objectives.*—This study investigated whether bariatric surgery is associated with a decreased rate of HF exacerbation.

*Methods.*—We performed a self-controlled case series study of obese patients with HF who underwent bariatric surgery, using the population-based emergency department (ED) and inpatient sample in California, Florida, and Nebraska. Primary outcome was ED visit or hospitalization for HF exacerbation from 2005 to 2011. We used conditional logistic regression to compare the outcome event rate during sequential 12-month periods, using pre-surgery months 13 to 24 as the reference period.

*Results.*—We identified 524 patients with HF who underwent bariatric surgery. During the reference period, 16.2% of patients had an ED visit or hospitalization for HF exacerbation. The rate remained unchanged in the subsequent 12-month pre-surgery period (15.3%; $p = 0.67$). In the first 12-month period after bariatric surgery, we observed a nonsignificantly reduced rate (12.0%; $p = 0.052$). However, the rate was significantly lower in the subsequent 13 to 24 months after bariatric surgery (9.9%; adjusted odds ratio: 0.57; $p = 0.003$). By contrast, there was no significant reduction in the rate of HF exacerbation among obese patients who underwent nonbariatric surgery (i.e., cholecystectomy, hysterectomy).

*Conclusions.*—Our findings indicate that bariatric surgery is associated with a decline in the rate of HF exacerbation requiring ED evaluation or hospitalization among obese patients with HF (Table 2).

▶ Obesity is a known risk factor for cardiovascular disease, and bariatric surgery provides a highly effective method of weight loss with substantial improvements in diabetes and lipid profiles. Although obesity is also a risk factor for incident heart failure (HF), the role for bariatric surgery in HF patients is less clear, particularly given that multiple studies have outlined an interesting

TABLE 2.—Rates of ED Visits or Hospitalizations for HF Exacerbation

| Time Interval and Outcome | Number of Patients (N = 524) | Rate, % (95% CI) | aOR (95% CI)* | *p* Value |
|---|---|---|---|---|
| 13–24 months before bariatric surgery | | | | |
| ED visit or hospitalization† | 85 | 16.2 (13.1–19.4) | Reference | — |
| ED visit‡ | 18 | 3.4 (1.9–5.0) | Reference | — |
| Hospitalization§ | 73 | 13.9 (11.0–16.9) | Reference | — |
| 1–12 months before bariatric surgery | | | | |
| ED visit or hospitalization† | 80 | 15.3 (12.2–18.4) | 0.93 (0.67–1.30) | 0.67 |
| ED visit‡ | 10 | 1.9 (0.7–3.1) | 0.51 (0.22–1.17) | 0.11 |
| Hospitalization§ | 75 | 14.3 (11.3–17.3) | 1.03 (0.73–1.46) | 0.86 |
| 0–12 months after bariatric surgery | | | | |
| ED visit or hospitalization† | 63 | 12.0 (9.2–14.8) | 0.71 (0.50–1.003) | 0.052 |
| ED visit‡ | 8 | 1.5 (0.5–2.6) | 0.40 (0.16–0.97) | 0.043 |
| Hospitalization§ | 58 | 11.1 (8.4–13.8) | 0.77 (0.53–1.11) | 0.16 |
| 13–24 months after bariatric surgery | | | | |
| ED visit or hospitalization† | 52 | 9.9 (7.4–12.5) | 0.57 (0.39–0.82) | 0.003 |
| ED visit‡ | 7 | 1.3 (0.3–2.3) | 0.34 (0.13–0.87) | 0.016 |
| Hospitalization§ | 48 | 9.2 (6.7–11.6) | 0.62 (0.42–0.91) | 0.025 |

aOR = adjusted odds ratio; CI = confidence interval; ED = emergency department; HF = heart failure.

*Adjusted odds ratios are for each 12-month period versus the reference period (13 to 24 months before the index bariatric surgery), as calculated with conditional logistic regression.

†Composite of at least 1 ED visit or hospitalization for HF exacerbation.

‡At least 1 ED visit for HF exacerbation, not resulting in hospitalization.

§At least 1 hospitalization for HF exacerbation.

survival advantage in obese HF patients, often referred to as the "obesity paradox." Whether this apparent survival advantage is secondary to earlier diagnosis in the obese and other forms of bias or a pathophysiologic process through which obesity is actually protective (ie, the avoidance of the negative effects of cardiac cachexia) has yet to be determined. As a result, whether aggressive weight loss in patients with HF will translate into a clinical benefit is unknown.

The authors used claims data from 3 states to examine the impact of bariatric surgery on emergency department visits and HF hospitalizations in obese HF patients. They report an impressive decline of nearly 50% in events from the presurgical period to 13 to 24 months postbariatric surgery (Table 2). Importantly, 40% of the patients included in this study had HF with reduced ejection fraction (EF), and 60% had HF with preserved EF. With the increasing numbers of obese HF patients set against the backdrop of limited treatments to prevent readmissions, these results have important potential implications on how we care for our patients. However, the study has significant limitations, the largest of which is the data source, and as such, these results must be interpreted with caution. There were no data on the amount of weight loss achieved, changes in cardiac performance or functional capacity, the potential adjustments made in medication therapy or improvements in comorbid conditions such as diabetes, hypertension, or renal dysfunction. Furthermore, given the overlap in symptoms between HF and obesity, including abdominal distension, edema, and shortness of breath, whether bariatric surgery merely attenuated symptoms of obesity incorrectly thought to be secondary to HF is unknown. Further prospective research is necessary to confirm the reported findings in this study, particularly given the lack of granular information available on each individual patient secondary to the study design.

**M. A. Brisco, MD, MSCE, FACC**

---

### Comparative Effectiveness of CRT-D Versus Defibrillator Alone in HF Patients With Moderate-to-Severe Chronic Kidney Disease

Friedman DJ, Singh JP, Curtis JP, et al (Duke Univ Hosp, Durham, NC; Massachusetts General Hosp, Boston; Yale Univ School of Medicine, New Haven, CT; et al)
*J Am Coll Cardiol* 66:2618-2629, 2015

---

*Background.*—Patients with moderate-to-severe chronic kidney disease (CKD) are poorly represented in clinical trials of cardiac resynchronization therapy (CRT).

*Objectives.*—This study sought to assess the real-world comparative effectiveness of CRT with defibrillator (CRT-D) versus implantable cardioverter-defibrillator (ICD) alone in CRT-eligible patients with moderate-to-severe CKD.

*Methods.*—We conducted an inverse probability-weighted analysis of 10,946 CRT-eligible patients (ejection fraction <35%, QRS >120 ms, New York Heart Association functional class III/IV) with stage 3 to 5 CKD in the National Cardiovascular Data Registry (NCDR) ICD Registry, comparing outcomes between patients who received CRT-D (n = 9,525) versus ICD only (n = 1,421). Outcomes were obtained via Medicare claims and censored at 3 years. The primary endpoint of heart failure (HF) hospitalization or death and the secondary endpoint of death were assessed with Cox proportional hazards models. HF hospitalization, device explant, and progression to end-stage renal disease were assessed using Fine-Gray models.

*Results.*—After risk adjustment, CRT-D use was associated with a reduction in HF hospitalization or death (hazard ratio [HR]: 0.84; 95% confidence interval [CI]: 0.78 to 0.91; $p < 0.0001$), death (HR: 0.85; 95% CI: 0.77 to 0.93; $p < 0.0004$), and HF hospitalization alone (subdistribution HR: 0.84; 95% CI: 0.76 to 0.93; $p < 0.009$). Subgroup analyses suggested that CRT was associated with a reduced risk of HF hospitalization and death across CKD classes. The incidence of in-hospital, short-term, and mid-term device-related complications did not vary across CKD stages.

*Conclusions.*—In a nationally representative population of HF and CRT-eligible patients, use of CRT-D was associated with a significantly lower risk of the composite endpoint of HF hospitalization or death

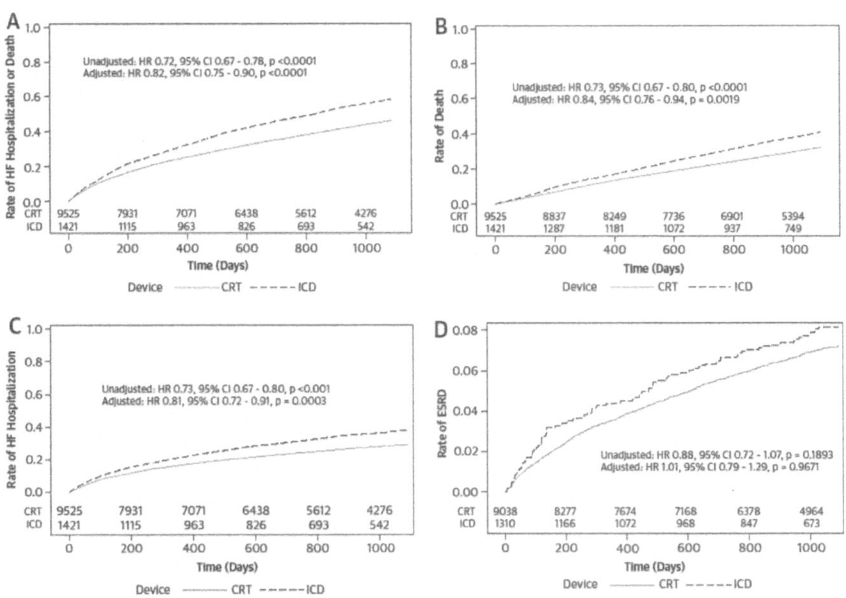


FIGURE 1.—Rates of HF hospitalization or death, death, HF hospitalization, and progression to ESRD among patients with CRT-D versus ICD alone. Kaplan-Meier curves are shown for heart failure (HF) hospitalization or death (**A**) and death (**B**). Cumulative incidence functions accounting for the competing risks of death for HF hospitalization (**C**) and progression to end-stage renal disease (ESRD) (**D**) are shown. CI = confidence interval; CRT = cardiac resynchronization therapy; CRT-D = cardiac resynchronization therapy with defibrillator; HR = hazard ratio; ICD = implantable cardioverter-defibrillator. (Reprinted from Friedman DJ, Singh JP, Curtis JP, et al. Comparative effectiveness of CRT-D versus defibrillator alone in HF patients with moderate-to-severe chronic kidney disease. *J Am Coll Cardiol.* 2015;66:2618-2629, with permission from the American College of Cardiology Foundation.)

among patients with moderate-to-severe CKD in the setting of acceptable complication rates (Fig 1).

▶ Implantable cardioverter defibrillators (ICDs) with or without cardiac resynchronization therapy (CRT) have been shown to reduce mortality in several high-risk cohorts including those with heart failure and a reduced ejection fraction. Risk assessment models have demonstrated that the benefit of ICD therapy may be diminished or eliminated in the presence of multiple competing comorbidities. One of the most consistent comorbidities associated with worse outcomes is renal failure. Moreover, patients with advanced renal failure are excluded from most large randomized device trials. Accordingly, the present analysis was designed to assess the impact of renal failure among patients eligible for ICD and CRT implantations. The National Cardiovascular Data Registry of Medicare recipients was used to evaluate retrospectively more than 10 000 patients with New York Heart Association III/IV CHF, left ventricular ejection fraction ≤35%, and QRS duration >120 msec. About 87% of patients received CRT ICDs (CRT-D) consistent with clinical guidelines. The composite end point of time to first heart failure hospitalization or death was decreased 18% after adjustment with CRT-D, which was similar to the magnitudes of the decrease in each of the component end points (Fig 1). The results were not affected by the degree of renal failure (chronic kidney disease stage III–V). These results support the strategy of implanting CRT-D devices in elderly patients with chronic kidney disease who meet current guidelines.

**M. Gold, MD, PhD**

---

**Early Detection of Anthracycline Cardiotoxicity and Improvement With Heart Failure Therapy**

Cardinale D, Colombo A, Bacchiani G, et al (European Inst of Oncology, Milan, Italy; et al)

*Circulation* 131:1981-1988, 2015

---

*Background.*—Three types of anthracycline-induced cardiotoxicities are currently recognized: acute, early-onset chronic, and late-onset chronic. However, data supporting this classification are lacking. We prospectively evaluated incidence, time of occurrence, clinical correlates, and response to heart failure therapy of cardiotoxicity.

*Methods and Results.*—We assessed left ventricular ejection fraction (LVEF), at baseline, every 3 months during chemotherapy and for the following year, every 6 months over the following 4 years, and yearly afterward in a heterogeneous cohort of 2625 patients receiving anthracycline-containing therapy. In case of cardiotoxicity (LVEF decrease >10 absolute points, and <50%), heart failure therapy was initiated. Recovery from cardiotoxicity was defined as partial (LVEF increase >5 absolute points and >50%) or full (LVEF increase to the baseline value). The median follow-up was 5.2 (quartile 1 to quartile 3, 2.6–8.0) years. The overall incidence of cardiotoxicity was 9% (n = 226). The median time elapsed between the end of chemotherapy and cardiotoxicity development was 3.5 (quartile 1 to quartile 3, 3–6) months. In 98% of cases (n = 221), cardiotoxicity occurred within the first year. Twenty-five (11%) patients had full recovery, and 160 (71%) patients had partial recovery. At multivariable analysis, end-chemotherapy LVEF (hazard ratio, 1.37; 95% confidence interval, 1.33–1.42 for each percent unit decrement) and cumulative doxorubicin dose (hazard ratio, 1.09; 95% confidence interval, 1.04–1.15 for each 50 mg/m$^2$ increment) were independent correlates of cardiotoxicity.

*Conclusions.*—Most cardiotoxicity after anthracycline-containing therapy occurs within the first year and is associated with anthracycline dose and LVEF at the end of treatment. Early detection and prompt therapy of cardiotoxicity appear crucial for substantial recovery of cardiac function (Fig 1).

▶ Cardinale and colleagues present data on anthracycline-induced cardiotoxicity from more than 2500 patients over a period of nearly 20 years with a median follow-up of 5.2 years. Anthracycline cardiotoxicity, defined as a greater than 10% reduction in ejection fraction occurred in 9% of the population. One of the most important findings from this study is the timing of anthracycline-induced cardiotoxicity because almost all cardiotoxicity occurs within the first year and is often in the form of asymptomatic left ventricular dysfunction (Fig 1). This finding potentially explains why prior retrospective studies of anthracycline cardiotoxicity in patients with symptomatic heart failure surmised a longer period from

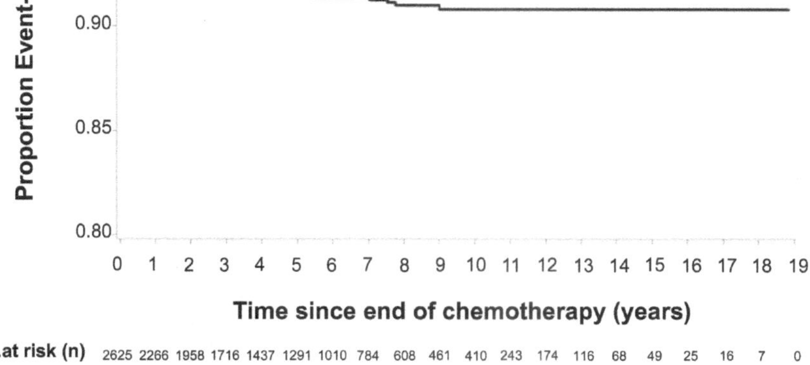


FIGURE 1.—Kaplan–Meier curve showing the cumulative incidence of cardiotoxicity in the study population. Pts. indicates patients. (Reprinted from Cardinale D, Colombo A, Bacchiani G, et al. Early detection of anthracycline cardiotoxicity and improvement with heart failure therapy. *Circulation.* 2015;131:1981-1988, with permission from American Heart Association, Inc.)

treatment to heart failure onset. The early onset of cardiotoxicity as outlined by the authors has important diagnostic and treatment implications. Although no current official screening recommendations exist, a commonly used approach to screening for cardiotoxicity was based on the previous assumption that an individual patients risk was more evenly distributed over the first few years after therapy and that cardiotoxicity could develop as late as 10 years after treatment. The time course outlined by Cardinale et al suggests screening should perhaps be more frequent in the first year following treatment with decay in surveillance thereafter.

From a treatment perspective, we know from the heart failure literature that earlier treatment is associated with a greater likelihood of myocardial recovery, and in the case of asymptomatic left ventricular dysfunction ACC Stage B Heart Failure, treatment with an angiotensin-converting enzyme inhibitor provides a mortality benefit. However, whether these factors apply to anthracycline-induced cardiotoxicity is unknown. The patients included in this longitudinal study all received treatment for left ventricular dysfunction, with 82% of those treated experiencing improvement in their cardiac function, and the authors acknowledge that whether the asymptomatic patients would have recovered without medication intervention is unknown. Still, the high percentage of patients with myocardial recovery with treatment suggests that anthracycline-induced cardiomyopathy is more reversible than previously believed and therefore the pathophysiology is not exclusively myocardial cell death.

Unfortunately, despite a rigorous longitudinal analysis with cardiac follow-up and treatment, what this article fails to outline is how best to balance the risks associated with anthracycline cardiotoxicity and the benefits of continued first-line cancer treatment. In total, 31% of patients died during follow-up with 97% of those deaths categorized as tumor related. Although not described by the authors, development of cardiotoxicity often results in discontinuation of the offending agent, potentially jeopardizing patient survival. If a life-saving cancer therapy is withheld for mild asymptomatic cardiotoxicity that may have resolved on its own, we may be doing a disservice. Future research is necessary to distinguish clinically meaningful cardiotoxicity and determine the safest treatment approach in each individual patient.

**M. A. Brisco, MD, MSCE, FACC**

---

**Bone marrow-derived mesenchymal stromal cell treatment in patients with severe ischaemic heart failure: a randomized placebo-controlled trial (MSC-HF trial)**

Mathiasen AB, Qayyum AA, Jørgensen E, et al (Copenhagen Univ Hosp, Denmark)

*Eur Heart J* 36:1744-1753, 2015

---

*Aims.*—Regenerative treatment with mesenchymal stromal cells (MSCs) has been promising in patients with ischaemic heart failure but needs confirmation in larger randomized trials. We aimed to study effects of intra-myocardial autologous bone marrow-derived MSC treatment in patients with severe ischaemic heart failure.

*Methods and Results.*—The MSC-HF trial is a randomized, double-blind, placebo-controlled trial. Patients were randomized 2:1 to intra-myocardial injections of MSC or placebo, respectively. The primary endpoint was change in left ventricular end-systolic volume (LVESV), measured by magnetic resonance imaging or computed tomography at 6 months follow-up. Sixty patients aged 30–80 years with severe ischaemic heart failure, New York Heart Association (NYHA) classes II–III, left ventricular ejection fraction (LVEF) <45% and no further treatment options were randomized. Fifty-five patients completed the 6-month follow-up (37 MSCs vs. 18 placebo). At 6 months, LVESV was reduced in the MSC group: −7.6 (95% CI −11.8 to −3.4) mL ($P = 0.001$), and increased in the placebo group: 5.4 (95% CI 20.4 to 11.2) mL ($P = 0.07$). The difference between groups was 13.0 (95% CI 5.9–20.1) mL ($P = 0.001$). Compared with placebo, there were also significant improvements in LVEF of 6.2% ($P < 0.0001$), stroke volume of 18.4 mL ($P < 0.0001$), and myocardial mass of 5.7 g ($P = 0.001$). No differences were found in NYHA class, 6-min walking test and Kansas City cardiomyopathy questionnaire. No side effects were identified.

*Conclusion.*—Intra-myocardial injections of autologous culture expanded MSCs were safe and improved myocardial function in patients with severe ischaemic heart failure.

*Study Registration Number.*—NCT00644410 (ClinicalTrials.gov) (Fig 2).

▶ Mathiasen and colleagues describe their results from a single-center, double-blind, placebo-controlled trial of mesenchymal stromal cells for the treatment of ischemic cardiomyopathy. Injections of a patient's own bone marrow–derived stem cells into the myocardium was associated with statistically significant decreases in end systolic volume and improvements in both ejection fraction and myocardial mass (Fig 2). Furthermore, these results appeared to be dose dependent as patients who received the largest amounts of injected cells experienced the greatest benefits. Importantly, the injection procedures were relatively safe and associated with adverse events in only 2 patients (ventricular tachycardia and minor stroke without deficit). Taken together, these results are congruous with other studies in the literature and suggest a possible role for mesenchymal stromal cells for the treatment of ischemic cardiomyopathy. This was also a well-controlled study with a placebo-injected control group, which addresses one of the criticisms of previous trials. Whether this particular cell type will ultimately prove to be the most suitable for this therapy remains to be seen as the field of cell therapy continues to develop.

Despite the statistically significant improvements in left ventricular function, there were no differences in quality of life, functional status, or exercise capacity. This may be due to the relatively small mean increase in ejection fraction (6.2%), which may not translate into clinically meaningful improvements appreciated by the patient. The investigators have shown that stem cells are

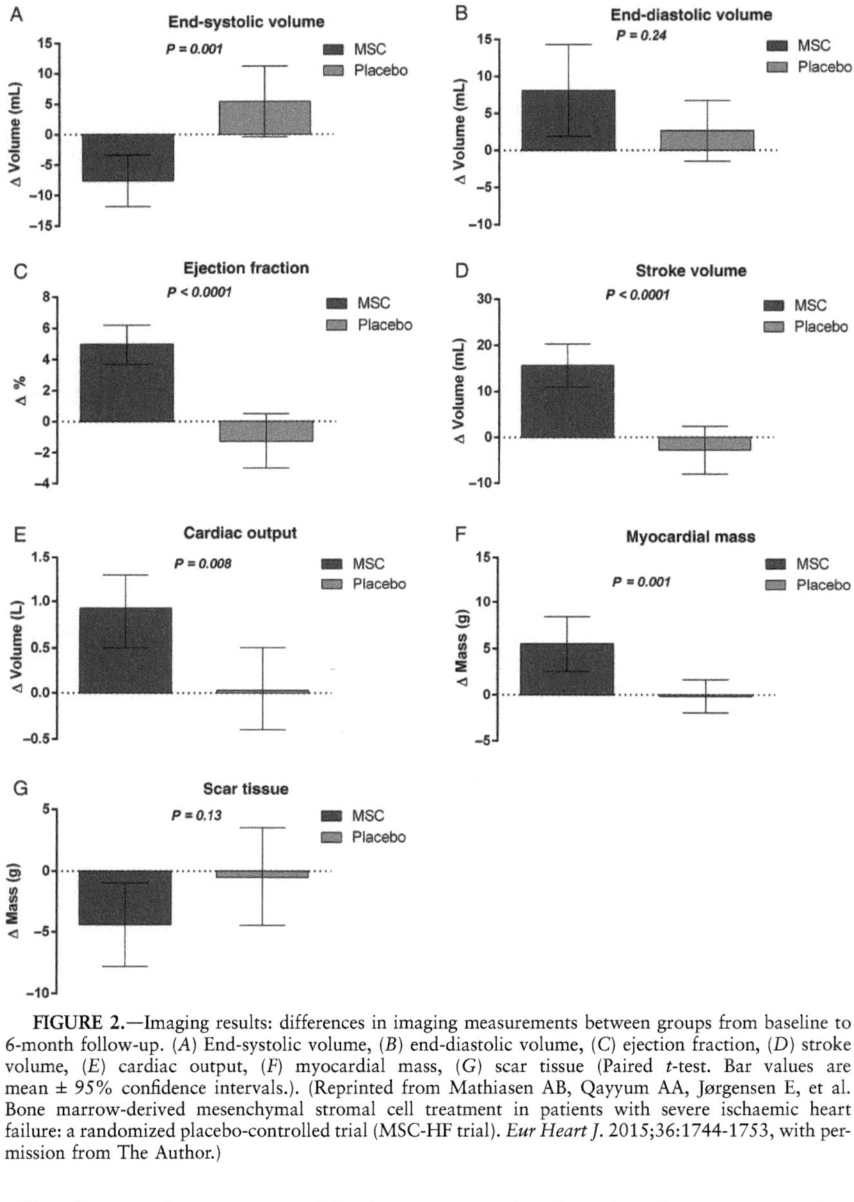


FIGURE 2.—Imaging results: differences in imaging measurements between groups from baseline to 6-month follow-up. (*A*) End-systolic volume, (*B*) end-diastolic volume, (C) ejection fraction, (*D*) stroke volume, (*E*) cardiac output, (*F*) myocardial mass, (*G*) scar tissue (Paired *t*-test. Bar values are mean ± 95% confidence intervals.). (Reprinted from Mathiasen AB, Qayyum AA, Jørgensen E, et al. Bone marrow-derived mesenchymal stromal cell treatment in patients with severe ischaemic heart failure: a randomized placebo-controlled trial (MSC-HF trial). *Eur Heart J.* 2015;36:1744-1753, with permission from The Author.)

efficacious and can successfully increase cardiac function; however, moving forward, the success of this therapy hinges on the magnitude of the benefit and associated clinical improvement.

**M. A. Brisco, MD, MSCE, FACC**

# 39 Chronic Coronary Artery Disease

**Alcohol consumption and cardiovascular disease, cancer, injury, admission to hospital, and mortality: a prospective cohort study**

Smyth A, on behalf of the PURE Investigators (McMaster Univ and Hamilton Health Sciences, Ontario, Canada; et al)

*Lancet* 386:1945-1954, 2015

*Background.*—Alcohol consumption is proposed to be the third most important modifiable risk factor for death and disability. However, alcohol consumption has been associated with both benefits and harms, and previous studies were mostly done in high-income countries. We investigated associations between alcohol consumption and outcomes in a prospective cohort of countries at different economic levels in five continents.

*Methods.*—We included information from 12 countries participating in the Prospective Urban Rural Epidemiological (PURE) study, a prospective cohort study of individuals aged 35–70 years. We used Cox proportional hazards regression to study associations with mortality (n = 2723), cardiovascular disease (n = 2742), myocardial infarction (n = 979), stroke (n = 817), alcohol-related cancer (n = 764), injury (n = 824), admission to hospital (n = 8786), and for a composite of these outcomes (n = 11 963).

*Findings.*—We included 114 970 adults, of whom 12 904 (11%) were from high-income countries (HICs), 24 408 (21%) were from upper-middle-income countries (UMICs), 48 845 (43%) were from lower-middle-income countries (LMICs), and 28 813 (25%) were from low-income countries (LICs). Median follow-up was 4·3 years (IQR 3·0–6·0). Current drinking was reported by 36 030 (31%) individuals, and was associated with reduced myocardial infarction (hazard ratio [HR] 0·76 [95% CI 0·63–0·93]), but increased alcohol-related cancers (HR 1·51 [1·22–1·89]) and injury (HR 1·29 [1·04–1·61]). High intake was associated with increased mortality (HR 1·31 [1·04–1·66]). Compared with never drinkers, we identified significantly reduced hazards for the composite outcome for current drinkers in HICs and UMICs (HR 084 [077–092]), but not in LMICs and LICs, for which we identified no reductions in this outcome (HR 1·07 [0·95–1·21]; $P_{interaction}$<0·0001).

*Interpretation.*—Current alcohol consumption had differing associations by clinical outcome, and differing associations by income region.

However, we identified sufficient commonalities to support global health strategies and national initiatives to reduce harmful alcohol use.

▶ Alcohol consumption is associated with many adverse effects, but it is often cited as being protective from coronary artery disease. The results of studies have varied, possibly because of heterogeneous populations. To address some of these issues, the PURE study was a prospective observational, multinational trial involving more than 114 970 subjects across different economic levels and geographies. There was a higher incidence of alcohol use in higher income countries. In addition, alcohol use was associated with a lower risk of myocardial infarction but higher risk of cancers and injury. High alcohol consumption was associated with increased mortality. Most interesting, alcohol consumption was associated with a decreased composite end point of mortality, cardiovascular disease, myocardial infarction, stroke, alcohol-related cancer, injury, or hospital admission. However, this relationship was only observed in higher income countries. These findings highlight the complex and interrelated impact of alcohol on survival and clinical outcomes and emphasizes the variability of these associations based on economic status. This suggests that different strategies are needed in different societies to affect the impact of alcohol and population health.

**M. Gold, MD, PhD**

---

**Troponin and Cardiac Events in Stable Ischemic Heart Disease and Diabetes**

Everett BM, for the BARI 2D Study Group (Brigham and Women's Hosp and Harvard Med School, Boston, MA; et al)
*N Engl J Med* 373:610-620, 2015

---

*Background.*—Cardiac troponin concentrations are used to identify patients who would benefit from urgent revascularization for acute coronary syndromes. We hypothesized that they might be used in patients with stable ischemic heart disease to identify those at high risk for cardiovascular events who might also benefit from prompt coronary revascularization.

*Methods.*—We measured the cardiac troponin T concentration at baseline with a high-sensitivity assay in 2285 patients who had both type 2 diabetes and stable ischemic heart disease and were enrolled in the Bypass Angioplasty Revascularization Investigation in Type 2 Diabetes trial. We tested for an association between the troponin T concentration and a composite end point of death from cardiovascular causes, myocardial infarction, or stroke; we then evaluated whether random assignment to prompt revascularization reduced the rate of the composite end point in patients with an abnormal troponin T concentration (≥14 ng per liter) as compared with those with a normal troponin T concentration (<14 ng per liter).

*Results.*—Of the 2285 patients, 2277 (99.6%) had detectable (≥3 ng per liter) troponin T concentrations and 897 (39.3%) had abnormal troponin T concentrations at baseline. The 5-year rate of the composite end point was 27.1% among the patients who had had abnormal troponin T concentrations at baseline, as compared with 12.9% among those who had had normal baseline troponin T concentrations. In models that were adjusted for cardiovascular risk factors, severity of diabetes, electrocardiographic abnormalities, and coronary anatomy, the hazard ratio for the composite end point among patients with abnormal troponin T concentrations was 1.85 (95% confidence interval [CI], 1.48 to 2.32; $P < 0.001$). Among patients with abnormal troponin T concentrations, random assignment to prompt revascularization, as compared with medical therapy alone, did not result in a significant reduction in the rate of the composite end point (hazard ratio, 0.96; 95% CI, 0.74 to 1.25).

*Conclusions.*—The cardiac troponin T concentration was an independent predictor of death from cardiovascular causes, myocardial infarction, or stroke in patients who had both type 2 diabetes and stable ischemic heart disease. An abnormal troponin T value of 14 ng per liter or higher did not identify a subgroup of patients who benefited from random assignment to prompt coronary revascularization. (Funded by the National Institutes of Health and Roche Diagnostics; BARI 2D ClinicalTrials.gov number, NCT00006305.)

▶ Elevated serum troponin concentrations are used to determine patients who may benefit most from early revascularization in the setting of acute coronary syndrome. However, use of troponin in patients with stable coronary artery disease to direct revascularization is not well defined. A subset, consisting of 2285 patients from the Bypass Angioplasty Revascularization Investigation in Type 2 Diabetes (BARI 2D) trial, was investigated using high-sensitivity troponin T assays. All patients were determined to have stable coronary/ischemic heart disease as well as type 2 diabetes. Baseline serum concentrations of high-sensitivity troponin T were measured and deemed classified as detectable at a level of ≥3 ng/L, normal ≤14 ng/L, or abnormal ≥14 ng/L. In addition, follow-up levels at 1 year were available for 1984 patients. Association between troponin T concentrations and the composite end point of death from cardiovascular causes, myocardial infarction (MI), or stroke was evaluated. Additionally the effect of randomization to early revascularization on the composite end point was investigated. Within the study population 99.6% of patients had detectable levels (≥3 ng/L) of troponin T, whereas 39.3% had abnormal (≥14 ng/L) levels. The composite end point was observed in 27.1% of the patients with abnormal troponin T concentrations compared with only 12.9% of those with normal baseline levels. There were differences in the baseline characteristics of the 2 groups with respect to factors such as age, sex, history of MI, history of congestive heart failure (CHF), chronic kidney disease, estimated glomerular filtration rate (GFR), NT-pro B-type natriuretic peptide level, and number of vessels with lesions of greater than 50%. However, when adjusted for diabetes severity, ejection fraction, GFR, and number of coronary lesions, the hazard ratio remained statistically significant at 1.48 to 2.32 ($P < .001$). It was also noted that in patients whom had an increase of more than 25% in their baseline troponin

T level at 1 year had higher rates of MI, stroke, or heart failure. Thus, elevated baseline levels of high sensitivity troponin T appeared to identify patients at higher risk of adverse outcomes. However, randomization to early revascularization did not appear to reduce event rates. When compared with medical management alone, early revascularization yielded a hazard ratio of 0.98. This was consistent between both patients with normal and elevated baseline troponin T concentrations. In conclusion, baseline elevation and/or an increase in baseline troponin T levels of >25% appears to identify patients at higher risk of adverse outcomes. However, given the lack of effect of revascularization, these changes should not be used to identify patients who would benefit from invasive management strategies.

**R. Bayer II, MD**

---

**Effect of PCI on Long-Term Survival in Patients with Stable Ischemic Heart Disease**

Sedlis SP, for the COURAGE Trial Investigators (New York Veterans Affairs (VA) Healthcare Network; et al)
*N Engl J Med* 373:1937-1946, 2015

---

*Background.*—Percutaneous coronary intervention (PCI) relieves angina in patients with stable ischemic heart disease, but clinical trials have not shown that it improves survival. Between June 1999 and January 2004, we randomly assigned 2287 patients with stable ischemic heart disease to an initial management strategy of optimal medical therapy alone (medical-therapy group) or optimal medical therapy plus PCI (PCI group) and did not find a significant difference in the rate of survival during a median follow-up of 4.6 years. We now report the rate of survival among the patients who were followed for up to 15 years.

*Methods.*—We obtained permission from the patients at the Department of Veterans Affairs (VA) sites and some non-VA sites in the United States to use their Social Security numbers to track their survival after the original trial period ended. We searched the VA national Corporate Data Warehouse and the National Death Index for survival information and the dates of death from any cause. We calculated survival according to the Kaplan–Meier method and used a Cox proportional-hazards model to adjust for significant between-group differences in baseline characteristics.

*Results.*—Extended survival information was available for 1211 patients (53% of the original population). The median duration of follow-up for all patients was 6.2 years (range, 0 to 15); the median duration of follow-up for patients at the sites that permitted survival tracking was 11.9 years (range, 0 to 15). A total of 561 deaths (180 during the follow-up period in the original trial and 381 during the extended follow-up period) occurred: 284 deaths (25%) in the PCI group and 277 (24%) in the medical-therapy group (adjusted hazard ratio, 1.03; 95% confidence interval, 0.83 to 1.21; $P = 0.76$).

*Conclusions.*—During an extended-follow-up of up to 15 years, we did not find a difference in survival between an initial strategy of PCI plus medical therapy and medical therapy alone in patients with stable ischemic heart disease. (Funded by the VA Cooperative Studies Program and others; COURAGE ClinicalTrials.gov number, NCT00007657.)

▶ The Clinical Outcomes Utilizing Revascularization and Aggressive Drug Evaluation (COURAGE) compared initial management strategy alone with optimal medical therapy plus percutaneous coronary intervention (PCI) among patients with stable ischemic heart disease. The results have been previously published and showed no significant difference between treatment groups with respect to survival during a median follow-up of 4.6 years. In the present study, the authors perform an extended survival analysis on a subset of patients in the original COURAGE patient population. As part of the initial informed-consent process, patients in the United States were asked to provide their Social Security numbers for survival tracking. The "extended follow-up" cohort consisted of patients (53% of the original study population). The median duration of follow-up in the "extended follow-up" cohort was 11.9 years (mean 10.5 years; range 0-15.3 years). A total of 561 (25%) patients died during follow-up (180 during follow-up of the original trial and an additional 381 deaths during the extended follow-up period). There is no difference in survival between treatment strategy of PCI plus medical therapy and medical therapy alone (adjusted hazard ratio [HR] 1.03; 95% confidence interval [CI] 0.83-1.21; $P = .76$). Survival curves for the entire study cohort and the extended follow-up cohort are shown in Fig 2A, B in the original article, respectively. In the original trial, the survival curves appeared to separate at 5 years in favor of PCI (HR 0.87; 95% CI, 0.65-1.13), suggesting a late survival benefit; however, this was not seen in the extended follow-up study. One major limitation of this analysis is that the extended follow-up included only a little more than half of the original population. Also, the extended follow-up cohort was mostly veterans and only a small number of non-VA trial participants. Nevertheless, these data again question the routine use of aggressive revascularization for clinically stable coronary artery disease.

**T. M. Todoran, MD, MSc**

---

**Effects of Ranolazine on Angina and Quality of Life After Percutaneous Coronary Intervention With Incomplete Revascularization: Results From the Ranolazine for Incomplete Vessel Revascularization (RIVER-PCI) Trial**

Alexander KP, Weisz G, Prather K, et al (Duke Clinical Res Inst and Duke Univ, Durham, NC; Shaare Zedek Med Ctr, Jerusalem, Israel; et al)

*Circulation* 133:39-47, 2016

---

*Background.*—Angina often persists or returns in populations following percutaneous coronary intervention (PCI). We hypothesized that ranolazine would be effective in reducing angina and improving quality of life (QOL) in incomplete revascularization (ICR) post-PCI patients.

*Methods and Results.*—In RIVER-PCI, 2604 patients with a history of chronic angina who had ICR post-PCI were randomized 1:1 to oral ranolazine versus placebo; QOL analyses included 2389 randomized subjects. Angina and QOL questionnaires were collected at baseline and months 1, 6, and 12. Ranolazine patients were more likely than placebo to discontinue study drug by month 6 (20.4% versus 14.1%, $P < 0.001$) and 12 (27.2% versus 21.3%, $P < 0.001$). Following qualifying index PCI, the primary QOL outcome (Seattle Angina Questionnaire [SAQ] angina frequency score) improved markedly, but similarly, in the ranolazine and placebo groups, respectively, from baseline (67.3 ± 24.5 versus 69.7 ± 24.0, $P = 0.01$) to month 1 (86.6 ± 18.1 versus 85.8 ± 18.5, $P = 0.27$) and month 12 (88.4 ± 17.8 versus 88.5 ± 17.8, $P = 0.94$). SAQ angina frequency repeated measures did not differ in adjusted analysis between groups post baseline (mean difference 1.0; 95% CI -0.2, 2.2; $P = 0.11$). Improvement in SAQ angina frequency was observed with ranolazine at month 6 among diabetics (mean difference 3.3; 95% CI 0.6, 6.1; $P = 0.02$) and those with more angina (baseline SAQ angina frequency ≤60; mean difference 3.4; 95% CI 0.6, 6.2; $P = 0.02$), but was not maintained at month 12.

*Conclusions.*—Despite ICR following PCI, there was no incremental benefit in angina or QOL measures by adding ranolazine in this angiographically-identified population. These measures markedly improved within 1 month of PCI and persisted up to 1 year in both treatment arms.

*Clinical Trial Registration.*—URL: http://www.clinicaltrials.gov. Unique identifier: NCT01442038 (Fig 1).

▶ Despite revascularization, patients with coronary artery disease frequently develop recurrent angina. Ranolazine, which inhibits late sodium current, is able to reduce angina frequency and improve exercise tolerance by modulating the effect of intracellular sodium and calcium concentrations in ischemic cardiac myocytes. RIVER-PCI investigated the effects of addition of ranolazine compared with placebo in 2604 patients with chronic angina (≥2 episodes of angina between 30 days and 1 year before index percutaneous coronary intervention [PCI]) who were deemed to have undergone incomplete revascularization (ICR; ≥50% stenosis in a coronary artery with a reference vessel diameter of ≥2.0 mm). Effects of ranolazine were measured using quality of life (QOL) scores from the Seattle Angina Questionnaire (SAQ) angina frequency as the primary end point with secondary end points using the SAQ treatment satisfaction and Duke Activity Status Index (DASI) scores. The QOL measures were collected at baseline and months 1, 6, and 12, respectively. With both placebo and ranolazine there was significant improvement above baseline QOL scores at all time points following index PCI in regards to the primary and both secondary end points. There effects were similar between the 2 groups (Fig 1). In a subgroup analysis there was a significant difference in favor of ranolazine at 6 months in diabetics and those with high baseline SAQ angina frequency score; however, this difference was not maintained at the 12-month follow-up. Interestingly, although patients had to be characterized as being

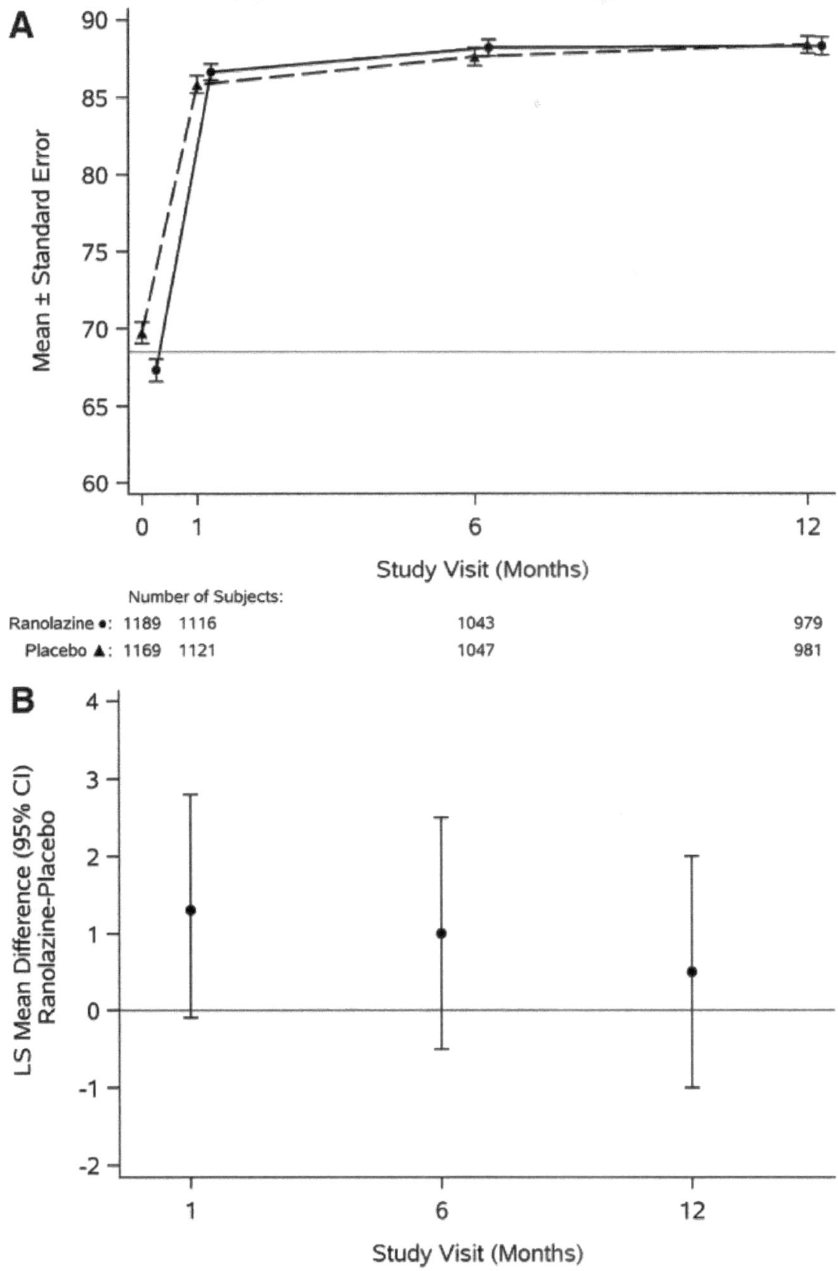


FIGURE 1.—SAQ angina frequency (A) by treatment arm at baseline, month 1, month 6, month 12 and (B) adjusted mean difference and standard error between treatment arms controlling for baseline score and covariates. CI indicates confidence interval; LS, least squares; and SAQ, Seattle Angina Questionnaire. (Reprinted from Alexander KP, Weisz G, Prather K, et al. Effects of ranolazine on angina and quality of life after percutaneous coronary intervention with incomplete revascularization: results from the ranolazine for incomplete vessel revascularization (RIVER-PCI) trial. *Circulation.* 2016; 133:39-47, with permission from American Heart Association, Inc.)

incompletely revascularized for inclusion in the study, this was evaluated using visual estimation of stenosis severity only and did not include functional analysis. It has been previously well described that visual estimation of coronary stenosis has poor correlation to functional significance.[1] Given that there was a low incidence of recurrent angina in the placebo group post–index PCI, there is a question as to the degree of true functional significance of lesions that were deemed to be incompletely revascularized. In conclusion, addition of ranolazine to standard optimal medical therapy in patients who undergo incomplete revascularization as determined by visual coronary stenosis assessment does not offer incremental benefit in QOL measures up to 1 year after index PCI.

**R. Bayer II, MD**

*Reference*

1. Fischer JJ, Samady H, McPherson JA, et al. Comparison between visual assessment and quantitative angiography versus fractional flow reserve for native coronary narrowings of moderate severity. *Am J Cardiol.* 2002;90:210-215.

## Atrial Fibrillation and Risk of ST-Segment–Elevation Versus Non–ST-Segment–Elevation Myocardial Infarction: The Atherosclerosis Risk in Communities (ARIC) Study

Soliman EZ, Lopez F, O'Neal WT, et al (Wake Forest School of Medicine, Winston Salem, NC; Univ of Minnesota, Minneapolis; et al)
*Circulation* 131:1843-1850, 2015

*Background.*—It has recently been reported that atrial fibrillation (AF) is associated with an increased risk of myocardial infarction (MI). However, the mechanism underlying this association is currently unknown. Further study of the relationship of AF with the type of MI (ST-segment–elevation MI [STEMI] versus non–ST-segment–elevation MI [NSTEMI]) might shed light on the potential mechanisms.

*Methods and Results.*—We examined the association between AF and incident MI in 14 462 participants (mean age, 54 years; 56% women; 26% blacks) from the Atherosclerosis Risk in Communities (ARIC) study who were free of coronary heart disease at baseline (1987–1989) with follow-up through December 31, 2010. AF cases were identified from study visit ECGs and by review of hospital discharge records. Incident MI and its types were ascertained by an independent adjudication committee. Over a median follow-up of 21.6 years, 1374 MI events occurred (829 NSTEMIs, 249 STEMIs, 296 unclassifiable MIs). In a multivariable-adjusted model, AF ($n = 1545$) as a time-varying variable was associated with a 63% increased risk of MI (hazard ratio, 1.63; 95% confidence interval, 1.32–2.02). However, AF was associated with NSTEMI (hazard ratio, 1.80; 95% confidence interval, 1.39–2.31) but not STEMI (hazard ratio, 0.49; 95% confidence interval, 0.18–1.34; $P$ for hazard ratio comparison $= 0.004$). Combining the unclassifiable MI group with either STEMI or NSTEMI did not change this conclusion.

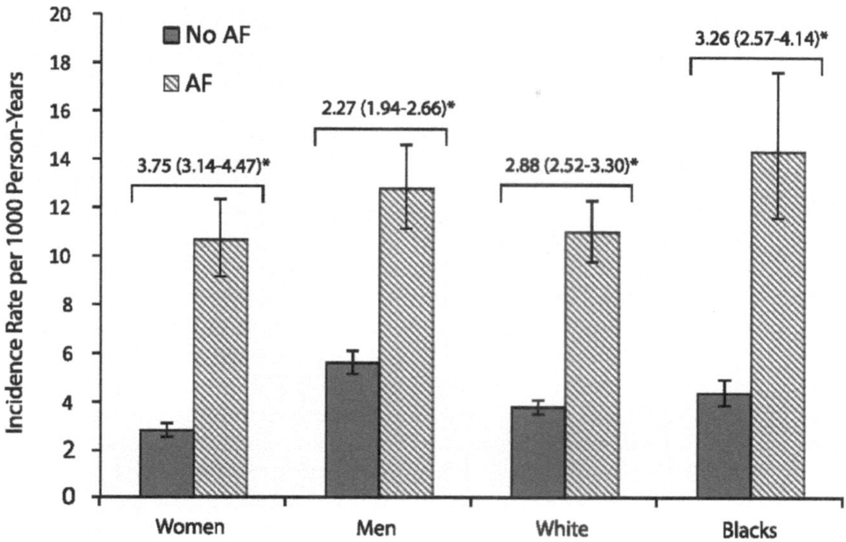


FIGURE 2.—Sex- and race-stratified age-adjusted incidence rates and incidence rate ratios of myocardial infarction by atrial fibrillation (AF) status. *Age-adjusted incidence rate ratio and incidence rates were based on the average age of the cohort (54 years). †Time to event in the AF group is the time from detection of AF, not the cohort inception. (Reprinted from Soliman EZ, Lopez F, O'Neal WT, et al. Atrial fibrillation and risk of ST-segment–elevation versus non–ST-segment–elevation myocardial infarction: the atherosclerosis risk in communities (ARIC) study. *Circulation.* 2015;131:1843-1850, with permission from American Heart Association, Inc.)

The association between AF and MI, total and NSTEMI, was stronger in women than in men (*P* for interaction <0.01 for both).

*Conclusions.*—AF is associated with an increased risk of incident MI, especially in women. However, this association is limited to NSTEMI (Fig 2).

▶ Previous studies have suggested that atrial fibrillation is associated with an increased risk of myocardial infarction (MI), especially in women and African Americans. This study evaluated 14 462 patients enrolled in the Atherosclerosis Risk in Communities trial over 21.6 years median follow-up. Among the 1545 (10.7%) patients who either previously had or subsequently developed atrial fibrillation, the incidence of MI was significantly higher than in those without atrial fibrillation (hazard ratio [HR] 2.93, 95% confidence interval [CI] 2.61-3.30), and it was particularly higher in women (HR, 3.75; 95% CI, 3.14-4.47) and African Americans (HR, 3.26; 95% CI, 2.57-4.14) (Fig 2) Of note, this difference appears to apply only to non–ST segment elevation myocardial infarction (STEMI; HR, 1.80; 95% CI, 1.39-2.31) and not STEMI (HR, 0.49; 95% CI, 0.18-1.34). Based on this study, atrial fibrillation is associated with myocardial infarction, particularly in women and African American patients, but atrial fibrillation is not associated with STEMI.

**D. Steinberg, MD**

**A Multicenter Trial of Remote Ischemic Preconditioning for Heart Surgery**

Meybohm P, for the RIPHeart Study Collaborators (Univ Hosp Frankfurt, Germany, et al)

*N Engl J Med* 373:1397-1407, 2015

*Background.*—Remote ischemic preconditioning (RIPC) is reported to reduce biomarkers of ischemic and reperfusion injury in patients undergoing cardiac surgery, but uncertainty about clinical outcomes remains.

*Methods.*—We conducted a prospective, double-blind, multicenter, randomized, controlled trial involving adults who were scheduled for elective cardiac surgery requiring cardiopulmonary bypass under total anesthesia with intravenous propofol. The trial compared upper-limb RIPC with a sham intervention. The primary end point was a composite of death, myocardial infarction, stroke, or acute renal failure up to the time of hospital discharge. Secondary end points included the occurrence of any individual component of the primary end point by day 90.

*Results.*—A total of 1403 patients underwent randomization. The full analysis set comprised 1385 patients (692 in the RIPC group and 693 in the sham-RIPC group). There was no significant between-group difference in the rate of the composite primary end point (99 patients [14.3%] in the RIPC group and 101 [14.6%] in the sham-RIPC group, $P = 0.89$) or of any of the individual components: death (9 patients [1.3%] and 4 [0.6%], respectively; $P = 0.21$), myocardial infarction (47 [6.8%] and 63 [9.1%], $P = 0.12$), stroke (14 [2.0%] and 15 [2.2%], $P = 0.79$), and acute renal failure (42 [6.1%] and 35 [5.1%], $P = 0.45$). The results were similar in the per-protocol analysis. No treatment effect was found in any subgroup analysis. No significant differences between the RIPC group and the sham-RIPC group were seen in the level of troponin release, the duration of mechanical ventilation, the length of stay in the intensive care unit or the hospital, new onset of atrial fibrillation, and the incidence of postoperative delirium. No RIPC-related adverse events were observed.

*Conclusions.*—Upper-limb RIPC performed while patients were under propofol-induced anesthesia did not show a relevant benefit among patients undergoing elective cardiac surgery. (Funded by the German Research Foundation; RIPHeart ClinicalTrials.gov number, NCT01067703.)

▶ Proof of concept studies in humans have suggested that remote ischemic preconditioning (RIPC) in patients undergoing coronary artery revascularization enhances the ability of vital organs, such as the heart, to withstand prolonged ischemic and reperfusion injury. Although RIPC has been shown to improve surrogate end points such as cardiac biomarkers, clinical outcomes were uncertain. This was evaluated in the present study, which was a prospective, double-blind, multicenter, randomized, controlled trial comparing upper-limb RIPC to sham intervention in 1403 patients undergoing elective cardiac surgery requiring cardiopulmonary bypass. RIPC was induced by 4 cycles of upper-limb ischemia consisting of 5-minute blood pressure cuff inflation to greater than or equal to 200 mm Hg, but at least 15 mm Hg higher than the patient's actual systolic arterial blood pressure, followed by 5-minute cuff deflation. A dummy arm was used for patients assigned to the sham procedure. The primary end point was a binary composite of death from any cause, nonfatal myocardial infarction, new stroke, or acute renal failure up to the time of hospital discharge or a maximum of 14 days if the hospital stay was longer. A significant proportion of patients were high risk based on New York Heart Association class III or IV symptoms (27.7%) or a EuroSCORE of 6 or higher (31.3%). There was no significant difference in the rate of primary end point between the RIPC group (14.3%) and the sham RIPC group (14.6%). Kaplan-Meier estimates of event-free survival were similar in each group at 30 and 90 days (Fig 2 in the original article). Only the EuroSCORE was prognostic for risk of primary end point event: 10.1%, 12.8%, and 20.6% for patients with a EuroSCORE of 0 to 2, 3 to 5, and 6 or higher, respectively ($P < .001$). Although preliminary data suggest RIPC to be beneficial, this randomized clinical trial demonstrated no difference in clinical outcomes.

**T. M. Todoran, MD, MSc**

---

**Coronary Artery Bypass Grafting in Patients 50 Years or Younger: A Swedish Nationwide Cohort Study**

Dalén M, Ivert T, Holzmann MJ, et al (Karolinska Univ Hosp, Stockholm, Sweden)

*Circulation* 131:1748-1754, 2015

---

*Background.*—There are limited data regarding long-term results after coronary artery bypass grafting (CABG) in young adults. We performed a nationwide population-based cohort study to analyze long-term survival, major adverse cardiovascular events, and factors associated with elevated risk in young adults undergoing CABG.

*Methods and Results.*—We included all adult patients ≤50 years of age who underwent primary isolated CABG in Sweden between 1997 and 2013 from the Swedish Web System for Enhancement and Development of Evidence-Based Care in Heart Disease Evaluated According to Recommended Therapies (SWEDEHEART) register. Patient data were linked from national Swedish health data registers to create a study database. We identified 4086 young adults with a mean age of 46 years and 18% women. During a median follow-up time of 10.9 years (interquartile range, 6.4–14.1) 490 (12%) patients died. Survival at 5, 10, and 15 years was 96% (95% CI, 95–96), 90% (95% CI, 89–91), and 82% (95% CI, 80–83), respectively, which was significantly better in comparison with patients aged 51 to 70 years and >70 years who underwent CABG during the same period. The cumulative incidence of death or a major adverse cardiovascular event during 17 years after CABG was mainly driven by myocardial infarction or the need for repeat revascularization. The most important risk factors for all-cause mortality were chronic kidney disease, reduced left ventricular ejection fraction, peripheral vascular disease, or chronic obstructive pulmonary disease.

*Conclusions.*—Long-term survival and freedom from major cardiovascular events after CABG was better in young adults than in older patients. Factors significantly associated with an elevated long-term risk of death or adverse outcome were similar to well-known risk factors for older age groups following CABG.

*Clinical Trial Registration.*—URL: http://www.clinicaltrials.gov. Unique identifier: NCT02276950 (Figs 1, 3 and 4).

▶ There are limited data on long-term outcomes in younger patients who undergo coronary artery bypass grafting (CABG). This study was an observational, population-based cohort study looking at the long-term survival, major adverse cardiovascular events, and factors associated with elevated risk in all adults ≤50 years of age undergoing primary isolated CABG in Sweden from 1997 to 2013. Patients >50 years of age who underwent primary isolated CABG during the same time period were included for comparison. Primary outcomes were all cause mortality and repeat hospitalization for myocardial infarction, heart failure, stroke, or repeat revascularization. From a total of 76 780 patients, 4086 patients age ≤50 years (5.3%), 36 446 patients age 51 to 70 years (47.5%), and 36 252 patients age >70 years identified from the SWEDEGEART register. During a median follow-up of 10.9 years mortality occurred in 12% (490/4086) of patients ≤50 years of age. Cause of death was classified as cardiovascular in 5.8%, noncardiovascular in 4.8%, and unknown in 1.8%. Survival at 5, 10, and 15 years was 96% (confidence interval [CI], 95–96),

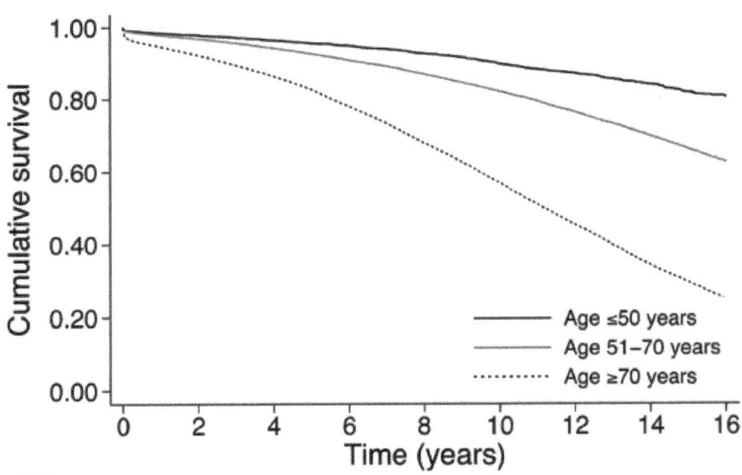


Number at risk

| | | | | | | | | | |
|---|---|---|---|---|---|---|---|---|---|
| Age ≤50 years | 4086 | 3830 | 3496 | 3153 | 2722 | 2291 | 1685 | 1037 | 415 |
| Age 51–70 years | 36442 | 33253 | 29889 | 25983 | 21484 | 16774 | 11529 | 6473 | 2187 |
| Age ≥70 years | 36252 | 31330 | 26923 | 21814 | 16436 | 11318 | 6545 | 2999 | 867 |

FIGURE 1.—Unadjusted overall survival in different age groups who underwent primary isolated CABG in Sweden between 1997 and 2013. CABG indicates coronary artery bypass grafting. (Reprinted from Dalén M, Ivert T, Holzmann MJ, et al. Coronary artery bypass grafting in patients 50 years or younger: a Swedish nationwide cohort study. *Circulation.* 2015;131:1748-1754, with permission from American Heart Association, Inc.)

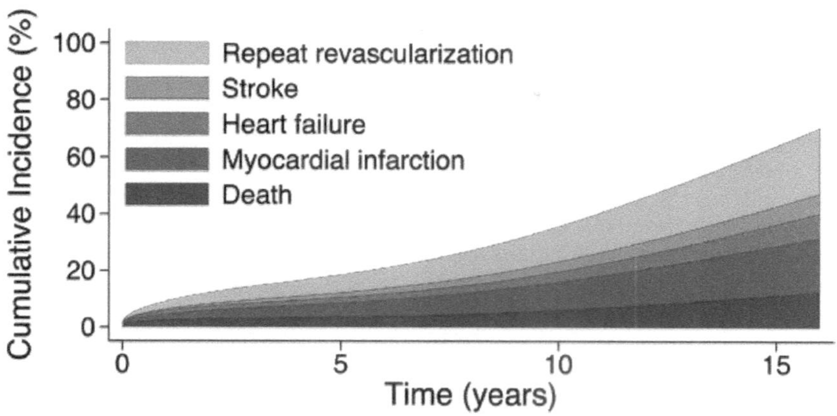


FIGURE 3.—Stacked cumulative incidence of death, myocardial infarction, heart failure, stroke, or repeat revascularization in 3996 patients ≤50 years of age who underwent primary isolated CABG in Sweden between 1997 and 2012. CABG indicates coronary artery bypass grafting. (Reprinted from Dalén M, Ivert T, Holzmann MJ, et al. Coronary artery bypass grafting in patients 50 years or younger: a Swedish nationwide cohort study. *Circulation.* 2015;131:1748-1754, with permission from American Heart Association, Inc.)

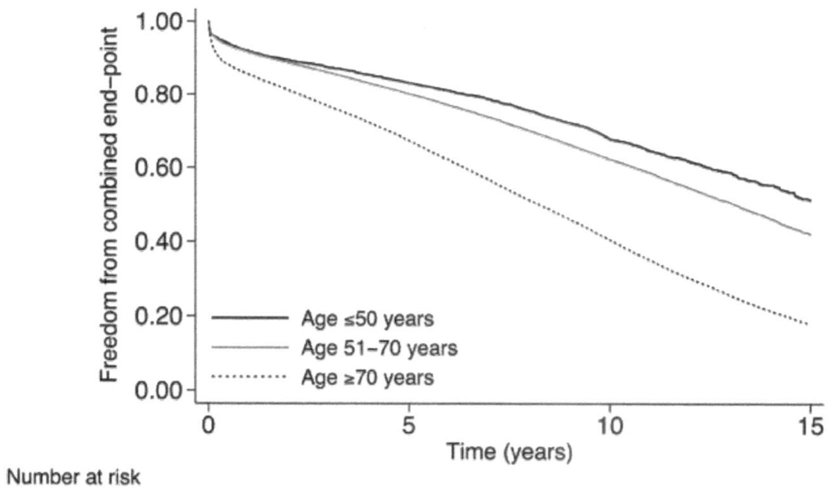


FIGURE 4.—Unadjusted overall freedom from a combination of myocardial infarction, heart failure, stroke, repeat revascularization, or death in different age groups who underwent primary isolated CABG in Sweden between 1997 and 2012. CABG indicates coronary artery bypass grafting. (Reprinted from Dalén M, Ivert T, Holzmann MJ, et al. Coronary artery bypass grafting in patients 50 years or younger: a Swedish nationwide cohort study. *Circulation.* 2015;131:1748-1754, with permission from American Heart Association, Inc.)

90% (CI, 89–91) and 82% (CI, 80–83), respectively (Fig 1). Survival was related to age with higher mortality among older age groups. Multivariate analysis showed impaired renal function, type-1 diabetes, peripheral vascular disease, chronic obstructive pulmonary disease, prior stroke, and reduced ejection fraction were independent risk factors for mortality. Freedom from a composite all-cause mortality, repeat revascularization, myocardial infarction, heart failure, stroke at 5, 10, and 15 years was 83% (CI, 82–84), 68% (CI, 66–69), and 51% (CI, 49–54), respectively (Fig 4). This study demonstrates that younger adults have better long-term survival and freedom from adverse cardiovascular events compared with older patients. Although younger adults have a lower long-term mortality and incidence of adverse cardiovascular events, 15 years after surgery combined outcomes occurred in more than half patients (Fig 3). This result was driven by repeat revascularization and myocardial infarction.

**T. M. Todoran, MD, MSc**

**Subclinical Cardiovascular Disease and Death, Dementia, and Coronary Heart Disease in Patients 80+ Years**

Kuller LH, Lopez OL, Mackey RH, et al (Univ of Pittsburgh, PA; et al)

*J Am Coll Cardiol* 67:1013-1022, 2016

*Background.*—The successful prevention and treatment of coronary heart disease (CHD) and stroke has resulted in a substantial increase in longevity, with subsequent growth in the population of older people at risk for dementia.

*Objectives.*—The authors evaluated the relationship of coronary and other peripheral atherosclerosis to risk of death, dementia, and CHD in the very elderly. Because the extent of vascular disease differs substantially between men and women, sex- and race-specific analyses were included, with a specific focus on women with low coronary artery calcium (CAC) Agatston scores.

*Methods.*—We evaluated the relationship between measures of subclinical cardiovascular disease (CAC, carotid intimal medial thickness, stenosis, and ankle brachial index) and risk of dementia, CHD, and total mortality in 532 participants of the Cardiovascular Health Study-Cognition Study from 1998/1999 (mean age, 80 years) to 2012/2013 (mean age, 93 years).

*Results.*—Thirty-six percent of participants had CAC scores >400. Women and African-Americans had lower CAC scores. Few men had low CAC scores. CAC score and number of coronary calcifications were directly related to age-adjusted total mortality and CHD. The age-specific incidence of dementia was higher than for CHD. Only about 25% of deaths were caused by CHD and 16% by dementia. Approximately 64% of those who died had a prior diagnosis of dementia. White women with low CAC scores had a significantly decreased incidence of dementia.

*Conclusions.*—In subjects 80+ years of age, there is a greater incidence of dementia than of CHD. CAC, as a marker of atherosclerosis, is a determinant of mortality, and risk of CHD and myocardial infarction. White women with low CAC scores had a significantly decreased risk of dementia. A very important unanswered question, especially in the very elderly, is whether prevention of atherosclerosis and its complications is associated with less Alzheimer disease pathology and dementia. (Cardiovascular Health Study [CHS]; NCT00005133) (Image 1 and Fig. 2).

▶ There are limited data evaluating the relationship between coronary artery calcium (CAC) and risk of dementia. In this study the authors examined the relationship of subclinical cardiovascular disease (CVD), CAC, carotid intimal thickness, carotid stenosis, and ankle-brachial index, to the risk of dementia, coronary heart disease, and total mortality in 532 participants of the Cardiovascular Health Study-Cognition Study from 1998–1999 to 2012–2013. The analysis was restricted to 311 participants free from clinical coronary artery disease. CAC >400 and <10 were independent predictor of total mortality (hazard ratio 1.73; 95% confidence interval: 1.18–2.54). The incidence of dementia was similar for men and women. Among white women, the incidence of dementia with a CAC score of 0 was approximately one-third the rate of dementia with a CAC score >400 (*P*=.04; Central Illustration). There were no significant trends for CAC and risk of dementia for white men or African American men and women. The age-specific incidence of dementia was higher than CHD at all ages for women and at older ages for men. The cumulative incidence of CHD was higher in men than women and both white men and women with lower calcium scores have reduced risk of CHD (Fig 2). In summary, this study shows the incidence of dementia in participants >80 years of age is greater than for CHD, especially for women. Approximately 25% of deaths were attributed to CAD and 16% to dementia. These results suggest that the

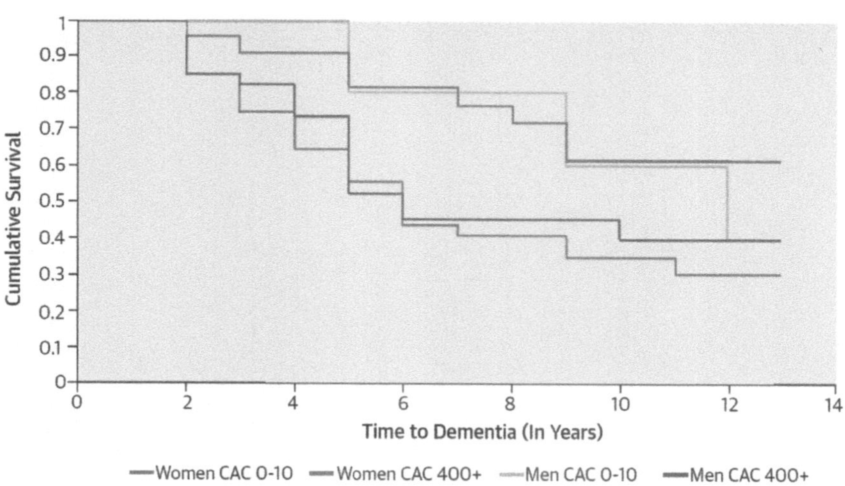


**IMAGE 1.**—Coronary Artery Calcium and Risk of Dementia: Cumulative Incidence of Dementia, 1998/1999 to 2013 for White Women and Men by CAC Score 0 to 10 and 400+. The incidence of dementia is similar in men and women. Men with low CAC scores from 0 to 10 have a low cumulative incidence of dementia. CAC = coronary artery calcium. (Reprinted from Kuller LH, Lopez OL, Mackey RH, et al. Subclinical cardiovascular disease and death, dementia, and coronary heart disease in patients 80+ years. J Am Coll Cardiol. 2016;67:1013-1022, with permission from the American College of Cardiology Foundation.)

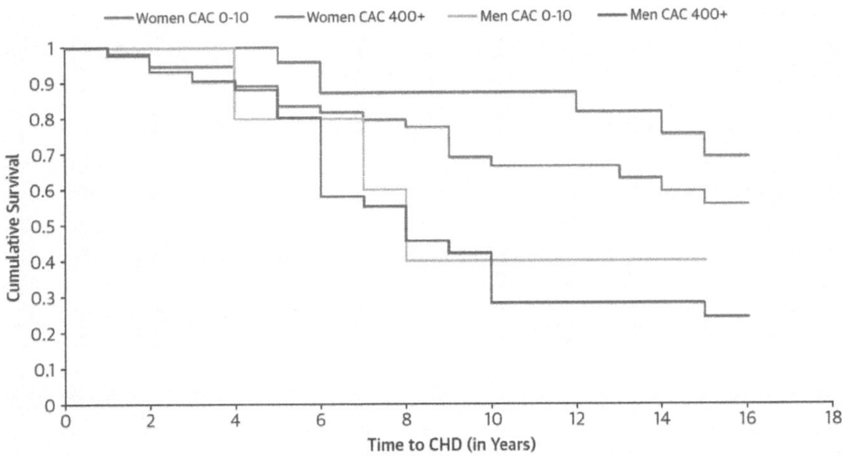


**FIGURE 2.**—Cumulative incidence of CHD, 1998/1999 to 2013 for white women and men by CAC scores 0 to 10 and 400+ cumulative incidence of CHD is higher in men than women. Both white men and women with lower CAC scores have reduced risk of CHD. Abbreviations as in Figure 1. (Reprinted from Kuller LH, Lopez OL, Mackey RH, et al. Subclinical cardiovascular disease and death, dementia, and coronary heart disease in patients 80+ years. *J Am Coll Cardiol.* 2016;67:1013-1022, with permission from the American College of Cardiology Foundation.)

prevalence of dementia in older patients will continue to increase with increasing longevity, and zero or low CAC was associated with lower incidence of dementia among women. This study is limited in that is it an observational study with a small sample size.

**T. M. Todoran, MD, MSc**

# 40 Coronary Intervention Procedures

**Everolimus-Eluting Bioresorbable Scaffolds for Coronary Artery Disease**
Ellis SG, for the ABSORB III Investigators (Cleveland Clinic, OH; et al)
*N Engl J Med* 373:1905-1915, 2015

*Background.*—In patients with coronary artery disease who receive metallic drug-eluting coronary stents, adverse events such as late target-lesion failure may be related in part to the persistent presence of the metallic stent frame in the coronary-vessel wall. Bioresorbable vascular scaffolds have been developed to attempt to improve long-term outcomes.

*Methods.*—In this large, multicenter, randomized trial, 2008 patients with stable or unstable angina were randomly assigned in a 2:1 ratio to receive an everolimus-eluting bioresorbable vascular (Absorb) scaffold (1322 patients) or an everolimus-eluting cobalt–chromium (Xience) stent (686 patients). The primary end point, which was tested for both noninferiority (margin, 4.5 percentage points for the risk difference) and superiority, was target-lesion failure (cardiac death, target-vessel myocardial infarction, or ischemia-driven target-lesion revascularization) at 1 year.

*Results.*—Target-lesion failure at 1 year occurred in 7.8% of patients in the Absorb group and in 6.1% of patients in the Xience group (difference, 1.7 percentage points; 95% confidence interval, −0.5 to 3.9; $P = 0.007$ for noninferiority and $P = 0.16$ for superiority). There was no significant difference between the Absorb group and the Xience group in rates of cardiac death (0.6% and 0.1%, respectively; $P = 0.29$), target-vessel myocardial infarction (6.0% and 4.6%, respectively; $P = 0.18$), or ischemia-driven target-lesion revascularization (3.0% and 2.5%, respectively; $P = 0.50$). Device thrombosis within 1 year occurred in 1.5% of patients in the Absorb group and in 0.7% of patients in the Xience group ($P = 0.13$).

*Conclusions.*—In this large-scale, randomized trial, treatment of noncomplex obstructive coronary artery disease with an everolimus-eluting bioresorbable vascular scaffold, as compared with an everolimus-eluting cobalt–chromium stent, was within the prespecified margin for noninferiority with respect to target-lesion failure at 1 year. (Funded by Abbott Vascular; ABSORB III ClinicalTrials.gov number, NCT01751906.)

▶ For patients undergoing percutaneous coronary intervention (PCI), both the efficacy and the safety of drug-eluting stents have evolved significantly. With current device iterations, restenosis rates of less than 5% and thrombosis rates of less than 1% can be expected across a large spectrum of patient and lesion subsets. Nevertheless, the permanent nature of both the stent scaffold and the polymer remain potential safety concerns; for this reason, bioabsorbable stents have intuitive attractiveness. The current study compared the Absorb bioabsorbable stent with the Xience drug-eluting stent in 2008 patients with stable or unstable angina undergoing PCI with a primary end point of target lesion failure (cardiac death, target vessel myocardial infarction or target lesion revascularization) at 1 year. The study had both noninferior and superiority design. As shown in Fig 1 of the original article, target lesion failure rates were similar between groups (7.8% Absorb vs 6.1% Xience, difference 1.7% (−0.5-3.9), $P = 007$ noninferiority and 0.16 superiority) as was cardiac death (0.6% Absorb vs 0.1% Xience, $P = .29$) myocardial infarction (6.0% Absorb vs 4.6% Xience, $P = .18$) and revascularization (3.0% Absorb vs 2.5% Xience, $P = .50$). Importantly, device thrombosis was also similar between groups (1.5% Absorb vs 0.7% Xience, $P = .13$). Taken together, these results suggest that the Absorb stent is both safe and effective for patients undergoing PCI.

**D. Steinberg, MD**

## Stopping vs. Continuing Aspirin before Coronary Artery Surgery

Myles PS, for the ATACAS Investigators of the ANZCA Clinical Trials Network (Alfred Hosp, Melbourne, Victoria, Australia; et al)
*N Engl J Med* 374:728-737, 2016

*Background.*—Most patients with coronary artery disease receive aspirin for primary or secondary prevention of myocardial infarction, stroke, and death. Aspirin poses a risk of bleeding in patients undergoing surgery, but it is unclear whether aspirin should be stopped before coronary artery surgery.

*Methods.*—We used a 2-by-2 factorial trial design to randomly assign patients who were scheduled to undergo coronary artery surgery and were at risk for perioperative complications to receive aspirin or placebo and tranexamic acid or placebo. The results of the aspirin trial are reported here. Patients were randomly assigned to receive 100 mg of aspirin or matched placebo preoperatively. The primary outcome was a composite of death and thrombotic complications (nonfatal myocardial infarction, stroke, pulmonary embolism, renal failure, or bowel infarction) within 30 days after surgery.

*Results.*—Among 5784 eligible patients, 2100 were enrolled; 1047 were randomly assigned to receive aspirin and 1053 to receive placebo. A primary outcome event occurred in 202 patients in the aspirin group

(19.3%) and in 215 patients in the placebo group (20.4%) (relative risk, 0.94; 95% confidence interval, 0.80 to 1.12; $P = 0.55$). Major hemorrhage leading to reoperation occurred in 1.8% of patients in the aspirin group and in 2.1% of patients in the placebo group ($P = 0.75$), and cardiac tamponade occurred at rates of 1.1% and 0.4%, respectively ($P = 0.08$).

*Conclusions.*—Among patients undergoing coronary artery surgery, the administration of preoperative aspirin resulted in neither a lower risk of death or thrombotic complications nor a higher risk of bleeding than that with placebo. (Funded by the Australian National Health and Medical Research Council and others; Australia New Zealand Clinical Trials Registry number, ACTRN12605000557639.)

▶ Aspirin is a commonly used drug for both primary and secondary prevention in patients with coronary artery disease. However, the antiplatelet effects of aspirin can also result in an increased risk of bleeding in the perioperative setting. The relative risk versus benefit of aspirin in the immediate preoperative period before coronary artery bypass (CABG) surgery has not been specifically defined.

This trial enrolled 2000 patients who were randomized to 100 mg of enteric-coated aspirin or placebo administered 1 to 2 hours before CABG. Other antiplatelets, such as clopidogrel and warfarin were discontinued at least 7 days before surgery. Patients could not have been taking aspirin in the 4 days before CABG. Procedural specifics were left to the discretion of the surgeon, including choice of on or off pump, conduits, inotrope therapy, and all postoperative care. The primary end point was a composite of death, nonfatal myocardial infarction, stroke, pulmonary embolism, renal failure, and bowel infarction in the initial 30 days postoperatively. Secondary outcomes included death, nonfatal myocardial infarction, major hemorrhage, cardiac tamponade, and need for transfusion.

There were no significant differences in either the primary or secondary outcomes between the 2 groups. In addition, subgroup analysis based on sex, age, left ventricular systolic function, risk of bleeding, surgical subtype, or previous exposure to aspirin also revealed no difference between the 2 groups. This study seems to contradict other studies that have indicated a benefit to aspirin preoperatively in regard to thrombotic complications at the expense of a higher risk of bleeding. It should be noted that this trial did not include patients whom has been maintained on aspirin continuously because they had to be off aspirin at least 4 days before to meet enrollment criteria. This may have affected both the benefit and risk that was seen as many patients with CAD proceeding with CABG are on aspirin leading into CABG. Administration 1 to 2 hours before surgery may not have the same antiplatelet effect than being maintained on aspirin continuously leading into CABG.

**R. Bayer II, MD**

# 41 Risk Factors

---

**Fresh Fruit Consumption and Major Cardiovascular Disease in China**

Du H, for the China Kadoorie Biobank Study (Univ of Oxford, UK; Peking Univ Health Science Ctr, Beijing, China; et al)

*N Engl J Med* 374:1332-1343, 2016

---

*Background.*—In Western populations, a higher level of fruit consumption has been associated with a lower risk of cardiovascular disease, but little is known about such associations in China, where the consumption level is low and rates of stroke are high.

*Methods.*—Between 2004 and 2008, we recruited 512,891 adults, 30 to 79 years of age, from 10 diverse localities in China. During 3.2 million person-years of follow-up, 5173 deaths from cardiovascular disease, 2551 incident major coronary events (fatal or nonfatal), 14,579 ischemic strokes, and 3523 intracerebral hemorrhages were recorded among the 451,665 participants who did not have a history of cardiovascular disease or antihypertensive treatments at baseline. Cox regression yielded adjusted hazard ratios relating fresh fruit consumption to disease rates.

*Results.*—Overall, 18.0% of participants reported consuming fresh fruit daily. As compared with participants who never or rarely consumed fresh fruit (the "nonconsumption" category), those who ate fresh fruit daily had lower systolic blood pressure (by 4.0 mm Hg) and blood glucose levels (by 0.5 mmol per liter [9.0 mg per deciliter]) ($P < 0.001$ for trend for both comparisons). The adjusted hazard ratios for daily consumption versus nonconsumption were 0.60 (95% confidence interval [CI], 0.54 to 0.67) for cardiovascular death, and 0.66 (95% CI, 0.58 to 0.75), 0.75 (95% CI, 0.72 to 0.79), and 0.64 (95% CI, 0.56 to 0.74), respectively, for incident major coronary events, ischemic stroke, and hemorrhagic stroke. There was a strong loglinear dose–response relationship between the incidence of each outcome and the amount of fresh fruit consumed. These associations were similar across the 10 study regions and in subgroups of participants defined by baseline characteristics.

*Conclusions.*—Among Chinese adults, a higher level of fruit consumption was associated with lower blood pressure and blood glucose levels and, largely independent of these and other dietary and nondietary factors, with significantly lower risks of major cardiovascular diseases. (Funded by the Wellcome Trust and others.)

▶ Cardiovascular disease has long been the leading cause of death in Western cultures. This has led to much research regarding preventative treatments that has led to a dramatic reduction in the incidence of cardiovascular mortality. This includes pharmacologic, interventional, and lifestyle approaches to the problem. In this regard, smoking cessation, increased exercise, and dietary changes have all occurred and are associated with significant improvements in outcomes. Paradoxically, during the period of declining cardiovascular mortality in Western societies, it has increased in Asian and many developing societies in part because of adoption of Western lifestyles. For instance, in China the incidence of cigarette smoking is now significantly higher than in the United States. However, little is known regarding the impact of diet on cardiovascular mortality in Asia. The China Kadoorie Biobank Study is a prospective observational study of more than a half million Chinese. Only about 18% of the population eat fresh fruit daily. However, this subgroup had lower blood pressure and glycemic control. Importantly, the consumption of fresh fruit was associated with a 40% reduction in cardiovascular mortality and similar reductions in stroke rates. This study reinforces the role and opportunity for lifestyle changes, and in particular dietary modification, to reduce cardiovascular disease in China and likely more globally.

**M. Gold, MD, PhD**

---

**Effect of Financial Incentives to Physicians, Patients, or Both on Lipid Levels: A Randomized Clinical Trial**

Asch DA, Troxel AB, Stewart WF, et al (Univ of Pennsylvania, Philadelphia; Sutter Health System, Sacramento, CA; et al)
*JAMA* 314:1926-1935, 2015

---

*Importance.*—Financial incentives to physicians or patients are increasingly used, but their effectiveness is not well established.

*Objective.*—To determine whether physician financial incentives, patient incentives, or shared physician and patient incentives are more effective than control in reducing levels of low-density lipoprotein cholesterol (LDL-C) among patients with high cardiovascular risk.

*Design, Setting, and Participants.*—Four-group, multicenter, cluster randomized clinical trial with a 12-month intervention conducted from 2011 to 2014 in 3 primary care practices in the northeastern United States. Three hundred forty eligible primary care physicians (PCPs) were enrolled from a pool of 421. Of 25 627 potentially eligible patients of those PCPs, 1503 enrolled. Patients aged 18 to 80 years were eligible if they had a 10-year Framingham Risk Score (FRS) of 20% or greater, had coronary artery disease equivalents with LDL-C levels of 120 mg/dL or greater, or had an FRS of 10% to 20% with LDL-C levels of 140 mg/dL or greater. Investigators were blinded to study group, but participants were not.

*Interventions.*—Primary care physicians were randomly assigned to control, physician incentives, patient incentives, or shared physician-patient incentives. Physicians in the physician incentives group were eligible to receive up to $1024 per enrolled patient meeting LDL-C goals. Patients in the patient incentives group were eligible for the same amount, distributed through daily lotteries tied to medication adherence. Physicians and patients in the shared incentives group shared these incentives. Physicians and patients in the control group received no incentives tied to outcomes, but all patient participants received up to $355 each for trial participation.

*Main Outcomes and Measures.*—Change in LDL-C level at 12 months.

*Results.*—Only patients in the shared physician-patient incentives group achieved reductions in LDL-C levels statistically different from those in the control group (8.5 mg/dL; 95% CI, 3.8-13.3; $P = .002$). For comparison of all 4 groups, $P < .001$.

| Low-Density Lipoprotein Cholesterol Level | Incentives Group | | | |
|---|---|---|---|---|
| | Shared | Physician | Patient | Control |
| Mean reduction (95% CI), mg/dL | 33.6 (30.1-37.1) | 27.9 (24.9-31.0) | 25.1 (21.6-28.5) | 25.1 (21.7-28.5) |
| Baseline, mg/dL | 160.1 | 159.9 | 160.6 | 161.5 |
| 12 Months, mg/dL | 126.4 | 132 | 135.5 | 136.4 |

*Conclusions and Relevance.*—In primary care practices, shared financial incentives for physicians and patients, but not incentives to physicians or patients alone, resulted in a statistically significant difference in reduction of LDL-C levels at 12 months. This reduction was modest, however, and further information is needed to understand whether this approach represents good value.

*Trial Registration.*—clinicaltrials.gov Identifier: NCT01346189.

▶ Although increasingly used, the efficacy of financial incentives for physicians or patients to achieve clinical goals or to improve medical adherence is not proven. To address this issue, the present study was a multicenter, cluster randomized clinical trial comparing 4 approaches to reduce low-density lipoprotein cholesterol (LDL-C) levels among primary care patients with hyperlipidemia and increased cardiovascular disease risk. Participating primary care centers were randomly assigned to 1 of 4 study groups: control, physician incentives, patient incentives, and shared patient-physician incentives. Physicians in the physician incentive group received up to $1024 per enrolled patient meeting LDL-C goals. Patients in the patient incentive group received the same amount that was tied to medication adherence. Physicians and patients in the control group received no incentives tied to outcomes. Three hundred forty physicians were randomized. Of 25 626 eligible patients of these physicians, 1503 enrolled and were allocated to the groups with their physicians. Enrolled patients had a mean baseline Framingham Risk Score of 20%, approximately 35% had coronary artery disease or equivalent, and approximately 50% were not taking statins at enrollment. The primary outcome was change in LDL-C level at 12 months. Patients in the control group, shared physician-patient incentives group, physician incentive group, and patient incentive group has a mean reduction in LDL-C levels of 25.1 mg/dL, 33.6 mg/dL, 27.9 mg/dL, and 25.1 mg/dL, respectively. Compared with the control group, only the shared physician-patient incentive group achieved reductions in LDL-C that were statistically lower (8.5 mg/dL, $P = .002$). At 12 months, more patients in the shared physician-patient incentive group reached their goal LDL-C ($P = .03$), had their medications intensified ($P = .004$), and more medication adherence ($P < .001$) compared with the other groups (Table 2 in the original article). This is the first randomized trial testing the efficacy of financial incentives suggesting that shared incentives among physicians and patients result in achievement of clinical goals compared with no incentives or individual incentives. The changes shown in this study were modest, and further investigation is necessary to determine clinical relevance.

**T. M. Todoran, MD, MSc**

# 42 Valvular Heart Disease

**Initial Surgical Versus Conservative Strategies in Patients With Asymptomatic Severe Aortic Stenosis**

Taniguchi T, on behalf of the CURRENT AS Registry Investigators (Kyoto Univ Graduate School of Medicine, Japan; et al)

*J Am Coll Cardiol* 66:2827-2838, 2015

*Background.*—Current guidelines generally recommend watchful waiting until symptoms emerge for aortic valve replacement (AVR) in asymptomatic patients with severe aortic stenosis (AS).

*Objectives.*—The study sought to compare the long-term outcomes of initial AVR versus conservative strategies following the diagnosis of asymptomatic severe AS.

*Methods.*—We used data from a large multicenter registry enrolling 3,815 consecutive patients with severe AS (peak aortic jet velocity >4.0 m/s, or mean aortic pressure gradient >40 mm Hg, or aortic valve area <1.0 cm$^2$) between January 2003 and December 2011. Among 1,808 asymptomatic patients, the initial AVR and conservative strategies were chosen in 291 patients, and 1,517 patients, respectively. Median follow-up was 1,361 days with 90% follow-up rate at 2 years. The propensity score–matched cohort of 582 patients (n = 291 in each group) was developed as the main analysis set for the current report.

*Results.*—Baseline characteristics of the propensity score–matched cohort were largely comparable, except for the slightly younger age and the greater AS severity in the initial AVR group. In the conservative group, AVR was performed in 41% of patients during follow-up. The cumulative 5-year incidences of all-cause death and heart failure hospitalization were significantly lower in the initial AVR group than in the conservative group (15.4% vs. 26.4%, $p = 0.009$; 3.8% vs. 19.9%, $p < 0.001$, respectively).

*Conclusions.*—The long-term outcome of asymptomatic patients with severe AS was dismal when managed conservatively in this real-world analysis and might be substantially improved by an initial AVR strategy.

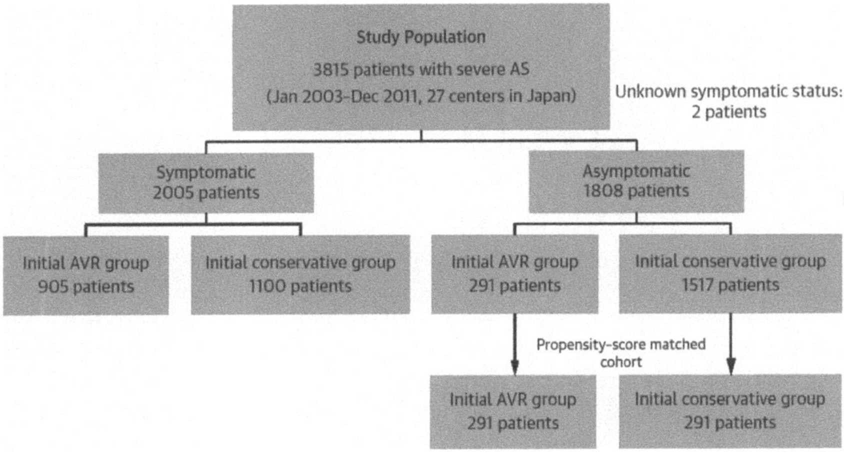


FIGURE 1.—Study flow. From a study population of 3,815 with severe aortic stenosis (AS), 291 of those patients who were asymptomatic underwent aortic valve replacement (AVR) and were compared to 291 managed with a conservative strategy in a propensity score-matched cohort study. (Reprinted from Taniguchi T, on behalf of the CURRENT AS Registry Investigators. Initial surgical versus conservative strategies in patients with asymptomatic severe aortic stenosis. *J Am Coll Cardiol.* 2015;66:2827-2838, with permission from the American College of Cardiology Foundation.)

(Contemporary Outcomes After Surgery and Medical Treatment in Patients With Severe Aortic Stenosis Registry; UMIN000012140) (Fig 1).

▶ For patients with severe aortic stenosis, the decision to pursue surgical aortic valve replacement is classically based on the onset of symptoms (angina, syncope, or congestive heart failure) because life expectancy is not believed to be affected until symptoms arise. The present study challenged that notion and compared outcomes in a propensity analysis of 582 patients with severe aortic stenosis undergoing strategies of initial surgery (n = 291) versus conservative management (n = 291). The primary end point was 5-year cumulative incidence of all-cause death and heart failure hospitalization. As shown in Fig 1, patients managed with initial surgery had a lower incidence of death (15.4% surgery vs 26.4% conservative, $P = .009$) and heart failure hospitalization (3.8% surgery vs 19.9% conservative, $P < .001$). Given a relatively predictable rate of progression with regard to both the severity of aortic stenosis and eventual onset of symptoms, these results suggest that early surgery may be appropriate for patients with asymptomatic severe aortic stenosis, and it provides impetus to rethink the initial treatment strategy.

**D. Steinberg, MD**

**Effect of Clopidogrel and Aspirin vs Aspirin Alone on Migraine Headaches After Transcatheter Atrial Septal Defect Closure: The CANOA Randomized Clinical Trial**

Rodés-Cabau J, Horlick E, Ibrahim R, et al (Quebec Heart and Lung Inst, Canada; Toronto General Hosp, Ontario, Canada; Montreal Heart Inst, Quebec, Canada; et al)

*JAMA* 314:2147-2154, 2015

*Importance.*—The occurrence of new-onset migraine attacks is a complication of transcatheter atrial septal defect (ASD) closure. It has been suggested that clopidogrel may reduce migraine attacks after ASD closure.

*Objective.*—To assess the efficacy of clopidogrel, used in addition to taking aspirin, for the prevention of migraine attacks following ASD closure.

*Design, Setting, and Participants.*—Randomized, double-blind clinical trial performed in 6 university hospitals in Canada. Participants were 171 patients with an indication for ASD closure and no history of migraine.

*Interventions.*—Patients were randomized (1:1) to receive dual antiplatelet therapy (aspirin + clopidogrel [the clopidogrel group], n = 84) vs single antiplatelet therapy (aspirin + placebo [the placebo group], n = 87) for 3 months following transcatheter ASD closure. The first patient was enrolled in December 2008, and the last follow-up was completed in February 2015.

*Main Outcomes and Measures.*—The primary efficacy outcome was the monthly number of migraine days within the 3 months following ASD closure in the entire study population. The incidence and severity of new-onset migraine attacks, as evaluated by the Migraine Disability Assessment questionnaire, were prespecified secondary end points. A zero-inflated Poisson regression model was used for data analysis.

*Results.*—The mean (SD) age of the participants was 49 (15) years and 62% (106) were women. Patients in the clopidogrel group had a reduced mean (SD) number of monthly migraine days within the 3 months following the procedure (0.4 [95% CI, 0.07 to 0.69] days) vs the placebo group (1.4 [95% CI, 0.54 to 2.26] days; difference, −1.02 days [95% CI, −1.94 to −0.10 days]; incident risk ratio [IRR], 0.61 [95% CI, 0.41 to 0.91]; $P = .04$) and a lower incidence of migraine attacks following ASD closure (9.5% for the clopidogrel group vs 21.8% for the placebo group; difference, −12.3% [95% CI, −23% to −1.6%]; odds ratio [OR], 0.38 [95% CI, 0.15 to 0.89]; $P = .03$). Among patients with migraines, those in the clopidogrel group had less-severe migraine attacks (zero patients with moderately or severely disabling migraine attacks vs 37% [7 patients] in the placebo group; difference, −36.8% [95% CI, −58.5% to −15.2%]; $P = .046$). There were no between-group differences in the rate of patients with at least 1 adverse event (16.7% [14 patients] in the clopidogrel group vs 21.8% [19 patients] in the placebo group; difference, −5.2% [95% CI, −17% to 6.6%]; $P = .44$).

*Conclusions and Relevance.*—Among patients who underwent transcatheter ASD closure, the use of clopidogrel and aspirin, compared with aspirin alone, resulted in a lower monthly frequency of migraine attacks over 3 months. Further studies are needed to assess generalizability and durability of this effect.

*Trial Registration.*—clinicaltrials.gov Identifier: NCT00799045

▶ It is well established that patients can develop migraine headaches after transcatheter atrial septal defect (ASD) closure. Although the mechanism is not fully elucidated, there is some thought that new-onset migraine headaches may be platelet-mediated and therefore potentially modifiable by antiplatelet therapy. This study randomized 171 patients to either aspirin and clopidogrel (n = 84) or aspirin and placebo (n = 87) for 3 months after transcatheter ASD closure. As shown in Table 2 in the original article, the patients treated with clopidogrel experienced a significant reduction in the onset of migraine headaches (9.5% clopidogrel vs 21.8% placebo group; odds ratio 0.38, 95% confidence interval [CI] 0.15-0.89; $P = .03$) as well as the number of migraine days per month 0.4 clopidogrel versus 1.4 days, relative risk 0.61, 95% CI 0.41 to 0.91; $P = .04$. These results suggest that 3 months of dual antiplatelet therapy after transcatheter ASD closure may reduce the incidence and frequency of migraine headaches after the procedure. However, it does not address the issue of whether ASD closure is useful for the treatment of migraines.

**D. Steinberg, MD**

# 43 Acute Coronary Syndromes

**Coronary CT Angiography for Suspected ACS in the Era of High-Sensitivity Troponins: Randomized Multicenter Study**

Dedic A, Lubbers MM, Schaap J, et al (Erasmus Univ Med Ctr, Rotterdam, the Netherlands; Amphia Ziekenhuis, Breda, the Netherlands; et al)

*J Am Coll Cardiol* 67:16-26, 2016

*Background.*—It is uncertain whether a diagnostic strategy supplemented by early coronary computed tomography angiography (CCTA) is superior to contemporary standard optimal care (SOC) encompassing high-sensitivity troponin assays (hs-troponins) for patients suspected of acute coronary syndrome (ACS) in the emergency department (ED).

*Objectives.*—This study assessed whether a diagnostic strategy supplemented by early CCTA improves clinical effectiveness compared with contemporary SOC.

*Methods.*—In a prospective, open-label, multicenter, randomized trial, we enrolled patients presenting with symptoms suggestive of an ACS at the ED of 5 community and 2 university hospitals in the Netherlands. Exclusion criteria included the need for urgent cardiac catheterization and history of ACS or coronary revascularization. The primary endpoint was the number of patients identified with significant coronary artery disease requiring revascularization within 30 days.

*Results.*—The study population consisted of 500 patients, of whom 236 (47%) were women (mean age 54 ± 10 years). There was no difference in the primary endpoint (22 [9%] patients underwent coronary revascularization within 30 days in the CCTA group and 17 [7%] in the SOC group [$p = 0.40$]). Discharge from the ED was not more frequent after CCTA (65% vs. 59%, $p = 0.16$), and length of stay was similar (6.3 h in both groups; $p = 0.80$). The CCTA group had lower direct medical costs (337 vs. 511, $p < 0.01$) and less outpatient testing after the index ED visit (10 [4%] vs. 26 [10%], p < 0.01). There was no difference in incidence of undetected ACS.

*Conclusions.*—CCTA, applied early in the work-up of suspected ACS, is safe and associated with less outpatient testing and lower costs. However, in the era of hs-troponins, CCTA does not identify more patients with sig-

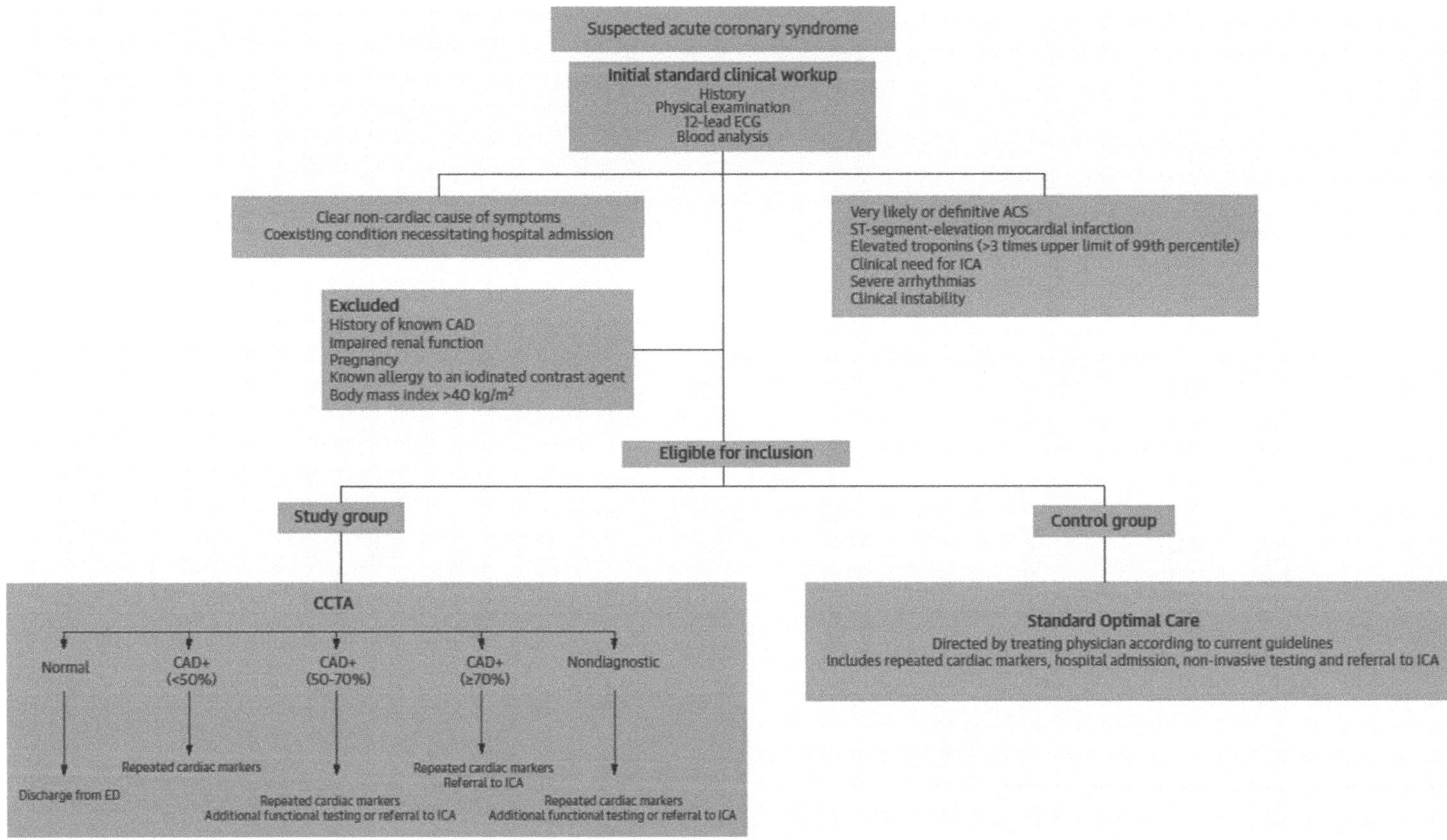


**FIGURE 1.**—Trial profile. In the study group, CCTA results were reported at the point of care, with imaging-based recommendations as displayed. However, the final decision regarding clinical work-up was left to the discretion of the treating physicians. Impaired renal function was classified as an estimated glomerular filtration rate <60% of the age-corrected normal values. ACS = acute coronary syndrome; CAD = coronary artery disease; CCTA = coronary computed tomography angiography; ECG = electrocardiogram; ED = emergency department; ICA = invasive coronary angiography. (Reprinted from Dedic A, Lubbers MM, Schaap J, et al. Coronary CT angiography for suspected ACS in the Era of high-sensitivity troponins randomized multicenter study. *J Am Coll Cardiol.* 2016;67:16-26, with permission from the American College of Cardiology Foundation.)

TABLE 3.—Diagnostic Testing and Resource Utilization

| | CCTA | SOC | *p* Value |
|---|---|---|---|
| Length of stay, h | 6.3 (4.8–11.1) | 6.3 (4.5–25.5) | 0.80 |
| Discharge status | | | 0.16 |
| Discharge from emergency department | 159 (65) | 144 (59) | |
| Admitted to hospital | 86 (35) | 101 (41) | |
| ExECG at index visit | 23 (9) | 130 (53) | <0.01 |
| ExECG <30 days | 32 (13) | 143 (58) | <0.01 |
| SPECT at index visit | 2 (1) | 7 (3) | 0.18 |
| SPECT <30 days | 2 (1) | 16 (7) | <0.01 |
| CMR at index | 1 (0) | 1 (0) | 1.00 |
| CMR <30 days | 1 (0) | 3 (1) | 0.62 |
| CCTA after index visit | 1 (0) | 2 (1) | 1.00 |
| Outpatient diagnostic testing <30 days* | 10 (4) | 26 (11) | <0.01 |
| Cost, | 337 (337–932) | 511 (309–916) | <0.01 |

Values are median (interquartile range) or n (%).

CMR = cardiac magnetic resonance imaging; ExECG = exercise electrocardiography; SPECT = single-photon emission computed tomography myocardial perfusion imaging; other abbreviations as in Table 1 of the original article.

*Total of ExECG, SPECT, CMR, and CCTA in an outpatient setting after index ED visit.

Reprinted from Dedic A, Lubbers MM, Schaap J, et al. Coronary CT angiography for suspected ACS in the Era of high-sensitivity troponins randomized multicenter study. *J Am Coll Cardiol.* 2016;67:16-26, with permission from the American College of Cardiology Foundation.

nificant CAD requiring coronary revascularization, shorten hospital stay, or allow for more direct discharge from the ED. (Better Evaluation of Acute Chest Pain with Computed Tomography Angiography [BEACON]; NCT01413282) (Fig 1, Table 3).

▶ Previous studies have demonstrated that the use of coronary computed tomography angiography (CCTA) as the initial test of choice for evaluation of chest pain in the emergency department (ED) may allow for faster time to diagnosis, shorter duration of ED stay, and reduced health care costs compared with the standard of care. However, in the era of high-sensitivity troponins, which allow for faster diagnosis of acute coronary syndrome (ACS), the incremental benefit of CCTA is less clear.

Accordingly, the addition of CCTA to standard of care (SOC), including high-sensitivity troponins, was investigated to assess whether this improved clinical effectiveness, length of stay, cost, and downstream testing. The study included 500 patients undergoing evaluation for suspected ACS at 5 community and 2 university hospitals in the Netherlands. Patients were excluded if they had clearly noncardiac causes of symptoms, history of coronary artery disease, need for urgent revascularization, a troponin level that exceeded 3× the upper limit of the 99th percentile of the assay, impaired renal function, contrast allergy, or obesity with a body mass index $>40\ kg/m^2$. All patients initially underwent a clinical evaluation, electrocardiogram, and serum markers. They were then subsequently randomized to SOC or SOC plus CCTA. There was no difference between the groups in regard to number of patients undergoing revascularization at 30 days, rate of discharge from the ED, or length of stay (central illustration). Patients in whom CCTA was performed did have lower direct medical costs and less downstream testing. However, they had greater radiation exposure.

This study suggests that use of CCTA in addition to SOC in the era of high-sensitivity troponins does not improve outcomes at 30 days in patients presenting to the ED for symptoms concerning for ACS. Both strategies allow for safe evaluation and discharge home with a low risk of adverse events at 30 days. In addition, it did not appear to affect rates of discharge from the ED or length of stay. It did, however, reduce total cost and use of downstream testing (Table 3). As attention currently continues to be directed at medical cost containment and resource utilization, use of CCTA may provide a way to reduce downstream resource utilization. In addition, it was shown that patients whom underwent CCTA were exposed to higher radiation doses. However, patients who had SOC alone underwent significantly more single-photon emission computed tomography (SPECT) perfusion imaging at 30 days. It was unclear whether this was figured into the radiation exposure of the SOC group. Because SPECT exposes patients to more radiation than standard CCTA examination, this could reduce the difference between the 2 groups.

**R. Bayer II, MD**

---

**Cyclosporine before PCI in Patients with Acute Myocardial Infarction**

Cung TT, Morel O, Cayla G, et al (Centre Hospitalier Universitaire (CHU) Arnaud de Villeneuve, France; Nouvel Hôpital Civil, Strasbourg, France; CHU de Nimes, France; et al)

*N Engl J Med* 373:1021-1031, 2015

---

*Background.*—Experimental and clinical evidence suggests that cyclosporine may attenuate reperfusion injury and reduce myocardial infarct size. We aimed to test whether cyclosporine would improve clinical outcomes and prevent adverse left ventricular remodeling.

*Methods.*—In a multicenter, double-blind, randomized trial, we assigned 970 patients with an acute anterior ST-segment elevation myocardial infarction (STEMI) who were undergoing percutaneous coronary intervention (PCI) within 12 hours after symptom onset and who had complete occlusion of the culprit coronary artery to receive a bolus injection of cyclosporine (administered intravenously at a dose of 2.5 mg per kilogram of body weight) or matching placebo before coronary recanalization. The primary outcome was a composite of death from any cause, worsening of heart failure during the initial hospitalization, rehospitalization for heart failure, or adverse left ventricular remodeling at 1 year. Adverse left ventricular remodeling was defined as an increase of 15% or more in the left ventricular end-diastolic volume.

*Results.*—A total of 395 patients in the cyclosporine group and 396 in the placebo group received the assigned study drug and had data that could be evaluated for the primary outcome at 1 year. The rate of the primary outcome was 59.0% in the cyclosporine group and 58.1% in the control group (odds ratio, 1.04; 95% confidence interval, 0.78 to 1.39;

$P = 0.77$). Cyclosporine did not reduce the incidence of the separate clinical components of the primary outcome or other events, including recurrent infarction, unstable angina, and stroke. No significant difference in the safety profile was observed between the two treatment groups.

*Conclusions.*—In patients with anterior STEMI who had been referred for primary PCI, intravenous cyclosporine did not result in better clinical outcomes than those with placebo and did not prevent adverse left ventricular remodeling at 1 year. (Funded by the French Ministry of Health and NeuroVive Pharmaceutical; CIRCUS ClinicalTrials.gov number, NCT01502774; EudraCT number, 2009-013713-99.)

▶ One of the primary goals of early revascularization in ST-segment elevation myocardial (STEMI) is to establish myocardial perfusion and limit infarction size. In addition to early revascularization, experimental evidence suggests that cyclosporine may further limit infarct size by attenuating reperfusion injury. This study evaluated 791 patients with anterior STEMI, randomizing them to either 2.5 mg/kg intravenous cyclosporine before percutaneous coronary intervention ($n = 395$) or to placebo ($n = 396$). The primary composite end point was death, heart failure during the index hospitalization, readmission for heart failure, or adverse left ventricular remodeling (> 15% increase in end-diastolic volume) at 1 year. As shown in Fig 2 of the original article, the primary end point occurred in 59% of the cyclosporine-treated patients and 58.1% of placebo-treated patients (odds ratio 1.04; 95% confidence interval 0.78-1.39; $P = .77$) with no significant differences in any of the components of the primary end point. Treatment with cyclosporine was of no clinical benefit, and there was no difference in adverse left ventricular remodeling at 1 year.

**D. Steinberg, MD**

---

**Complete revascularisation versus treatment of the culprit lesion only in patients with ST-segment elevation myocardial infarction and multivessel disease (DANAMI-3—PRIMULTI): an open-label, randomised controlled trial**

Engstrøm T, for the DANAMI-3—PRIMULTI Investigators (Univ of Copenhagen, Denmark; et al)

*Lancet* 386:665-671, 2015

---

*Background.*—Patients with acute ST-segment elevation myocardial infarction (STEMI) and multivessel coronary disease have a worse prognosis compared with individuals with single-vessel disease. We aimed to study the clinical outcome of patients with STEMI treated with fractional flow reserve (FFR)-guided complete revascularisation versus treatment of the infarct-related artery only.

*Methods.*—We undertook an open-label, randomised controlled trial at two university hospitals in Denmark. Patients presenting with STEMI who had one or more clinically significant coronary stenosis in addition to the lesion in the infarct-related artery were included. After successful percutaneous coronary intervention (PCI) of the infarct-related artery, patients were randomly allocated (in a 1:1 ratio) either no further invasive treatment or complete FFR-guided revascularisation before discharge. Randomisation was done electronically via a web-based system in permuted blocks of varying size by the clinician who did the primary PCI. All patients received best medical treatment. The primary endpoint was a composite of all-cause mortality, non-fatal reinfarction, and ischaemia-driven revascularisation of lesions in non-infarct-related arteries and was assessed when the last enrolled patient had been followed up for 1 year. Analysis was on an intention-to-treat basis. This trial is registered with ClinicalTrials.gov, number NCT01960933.

*Findings.*—From March, 2011, to February, 2014, we enrolled 627 patients to the trial; 313 were allocated no further invasive treatment after primary PCI of the infarct-related artery only and 314 were assigned complete revascularisation guided by FFR values. Median follow-up was 27 months (range 12–44 months). Events comprising the primary endpoint were recorded in 68 (22%) patients who had PCI of the infarct-related artery only and in 40 (13%) patients who had complete revascularisation (hazard ratio 056, 95% CI 038–083; $p = 0004$).

*Interpretation.*—In patients with STEMI and multivessel disease, complete revascularisation guided by FFR measurements significantly reduces the risk of future events compared with no further invasive intervention after primary PCI. This effect is driven by significantly fewer repeat revascularisations, because all-cause mortality and non-fatal reinfarction did not differ between groups. Thus, to avoid repeat revascularisation, patients can safely have all their lesions treated during the index admission. Future studies should clarify whether complete revascularisation should be done acutely during the index procedure or at later time and whether it has an effect on hard endpoints. (Fig 2)

▶ The optimal treatment of patients with ST-segment elevation myocardial infarction (STEMI) and multivessel disease is controversial. Multiple previous registries showed lack of benefit, or even harm, associated with complete revascularization versus treatment of the infarct artery only. This study evaluated outcomes in 627 patients with STEMI randomized to either fractional flow reserve (FFR)-guided complete revascularization during the index hospitalization ($n = 314$) or treatment of the infarct artery alone ($n = 313$). All patients were followed for at least 1 year with a primary composite end point of all-cause mortality, nonfatal reinfarction, or ischemia-driven revascularization. As shown in Fig 2, over a median follow-up of 27 months, patients with FFR-guided complete revascularization had a lower risk of events than those undergoing infarct artery treatment alone (13% vs 22%, hazard ratio 0.56, 95% confidence interval 0.38–0.83; $P = .004$). The reduction of events was driven primarily by revascularization, and there was no significant difference regarding either mortality or nonfatal reinfarction. This study suggests that patients with STEMI and multivessel

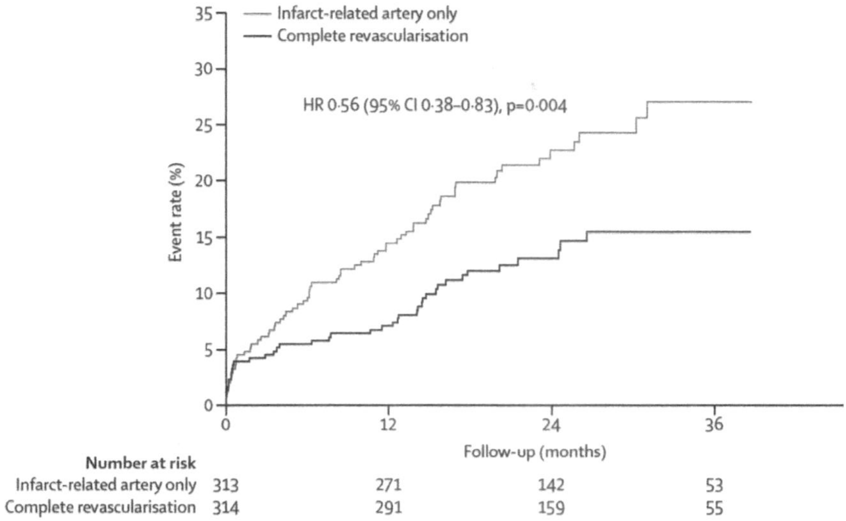


FIGURE 2.—Event rates of the combined primary endpoint. Follow-up was for 44 months after primary percutaneous coronary intervention. HR=hazard ratio. (Reprinted from Engstrøm T, for the DANAMI-3—PRIMULTI Investigators. Complete revascularisation versus treatment of the culprit lesion only in patients with ST-segment elevation myocardial infarction and multivessel disease (DANAMI-3—PRIMULTI): an open-label, randomised controlled trial. *Lancet.* 2015;386:665-671.)

coronary artery disease may benefit from a strategy of complete revascularization during the index hospitalization.

**D. Steinberg, MD**

---

**Association of Admission to Veterans Affairs Hospitals vs Non-Veterans Affairs Hospitals With Mortality and Readmission Rates Among Older Men Hospitalized With Acute Myocardial Infarction, Heart Failure, or Pneumonia**

Nuti SV, Qin L, Rumsfeld JS, et al (Yale–New Haven Hosp, CT; The VA Eastern Colorado Healthcare System, Denver; et al)

*JAMA* 315:582-592, 2016

---

*Importance.*—Little contemporary information is available about comparative performance between Veterans Affairs (VA) and non-VA hospitals, particularly related to mortality and readmission rates, 2 important outcomes of care.

*Objective.*—To assess and compare mortality and readmission rates among men in VA and non-VA hospitals.

*Design, Setting, and Participants.*—Cross-sectional analysis involving male Medicare fee-for-service beneficiaries aged 65 years or older hospitalized between 2010 and 2013 in VA and non-VA acute care hospitals for acute myocardial infarction (AMI), heart failure (HF), or pneumonia using the Medicare Standard Analytic Files and Enrollment Database together with VA administrative claims data. To avoid confounding geographic effects with health care system effects, we studied VA and non-VA hospitals within the same metropolitan statistical area (MSA).

*Exposures.*—Hospitalization in a VA or non-VA hospital in MSAs that contained at least 1 VA and non-VA hospital.

*Main Outcomes and Measures.*—For each condition, 30-day risk-standardized mortality rates and risk-standardized readmission rates for VA and non-VA hospitals. Mean aggregated within-MSA differences in mortality and readmission rates were also assessed.

*Results.*—We studied 104 VA and 1513 non-VA hospitals, with each condition-outcome analysis cohort for VA and non-VA hospitals containing at least 7900 patients (men; ≥65 years), in 92 MSAs. Mortality rates were lower in VA hospitals than non-VA hospitals for AMI (13.5% vs 13.7%, $P = .02$; −0.2 percentage-point difference) and HF (11.4%vs 11.9%, $P = .008$; −0.5 percentage-point difference), but higher for pneumonia (12.6% vs 12.2%, $P = .045$; 0.4 percentage-point difference). In contrast, readmission rates were higher in VA hospitals for all 3 conditions (AMI, 17.8% vs 17.2%, 0.6 percentage-point difference; HF, 24.7% vs 23.5%, 1.2 percentage-point difference; pneumonia, 19.4% vs 18.7%, 0.7 percentage-point difference, all $P < .001$). In within-MSA comparisons, VA hospitals had lower mortality rates for AMI (percentage-point difference, −0.22; 95% CI, −0.40 to −0.04) and HF (−0.63; 95% CI, −0.95 to −0.31), and mortality rates for pneumonia were not significantly different (−0.03; 95% CI, −0.46 to 0.40); however, VA hospitals had higher readmission rates for AMI (0.62; 95% CI, 0.48 to 0.75), HF (0.97; 95%CI, 0.59 to 1.34), or pneumonia (0.66; 95% CI, 0.41 to 0.91).

*Conclusions and Relevance.*—Among older men with AMI, HF, or pneumonia, hospitalization at VA hospitals, compared with hospitalization at non-VA hospitals, was associated with lower 30-day risk-standardized all-cause mortality rates for AMI and HF, and higher 30-day risk-standardized all-cause readmission rates for all 3 conditions, both nationally and within similar geographic areas, although absolute differences between these outcomes at VA and non-VA hospitals were small.

▶ Public reporting of hospital outcomes and readmission rates have garnered increase public attention. In addition, the Center for Medicare and Medicaid Services (CMS) instituted a program in 2012 to reduce 30-day hospital readmission rates in non-Veterans Affairs (VA) hospitals through financial penalties. This study sought to compare the performance of VA and non-VA hospitals in regard to mortality and 30-day readmission rates for patients with a discharge diagnosis of acute myocardial infarction (AMI), heart failure (HF), and pneumonia (PNA). The study population included only men aged >65 whom were Medicare fee-for-service beneficiaries. The study population was selected in metropolitan areas where there was at least 1 VA hospital and 1 non-VA hospital. In all 388 metropolitan areas in the United States were included, which encompassed 104 VA hospitals and 1513 non-VA hospitals. For the diagnostic categories of AMI and HF patients admitted to VA hospital had lower mortality rates when compared with non-VA hospitals (13.5% vs 13.7% and 11.4% vs 11.9%, respectively). This difference persisted even after risk-adjusted mortality was calculated. However, in regard to PNA, mortality rates at VA hospitals was higher than other non-VA hospitals (12.6% vs 12.2%). For all 3 diagnoses, 30-day readmission rates were higher for VA hospitals. In conclusion, although there did appear to be differences in both hospital mortality as well as readmission rates between VA and non-VA hospitals, these differences were quite small and unlikely to affect decisions regarding in these different institutions.

**R. Bayer II, MD**

PART SIX

# THE DIGESTIVE SYSTEM

KENNETH R. DEVAULT, MD, FACG

# Introduction

This has been another remarkable year in the literature for gastroenterology and hepatology. Practice guidelines are often well-researched documents and this year we highlighted guidelines in functional heartburn, Barrett's esophagus, Helicobacter pylori, small bowel bleeding, microscopic colitis, colon cancer screening and liver disease during pregnancy. In the esophagus and stomach, it has become clear that opioids adversely affect esophageal function in addition to their known gastric and colon affects. Celiac disease remains a large concern with papers calling some of our wide-spread testing into question. Advances in both diet and medication for IBS were published this year. Colon cancer screening continues to have a high importance and we have highlighted a few important studies. Important papers were selected in the pancreatic/biliary system and liver. Obesity remains a major health concern in both the young and old. Finally, a controversial association between proton pump inhibitor use and dementia was reviewed.

**Kenneth R. DeVault, MD, FACG**

# 44 Esophagus

**Lifestyle Intervention in Gastroesophageal Reflux Disease**

Ness-Jensen E, Hveem K, El-Serag H, et al (Karolinska Institutet, Stockholm, Sweden; Norwegian Univ of Science and Technology, Levanger, Norway)

*Clin Gastroenterol Hepatol* 14:175-182.e1-3, 2016

*Background & Aims.*—Gastroesophageal reflux disease (GERD) affects up to 30% of adults in Western populations and is increasing in prevalence. GERD is associated with lifestyle factors, particularly obesity and tobacco smoking, which also threatens the patient's general health. GERD carries the risk of several adverse outcomes and there is widespread use of potent acid-inhibitors, which are associated with long-term adverse effects. The aim of this systematic review was to assess the role of lifestyle intervention in the treatment of GERD.

*Methods.*—Literature searches were performed in PubMed (from 1946), EMBASE (from 1980), and the Cochrane Library (no start date) to October 1, 2014. Meta-analyses, systematic reviews, randomized clinical trials (RCTs), and prospective observational studies were included.

*Results.*—Weight loss was followed by decreased time with esophageal acid exposure in 2 RCTs (from 5.6% to 3.7% and from 8.0% to 5.5%), and reduced reflux symptoms in prospective observational studies. Tobacco smoking cessation reduced reflux symptoms in normal-weight individuals in a large prospective cohort study (odds ratio, 5.67). In RCTs, late evening meals increased time with supine acid exposure compared with early meals (5.2% point change), and head-of-the-bed elevation decreased time with supine acid exposure compared with a flat position (from 21% to 15%).

*Conclusions.*—Weight loss and tobacco smoking cessation should be recommended to GERD patients who are obese and smoke, respectively. Avoiding late evening meals and head-of-the-bed elevation is effective in nocturnal GERD.

▶ Gastroesophageal reflux disease is a common disorder. Lifestyle intervention is often suggested as the first step in treatment and is also advocated as an adjunct to medical therapy. Recent concern about the safety of proton pump inhibitor therapy has created added interest in nonpharmacologic therapy. This systematic review found that tobacco smoking should be eliminated and that weight loss should be suggested in obese patients. Elevation of the head of the bed and avoidance of late meals should be suggested in those with nocturnal symptoms. How much can be expected from these interventions? The data on weight loss are most robust for obese patients who loose a great deal of weight, but smaller, yet still significant, effects are seen when overweight or even normal weight patients lose weight, although this has not been seen in all studies. The data for smoking cessation are weaker but still supportable given the modest effect on reflux and the more important effect on other health factors. Many other diet and lifestyle interventions have been studied with pH testing, but the best clinical data were with avoiding late night meals and elevation of the head of the bed, both of which were only beneficial in patients with nighttime symptoms. Otherwise, a discussion with each patient about individual "trigger" symptoms will potentially result in improvement without creating unnecessary stress and lifestyle disruption.

**K. R. DeVault, MD**

## Opioid-Induced Esophageal Dysfunction (OIED) in Patients on Chronic Opioids

Ratuapli SK, Crowell MD, DiBaise JK, et al (Mayo Clinic, Scottsdale, AZ; et al)
*Am J Gastroenterol* 110:979-984, 2015

*Objectives.*—Bowel dysfunction has been recognized as a predominant side effect of opioid use. Even though the effects of opioids on the stomach and small and large intestines have been well studied, there are limited data on opioid effects on esophageal function. The aim of this study was to compare esophageal pressure topography (EPT) of patients taking opioids at the time of the EPT (≤24 h) with chronic opioid users who were studied off opioid medications for at least 24 h using the Chicago classification v3.0.

*Methods.*—A retrospective review identified 121 chronic opioid users who completed EPT between March 2010 and August 2012. Demographic and manometric data were compared between the two groups using general linear models or $\chi^2$.

*Results.*—Of the 121 chronic opioid users, 66 were studied on opioid medications (≤24 h) and 55 were studied off opioid medications for at least 24 h. Esophagogastric junction (EGJ) outflow obstruction was significantly more prevalent in patients using opioids within 24 h compared with those who did not (27% vs. 7%, $P = 0.004$). Mean 4 s integrated relaxation pressure was also significantly higher in patients studied on opioids (10.71 vs. 6.6 mm Hg, $P = 0.025$). Resting lower esophageal sphincter pressures tended to be higher on opioids (31.61 vs. 26.98 mm Hg, $P = 0.25$). Distal latency was significantly lower in patients studied on opioids (6.15 vs. 6.74 s, $P = 0.044$).

*Conclusions.*—Opioid use within 24 h of EPT is associated with more frequent EGJ outflow obstruction and spastic peristalsis compared with when opioid use is stopped for at least 24 h before the study.

▶ It has long been accepted that opioids result in motility problems in the gastrointestinal tract, including delayed gastric emptying and constipation. This article highlights the fact that the esophagus is not immune to opioid-induced dysmotility. The major finding was evidence of lower esophageal sphincter dysfunction (esophagogastric junction outflow obstruction). This did not seem to be case in patients in whom opioids were held 24 hours before the study.

How can this help me in clinical practice? First, if a patient on chronic opioids presents with dysphagia, obstructive and other mechanical causes still need to be excluded. Once those are excluded, opioid-induced dysfunction should be considered. This can be confirmed with manometry, but if the patient seems a candidate for pain rehabilitation and opioid elimination, then it is reasonable to go directly to that step. Although many patients have mild disorders, others may have more severe disorders, even an achalasia-like appearance including some of the patients in this study. Care should therefore be taken when diagnosing motility disorders with patients who are on narcotics. I would not go so far as to say don't test on narcotics, but would reconsider the diagnosis before surgical or endoscopic intervention. This article would suggest that stopping for 24 hours may be enough to allow the esophagus to recover, although there is still a possibility that the 2 groups were not well matched. They did not have paired studies (on and off narcotics), which would certainly be helpful. Other medications that could affect esophageal function include nitrates, calcium channel blockers, anticholinergics, and phosphodiesterase inhibitors.

**K. R. DeVault, MD**

---

**Diagnosis and Management of Functional Heartburn**

Hachem C, Shaheen NJ (St Louis Univ, MO; Univ of North Carolina at Chapel Hill)

*Am J Gastroenterol* 111:53-61, 2016

---

Heartburn is among the most common gastrointestinal symptoms presenting to both generalist physicians and gastroenterologists. Heartburn that does not respond to traditional acid suppression is a diagnostic and therapeutic dilemma. In the era of high utilization of proton pump inhibitors, a substantial proportion of patients presenting to the gastroenterologist with chronic symptoms of heartburn do not have a reflux-mediated disease. Subjects without objective evidence of reflux as a cause of their symptoms have "functional heartburn". The diagnostic role of endoscopy, reflux and motility testing in functional heartburn (FH) patients is discussed. Lifestyle modifications, pharmacological interventions, and alternative therapies for FH are also presented. Recognition of patients with FH allows earlier assignment of these patients to different treatment algorithms, which may allow greater likelihood of success of treatment, diminished resource utilization and improved quality of life. Further data on this large and understudied group of patients is necessary to allow improvement in treatment algorithms and a more evidence-based approach to care of these patients.

▶ Many functional disorders of the gastrointestinal tract have been defined, including noncardiac chest pain, dyspepsia, and irritable bowel syndrome. Functional heartburn (FH) is another, important syndrome to understand. A series of steps are required to come to the diagnosis of FH. First, the patient should have Barrett's esophagus and esophagitis excluded with endoscopy; second, a pH test is used to segregate the endoscopy negative patients into the following:

1. Nonerosive reflux disease (NERD): excess acid exposure but no esophagitis.
2. Esophageal hypersensitivity (EH): normal acid exposure but positive symptom correlation between esophageal acid and heartburn.
3. Functional heartburn (FH): normal acid exposure, negative symptom association and other etiologies for the symptoms excluded.

The authors suggest that around 15% of patients presenting with heartburn will be classified as FH. There are substantial challenges in the diagnosis of FH, including that most endoscopies are done on acid blockers, making it impossible to know whether the patient ever had esophagitis or truly has NERD, EH, or FH; the role of symptom index and symptom association probability in defining EH is incompletely defined; and finally, there are data suggesting a great deal of day-to-day variability in reflux testing.

Assuming we can diagnose FH, what do we know about treatment? Diet and lifestyle changes have not been well studied, but it is reasonable for patients to avoid triggering factors. There are also data suggesting increased esophageal sensitivity with loss of sleep and increased stress, so attempting to improve those factors is reasonable. Despite the negative testing, some patients still respond to acid suppression. The reason for this is not clear, but the overlap with dyspepsia and high placebo response are possibilities. Attempts at altering pain perception are part of the approach to most functional disorders. Melatonin, tricyclic antidepressants, and serotonin reuptake inhibitors have all been tried with some success.

**K. R. DeVault, MD**

---

**Imipramine for Treatment of Esophageal Hypersensitivity and Functional Heartburn: A Randomized Placebo-Controlled Trial**

Limsrivilai J, Charatcharoenwitthaya P, Pausawasdi N, et al (Mahidol Univ, Bangkok, Thailand)

*Am J Gastroenterol* 111:217-224, 2016

---

*Objectives.*—Tricyclic antidepressants could be effective in the treatment of symptoms related to hypersensitive esophagus through their pain-modulating effect. We therefore assessed the benefit of imipramine in patients with esophageal hypersensitivity and functional heartburn.

*Methods.*—Patients with normal endoscopy findings and typical reflux symptoms despite standard-dose proton-pump inhibitor therapy underwent 24-h pH-impedance monitoring. Patients with established esophageal hypersensitivity or functional heartburn were randomly assigned to receive 8 weeks of either once-daily imipramine 25 mg ($n = 43$) or placebo ($n = 40$). The primary end point was satisfactory relief of reflux symptoms, defined as a >50% reduction in the gastroesophageal reflux disease score. The secondary end point was improvement in quality-of-life (QoL) as assessed by the 36-Item Short Form Health Survey score.

*Results.*—Patients receiving imipramine did not achieve a higher rate of satisfactory relief of reflux symptoms than did patients receiving placebo (intention-to-treat (ITT) analysis: 37.2 vs. 37.5%, respectively; odds ratio (OR), 0.99; 95% confidence interval (CI), 0.41–2.41; per-protocol (PP) analysis: 45.5 vs. 41.2%, respectively; OR, 1.19; 95% CI, 0.45–3.13). Subgroup analysis to assess the efficacy of imipramine for either esophageal hypersensitivity or functional heartburn yielded similar results. Treatment with imipramine provided significant improvement of QoL by PP analysis (72 ± 17 and 61 ± 19, respectively; $P = 0.048$), but ITT analysis did not reveal any differences between imipramine and placebo (68 ± 19 and 61 ± 19, respectively; $P = 0.26$). Adverse events were similar in both groups; however, constipation was more common with imipramine than placebo (51.2 vs. 22.5%, respectively; $P = 0.01$).

*Conclusions.*—Although low-dose imipramine shows potential QoL benefits, it does not relieve symptoms more effectively than does placebo in patients with either esophageal hypersensitivity or functional heartburn.

▶ Antidepressant medications have long been advocated in the treatment of functional disorders of the gastrointestinal (GI) tract, including noncardiac chest pain, dyspepsia, and irritable bowel syndrome. This study looks the effect of imipramine in patients with esophageal hypersensitivity and functional heartburn. In contrast to studies of other "functional" GI diseases, low-dose imipramine was not superior to placebo in regard to symptoms, although quality of life improved more in the treated patients.

Why did this study fail to show a difference? First is the patient population. They had to have reflux symptoms, a normal endoscopy, manometry, and pH test. It is still possible that some of these patients had more traditional gastroesophageal reflux disease because there is a reasonable false-negative rate with a single 24-hour pH test. The symptom index (SI) was used to distinguish between esophageal sensitivity and functional heartburn, but both groups seemed to behave similarly in the study. It was not clear in the study how often the SI was related to acid or nonacid reflux. These may behave differently. Imipramine has anticholinergic activity, so there is some possibility that it actually increased reflux, which could more than offset any antinociceptive activity. This could be why the prior study of SSRIs was more successful. If I desired to suppress symptoms in this type of patient, this and other studies would support selective serotonin reuptake inhibitors over antidepressants with anticholinergic activity like imipramine. Trazodone might be another option, but it has not been studied in this group.

**K. R. DeVault, MD**

## ACG Clinical Guideline: Diagnosis and Management of Barrett's Esophagus

Shaheen NJ, Falk GW, Iyer PG, et al (Univ of North Carolina at Chapel Hill; Univ of Pennsylvania Perelman School of Medicine; Mayo Clinic Minnesota, Rochester; et al)

*Am J Gastroenterol* 111:30-50, 2016

Barrett's esophagus (BE) is among the most common conditions encountered by the gastroenterologist. In this document, the American College of Gastroenterology updates its guidance for the best practices in caring for these patients. These guidelines continue to endorse screening of high-risk patients for BE; however, routine screening is limited to men with reflux symptoms and multiple other risk factors. Acknowledging recent data on the low risk of malignant progression in patients with nondysplastic BE, endoscopic surveillance intervals are attenuated in this population; patients with nondysplastic BE should undergo endoscopic surveillance no more frequently than every 3–5 years. Neither routine use of biomarker panels nor advanced endoscopic imaging techniques (beyond high-definition endoscopy) is recommended at this time. Endoscopic ablative therapy is recommended for patients with BE and high-grade dysplasia, as well as T1a esophageal adenocarcinoma. Based on recent level 1 evidence, endoscopic ablative therapy is also recommended for patients with BE and low-grade dysplasia, although endoscopic surveillance continues to be an acceptable alternative. Given the relatively common recurrence of BE after ablation, we suggest postablation endoscopic surveillance intervals. Although many of the recommendations provided are based on weak evidence or expert opinion, this document provides a pragmatic framework for the care of the patient with BE.

▶ Barrett esophagus (BE) is a complication of gastroesophageal reflux disease that results in a small but real increase in the risk of esophageal adenocarcinoma (EAC). The American College of Gastroenterology has produced a guideline statement on the diagnosis and management of BE. Important or novel concepts from that guideline include the following:

1. BE remains a diagnosis that requires characteristic endoscopic findings (an extension of columnar mucosa into the body of the esophagus), along with biopsy-provided histological confirmation (intestinal metaplasia).
2. The important risk factors for BE and EAC are male sex, chronic ( > 5 years) reflux symptoms, very frequent symptoms, age > 50, Caucasian race, smoking, and family history.

3. Women are at lower risk and should not be screened without multiple of the preceding risk factors.
4. Additional endoscopy is not needed after a negative study except when patients have severe esophagitis. In that case, a repeat endoscopy after healing is reasonable to make sure BE has not been missed.
5. Patients with BE should undergo periodic surveillance endoscopy.
6. If biopsies show dysplasia, this finding should be confirmed with a second pathologist, ideally a BE expert.
7. For BE without histological dysplasia, the screening interval is 3–5 years.
8. If dysplasia is not clear (indefinite), the patient should be placed on acid blockers and endoscopy and biopsy repeated after 3 to 6 months of therapy.
9. Ablation should be considered in patients with confirmed low-grade dysplasia (this is a new, perhaps controversial guideline).
10. Endoscopic therapy (ablation, mucosal resection, or both) should be offered to patients with high-grade dysplasia. Details on the various methods are presented in the article.
11. Endoscopic surveillance must be continued even after ablation or mucosal resection.
12. Patients with BE should be on at least once-daily proton pump inhibitors. There is no proven role for aspirin or other chemopreventative agents.

**K. R. DeVault, MD**

---

**Length of Barrett's oesophagus and cancer risk: implications from a large sample of patients with early oesophageal adenocarcinoma**

Pohl H, Pech O, Arash H, et al (VA Medical Ctr, White River Junction, VT; Krankenhaus Barmherzige Brueder, Regensburg, Germany; HSK Wiesbaden, Germany; et al)

*Gut* 65:196-201, 2016

---

*Objective.*—Although it is well understood that the risk of oesophageal adenocarcinoma increases with Barrett length, transition risks for cancer associated with different Barrett lengths are unknown. We aimed to estimate annual cancer transition rates for patients with long-segment (≥3 cm), short-segment (≥1 to <3 cm) and ultra-short-segment (<1 cm) Barrett's oesophagus.

*Design.*—We used three data sources to estimate the annual cancer transition rates for each Barrett length category: (1) the distribution of long, short and ultra-short Barrett's oesophagus among a large German cohort with newly diagnosed T1 oesophageal adenocarcinoma; (2) population-based German incidence of oesophageal adenocarcinoma; and (3) published estimates of the population prevalence of Barrett's oesophagus for each Barrett length category.

*Results.*—Among 1017 patients with newly diagnosed T1 oesophageal adenocarcinoma, 573 (56%) had long-segment, 240 (24%) short-segment and 204 (20%) ultra-short-segment Barrett's oesophagus. The base-case estimates for the prevalence of Barrett's oesophagus among the general population were 1.5%, 5% and 14%, respectively. The annual cancer transition rates for patients with long, short and ultra-short Barrett's oesophagus were 0.22%, 0.03% and 0.01%, respectively. To detect one cancer, 450 patients with long-segment Barrett's oesophagus would need to undergo annual surveillance endoscopy; in short segment and ultra-short segment, the corresponding numbers of patients would be 3440 and 12 364. Similar results were obtained when applying US incidence data.

*Conclusions.*—The large number of patients, who need to undergo endoscopic surveillance to detect one cancer, raises questions about the value of surveillance endoscopy in patients with short segment or ultra-short segment of Barrett's oesophagus.

▶ Once diagnosed, patients with Barrett esophagus (BE) are routinely entered into surveillance programs with the goal of identifying dysplasia and cancer at an early stage. Risk stratification and screening intervals have been based on the presence or absence of dysplasia in endoscopically obtained biopsies. Whether the length (extent) of BE should be used as another criteria is unclear. This article looks at more than 1000 patients developing early stage (T1) cancer retrospectively to learn more about this subject. They found that 56% of the patients had a long segment of BE (LSBE; > 3 cm) before cancer diagnosis, 24% short-segment (SSBE; 1–3 cm), and 20% ultra short segment (uSSBE; < 1 cm). Because the length of BE is inversely related to prevalence of each group, the number of endoscopies required to find once cancer per year was 405 in LSBE, 3440 in SSBE and 12 365 in uSSBE.

It is apparent from these and other data that diagnosing and following patients with uSSBE and perhaps SSBE is unlikely to change the outcome of an individual patient, although one-fifth of the cancers are in uSSBE and almost half in the combination of SSBE and uSSBE. The dichotomy of this situation certainly makes decision making on who to survey and how often difficult. European guidelines currently suggest every 3-year surveillance for nondysplastic LSBE, 5 years for SSBE, and no surveillance for uSSBE. This has not become the standard in the United States, but if data like these continue to develop, current guidelines that do not take length into consideration should be reconsidered.

**K. R. DeVault, MD**

# 45 Stomach

**The Toronto Consensus for the Treatment of *Helicobacter pylori* Infection in Adults**

Fallone CA, Chiba N, van Zanten SV, et al (McGill Univ, Montreal, Quebec, Canada; Guelph GI and Surgery Clinic, Ontario, Canada; Univ of Alberta, Edmonton, Canada; et al)

*Gastroenterology* 151:51-69, 2016

*Background & Aims.*—*Helicobacter pylori* infection is increasingly difficult to treat. The purpose of these consensus statements is to provide a review of the literature and specific, updated recommendations for eradication therapy in adults.

*Methods.*—A systematic literature search identified studies on *H pylori* treatment. The quality of evidence and strength of recommendations were rated according to the Grading of Recommendation Assessment, Development and Evaluation (GRADE) approach. Statements were developed through an online platform, finalized, and voted on by an international working group of specialists chosen by the Canadian Association of Gastroenterology.

*Results.*—Because of increasing failure of therapy, the consensus group strongly recommends that all *H pylori* eradication regimens now be given for 14 days. Recommended first-line strategies include concomitant non-bismuth quadruple therapy (proton pump inhibitor [PPI] + amoxicillin + metronidazole + clarithromycin [PAMC]) and traditional bismuth quadruple therapy (PPI + bismuth + metronidazole + tetracycline [PBMT]). PPI triple therapy (PPI + clarithromycin + either amoxicillin or metronidazole) is restricted to areas with known low clarithromycin resistance or high eradication success with these regimens. Recommended rescue therapies include PBMT and levofloxacin-containing therapy (PPI + amoxicillin + levofloxacin). Rifabutin regimens should be restricted to patients who have failed to respond to at least 3 prior options.

*Conclusions.*—Optimal treatment of *H pylori* infection requires careful attention to local antibiotic resistance and eradication patterns. The quadruple therapies PAMC or PBMT should play a more prominent role in eradication of *H pylori* infection, and all treatments should be given for 14 days.

▶ *Helicobacter pylori* (HP) infection remains a cause of symptoms and mucosal damage related to the upper gastrointestinal tract. Simple, twice daily, clarithromycin-based therapy has been a mainstay of the approach to HP infection, but unfortunately antibiotic resistance has forced a change in approach with failure rates approaching 50% in some populations. This article supports quadruple therapies as first line and suggests that clarithromycin-based triple therapy only be used in areas with low resistance rates, which are actually rare and becoming more rare around the world. They also make suggestions for retreatment including the suggestion that rifabutin-based treatment be reserved for those who have failed at least 3 prior treatment attempts. All treatments should be given for 14 days.

Resistance has certainly made our job more difficult. Instead of a simple twice-daily regimen of 4 pills twice a day for 7 to 10 days, we now need to start with a more complicated group of medications, taken more frequently for 14 days. Triple therapy may work in some areas, and unfortunately, the local resistance rate is usually not known by prescribers. If unknown, it is probably best to assume that the resistance rate is high. Although using these longer, complicated treatments is clearly the right thing to do, compliance has always challenged the success of HP therapy and is likely inversely related to the complication and duration of the regimen.

**K. R. DeVault, MD**

# 46 Small Intestine

**Evidence Against Routine Testing of Patients With Functional Gastrointestinal Disorders for Celiac Disease: A Population-based Study**

Choung RS, Rubio-Tapia A, Lahr BD, et al (Mayo Clinic, Rochester, MN; et al)

*Clin Gastroenterol Hepatol* 13:1937-1943, 2015

*Background & Aims.*—Celiac disease has been linked to irritable bowel syndrome (IBS)–like symptoms in outpatient clinics. Guidelines recommend that all patients with IBS-like symptoms undergo serologic testing for celiac disease, but there is controversy over whether celiac disease is more prevalent in populations with IBS-like symptoms. We aimed to determine whether positive results from serologic tests for celiac disease are associated with IBS and other functional gastrointestinal disorders (FGIDs) in a large U.S. white population.

*Methods.*—Validated, self-report bowel disease questionnaires (BDQs) were sent to randomly selected cohorts of Olmsted County, Minnesota residents. In separate protocols, serum samples were collected from more than 47,000 Olmsted County residents without a prior diagnosis of celiac disease; we performed serologic tests for celiac disease on stored serum samples from residents who completed the BDQ. Logistic regression was used to test for the association between serologic markers of celiac disease (positive vs negative) and individual FGIDs.

*Results.*—A total of 3202 subjects completed the BDQ and had serum available for testing. IBS was identified in 13.6% of these subjects (95% confidence interval [CI], 12.4%–14.8%), and any gastrointestinal symptom occurred in 55.2% (95% CI, 53.5%–56.9%). The prevalence of celiac disease on the basis of serologic markers was 1.0% (95% CI, 0.7%–1.4%). IBS was less prevalent in patients with celiac disease (3%) than patients without celiac disease (14%), although the difference was not statistically significant (odds ratio, 0.2; 95% CI, 0.03–1.5). Abdominal pain, constipation, weight loss, and dyspepsia were the most frequent symptom groups in subjects who were seropositive for celiac disease, but none of the gastrointestinal symptoms or disorders were significantly associated with celiac disease serology.

*Conclusions.*—Symptoms indicative of FGIDs and seropositive celiac disease are relatively common in a U.S. white community. Testing for celiac disease in patients with IBS in the community may not have a significantly increased yield over population-based screening in the United States.

▶ Many guideline statements and expert opinion suggests serological testing for celiac disease (CD) in patients with irritable bowel syndrome (IBS) and in other "functional disorders." This population-based study calls that into question. In a survey of more than 3000 patients, they found 13.6% to have IBS symptoms (55% had some gastrointestinal symptom). Only 1% had serological evidence of CD, and CD was actually less common in those with IBS than those without.

Should these data change our practice and guidelines? The overall prevalence of CD at 1% means that a good number of patients regardless of their symptoms will be serologically positive. There are studies that suggest a gluten-free diet helps IBS, but it is less clear that serology predicts that response. The authors correctly point out that prior studies were, for the most part, based on patients presenting with symptoms and frequently were collected at tertiary referral centers. A small number of CD patients might have been missed in this study if they were already on a gluten-free diet and in the rare situation of immunoglobulin A deficiency, but I am sure that there would not be enough of these in the database to change the study outcomes. This study also may help to explain why an IBS patient who is serologically positive for CD might not improve with gluten avoidance. On the other hand, some gluten-sensitive, nonceliac patients may respond to gluten elimination despite negative CD testing. It is still reasonable to consider CD or even non-CD gluten sensitivity in a patient with IBS and diarrhea, but there also should be little surprise when that approach leads to minimal or no improvement in a substantial number of patients.

**K. R. DeVault, MD**

---

**Risk of Celiac Disease in the First- and Second-Degree Relatives of Patients With Celiac Disease: A Systematic Review and Meta-Analysis**

Singh P, Arora S, Lal S, et al (Massachusetts General Hosp, Boston; Brigham and Women's Hosp, Boston, MA; Max Healthcare, Gurgaon, India; et al)
*Am J Gastroenterol* 110:1539-1548, 2015

---

*Objectives.*—First-degree relatives (FDRs) of patients with celiac disease (CD) are at high risk for CD and prevalence among them varies from 1.6 to 38%. The risk of having CD among FDRs if the FDR is sister, brother, mother, father, son, or daughter of index patient with CD is not known. We conducted a meta-analysis and calculated pooled prevalence of CD among FDRs, second-degree relatives (SDRs), and specific relations with index patient.

*Methods.*—On search of literature, 2,259 articles appeared of which 54 articles were included in this metaanalysis. Diagnosis of CD was based on standard criteria.

*Results.*—Pooled prevalence of CD was 7.5% (95% confidence interval (CI) 6.3%, 8.8%) in 10,252 FDRs and 2.3% (95% CI 1.3%, 3.8%) in 642 SDRs. Pooled prevalence of CD was highest in siblings (8.9%), followed by offsprings (7.9%) and parents (3.0%). Female FDRs had higher prevalence than male FDRs (8.4% vs. 5.2%, $P = 0.047$). While sisters and daughters of index patient had the highest risk of having CD (1 in 7 and 1 in 8, respectively), the risk was 1 in 13 in sons, 1 in 16 in brothers, 1 in 32 in mothers, and 1 in 33 in fathers. There were also differences in the pooled prevalence of CD in FDRs according to their geographic location.

*Conclusions.*—Pooled prevalence of CD among FDRs is 7.5% and varies considerably with their relationship with the index patient. The risk of CD in FDRs also varies according to gender and geographical location.

▶ Celiac disease (CD) is an immune-mediated disease where exposure to gluten results in small bowel mucosal loss in genetically predisposed patients. This disease has been know for many years as a cause of diarrhea and malnutrition, but testing in less severely affected subjects has added an understanding that CD can present in many ways with varying degrees of severity. Current guidelines support testing for CD in all patients with chronic diarrhea, diarrhea-predominant IBS, and those with weight loss. This study adds to our understanding of the disorder by confirming an increased incidence of CD in relatives of CD patients.

How should this change practice? Just as family history of colon cancer can guide the use of colon screening, family history of CD should help guide who gets tested for CD. There are certainly problems with the testing because the available tests are most accurate when patients are consuming gluten. Patients who have a family member with CD may have already limited their gluten exposure, which can result in false-negative tests. In addition, many patients are gluten sensitive and do not have genetic CD, which may not be clear in a family history obtained from a relative. Another interesting finding in this study (and probably in other family studies) is that the detailed type of relationship is important rather than using the first- and second-degree label. For example, in first-degree relatives, the highest increased risk was if there was a female sibling or daughter with CD. Lower risks were seen with male siblings, sons, and parents.

**K. R. DeVault, MD**

---

**Diet Low in FODMAPs Reduces Symptoms of Irritable Bowel Syndrome as Well as Traditional Dietary Advice: A Randomized Controlled Trial**

Böhn L, Störsrud S, Liljebo T, et al (Univ of Gothenburg, Sweden; Karolinska Univ Hosp, Stockholm, Sweden; et al)

*Gastroenterology* 149:1399-1407.e2, 2015

---

*Background & Aims.*—A diet with reduced content of fermentable short-chain carbohydrates (fermentable oligo-, di-, monosaccharides, and polyols [FODMAPs]) has been reported to be effective in the treatment of patients with irritable bowel syndrome (IBS). However, there is no evidence of its superiority to traditional dietary advice for these patients. We compared the effects of a diet low in FODMAPs with traditional dietary advice in a randomized controlled trial of patients with IBS.

*Methods.*—We performed a multi-center, parallel, single-blind study of 75 patients who met Rome III criteria for IBS and were enrolled at gastroenterology outpatient clinics in Sweden. Subjects were randomly assigned to groups that ate specific diets for 4 weeks—a diet low in FODMAPs ($n = 38$) or a diet frequently recommended for patients with IBS (ie, a regular meal pattern; avoidance of large meals; and reduced intake of fat, insoluble fibers, caffeine, and gas-producing foods, such as beans, cabbage, and onions), with greater emphasis on how and when to eat rather than on what foods to ingest ($n = 37$). Symptom severity was assessed using the IBS Symptom Severity Scale, and patients completed a 4-day food diary before and at the end of the intervention.

*Results.*—A total of 67 patients completed the dietary intervention (33 completed the diet low in FODMAPs, 34 completed the traditional IBS diet). The severity of IBS symptoms was reduced in both groups during the intervention ($P < .0001$ in both groups before vs at the end of the 4-week diet), without a significant difference between the groups ($P = .62$). At the end of the 4-week diet period, 19 patients (50%) in the low-FODMAP group had reductions in IBS severity scores ≥50 compared with baseline vs 17 patients (46%) in the traditional IBS diet group ($P = .72$). Food diaries demonstrated good adherence to the dietary advice.

*Conclusions.*—A diet low in FODMAPs reduces IBS symptoms as well as traditional IBS dietary advice. Combining elements from these 2 strategies might further reduce symptoms of IBS. ClinicalTrials.gov ID NCT02107625.

▶ The treatment of irritable bowel syndrome (IBS) is challenging and often frustrating. Although many patients have diet triggers that worsen their symptoms, guidance for broad dietary advice in IBS has been lacking. A diet with reduced content of fermentable short-chain carbohydrates (fermentable oligo-, di-monosaccharides, and polyols [FODMAPs]) has recently been reported to improve IBS symptoms. Prior studies had compared the low FODMAPs diet to no dietary advice, while this study provided diet advice to both the low FODMAPs and the control group (patients received what the authors described as "standard" advice, which is outlined in the article). They found that both diets provided benefit but without a statistical difference between the two.

This study does not spell the end of the low FODMAPs diet for IBS. In fact, it suggests that dietary advice should play an important role in treating these patients. In addition, the interventions in both arms of this study were very practical and possible in routine clinical practice without intensive dietician-based intervention. Whether these data will hold in a larger sample is not known. In addition, it will be important to determine the tolerability and long-term success of each of these diets. It is also interesting that this study did not focus on any IBS subtype (patients could have diarrhea, constipation, or mixed type) with improvement seen in each group. Finally, patients in either treatment group lowered their caloric intake. This may have both beneficial and perhaps, in some cases, adverse affects. Monitoring intake and weight change is an important part of managing IBS patients on any type of restricted diet. These and other studies continue to expand our understanding of the role of food in IBS and other gastrointestinal disorders.

**K. R. DeVault, MD**

**ACG Clinical Guideline: Diagnosis and Management of Small Bowel Bleeding**

Gerson LB, Fidler JL, Cave DR, et al (Univ of California School of Medicine, San Francisco; Mayo Clinic School of Medicine, Rochester, MN; Univ of Massachusetts Med Ctr, Worcester; et al)

*Am J Gastroenterol* 110:1265-1287, 2015

Bleeding from the small intestine remains a relatively uncommon event, accounting for ~5–10% of all patients presenting with gastrointestinal (GI) bleeding. Given advances in small bowel imaging with video capsule endoscopy (VCE), deep enteroscopy, and radiographic imaging, the cause of bleeding in the small bowel can now be identified in most patients. The term small bowel bleeding is therefore proposed as a replacement for the previous classification of obscure GI bleeding (OGIB). We recommend that the term OGIB should be reserved for patients in whom a source of bleeding cannot be identified anywhere in the GI tract. A source of small bowel bleeding should be considered in patients with GI bleeding after performance of a normal upper and lower endoscopic examination. Second-look examinations using upper endoscopy, push enteroscopy, and/or colonoscopy can be performed if indicated before small bowel evaluation. VCE should be considered a first-line procedure for small bowel investigation. Any method of deep enteroscopy can be used when endoscopic evaluation and therapy are required. VCE should be performed before deep enteroscopy if there is no contraindication. Computed tomographic enterography should be performed in patients with suspected obstruction before VCE or after negative VCE examinations. When there is acute overt hemorrhage in the unstable patient, angiography should be performed emergently. In patients with occult hemorrhage or stable patients with active overt bleeding, multiphasic computed tomography should be performed after VCE or CTE to identify the source of bleeding and to guide further management. If a source of bleeding is identified in the small bowel that is associated with significant ongoing anemia and/or active bleeding, the patient should be managed with endoscopic therapy. Conservative management is recommended for patients without a source found after small bowel investigation, whereas repeat diagnostic investigations are recommended

**for patients with initial negative small bowel evaluations and ongoing overt or occult bleeding.**

▶ Bleeding from the small bowel is uncommon (5%–10% of all patients presenting with gastrointestinal bleeding), but often difficult to diagnosis and treat. The American College of Gastroenterology has produced a guideline statement on this issue. Major concepts from that guideline include the following:

1. Don't always trust the first endoscopy or colonoscopy. A "second" look may actually find the cause in many patients.
2. Video capsule endoscopy (VCE) is the method of choice for the initial evaluation of a possible bleeding site in the small intestine.
3. Deep enteroscopy uses a special endoscope to evaluate the small bowel. It should be used to confirm and treat lesions seen on VCE and in selected patients who have bleeding suggestive of a small bowel source even if the VCE is negative.
4. Barium studies are usually not helpful in the evaluation of small bowel bleeding.
5. CT enterography is superior to magnetic resonance enterography in this situation and is indicated before VCE in patients who are at increased risk of a mechanical issue in their small bowel.
6. In patients with massive small bowel bleeding, angiography is indicated.
7. In patients with significant but not massive bleeding, a CT angiogram may be helpful.
8. In patients with slower rates of bleeding, a tagged red blood cell scan may also help to localize the site of bleeding.
9. If a patient has significant anemia or ongoing bleeding, endoscopic therapy can be used to treat the lesion.
10. In the case of massive bleeding, surgical intervention may be required but will be more successful if guided by endoscopic or radiologic findings.
11. Patients with negative or minor findings and anemia that can be controlled with iron supplementation can be followed clinically.
12. Valve replacement should be considered in patients with aortic stenosis and bleeding angioectasia (Heyde syndrome).

**K. R. DeVault, MD**

---

**Short-term and Long-term Efficacy of Psychological Therapies for Irritable Bowel Syndrome: A Systematic Review and Meta-analysis**

Laird KT, Tanner-Smith EE, Russell AC, et al (Vanderbilt Univ, Nashville, TN)
*Clin Gastroenterol Hepatol* 14:937-947.e4, 2016

---

*Background & Aims.*—Several meta-analyses have demonstrated the efficacy of psychological therapies for reducing gastrointestinal (GI) symptoms in patients with irritable bowel syndrome (IBS). However, no meta-analysis has investigated the duration of these effects. We performed a meta-analysis to assess the immediate, short-term, and long-term efficacy of psychotherapy for reducing GI symptoms in adults with IBS.

*Methods.*—We searched PubMed, PsycINFO, Science Direct, and ProQuest Dissertations and Theses through August 15, 2015 for randomized controlled trials that compared psychological therapy with an active or non-active comparison (control) condition for treatment of GI symptoms in adults with IBS.

*Results.*—Forty-one trials were included in our meta-analysis, comprising data from 2290 individuals (1183 assigned to psychotherapy and 1107 assigned to a control condition). Compared with a mixed group of control conditions, psychological therapies had a medium effect on GI symptom severity ($d = 0.69$) immediately after treatment. On average, individuals who received psychotherapy had a greater reduction in GI symptoms after treatment than 75% of individuals assigned to a control condition. After short-term follow-up periods (1–6 months after treatment) and long-term follow-up periods (6–12 months after treatment), this effect remained significant and medium in magnitude ($d = 0.76$ and $d = 0.73$, respectively).

*Conclusions.*—Psychological therapies reduce GI symptoms in adults with IBS. These effects remained significant and medium in magnitude after short-term and long-term follow-up periods.

▶ Irritable bowel syndrome (IBS) remains a difficult to control and very expensive condition in both gastroenterology and primary care practices. There are a few new pharmacological approaches available, but all are expensive, have potential side effects, and, in general, provide a modest improvement over placebo. The stress-IBS connection has been known for years, and this meta-analysis looks at the effects of psychological therapies for IBS. They conclude that there are real but modest improvements in IBS symptoms generated by the psychological approach and that those improvements can persist long-term (6–12 months).

The most commonly studied approaches were cognitive therapy or cognitive behavior therapy with a smaller number of trials looking at relaxation and hypnosis. There were no differences between modality, but the sample sizes may have not been robust enough to make a definitive conclusion. Interestingly, in person and online therapy seemed to work similarly, as did individual versus group therapy. It seems that these maneuvers are at least as effective as some of the new medications. In addition, group and online therapy should be applicable at a favorable price point. Unfortunately, thus far there are limited programs available in many areas.

**K. R. DeVault, MD**

**Eluxadoline for Irritable Bowel Syndrome with Diarrhea**

Lembo AJ, Lacy BE, Zuckerman MJ, et al (Harvard Med School, Boston, MA; Geisel School of Medicine at Dartmouth, Hanover, NH; Texas Tech Univ Health Sciences Ctr, El Paso; et al)

*N Engl J Med* 374:242-253, 2016

*Background.*—Effective and safe treatments are needed for patients who have irritable bowel syndrome (IBS) with diarrhea. We conducted two phase 3 trials to assess the efficacy and safety of eluxadoline, a new oral agent with mixed opioid effects ($\mu$- and $\kappa$-opioid receptor agonist and $\delta$-opioid receptor antagonist), in patients with IBS with diarrhea.

*Methods.*—We randomly assigned 2427 adults who had IBS with diarrhea to eluxadoline (at a dose of 75 mg or 100 mg) or placebo twice daily for 26 weeks (IBS-3002 trial) or 52 weeks (IBS-3001 trial). The primary end point was the proportion of patients who had a composite response of decrease in abdominal pain and improvement in stool consistency on the same day for at least 50% of the days from weeks 1 through 12 and from weeks 1 through 26.

*Results.*—For weeks 1 through 12, more patients in the eluxadoline groups (75 mg and 100 mg) than in the placebo group reached the primary end point (IBS-3001 trial, 23.9% with the 75-mg dose and 25.1% with the 100-mg dose vs. 17.1% with placebo; $P = 0.01$ and $P = 0.004$, respectively; IBS-3002 trial, 28.9% and 29.6%, respectively, vs. 16.2%; $P < 0.001$ for both comparisons). For weeks 1 through 26, the corresponding rates in IBS-3001 were 23.4% and 29.3% versus 19.0% ($P = 0.11$ and $P < 0.001$, respectively), and the corresponding rates in IBS-3002 were 30.4% and 32.7% versus 20.2% ($P = 0.001$ and $P < 0.001$, respectively). The most common adverse events associated with 75 mg of eluxadoline and 100 mg of eluxadoline, as compared with placebo, were nausea (8.1% and 7.5% vs. 5.1%), constipation (7.4% and 8.6% vs. 2.5%), and abdominal pain (5.8% and 7.2% vs. 4.1%). Pancreatitis developed in 5 (2 in the 75-mg group and 3 in the 100-mg group) of the 1666 patients in the safety population (0.3%).

*Conclusions.*—Eluxadoline is a new therapeutic agent that reduced symptoms of IBS with diarrhea in men and women, with sustained efficacy over 6 months in patients who received the 100-mg dose twice daily. (Funded by Furiex Pharmaceuticals, an affiliate of Allergan; IBS-3001 and IBS-3002 ClinicalTrials.gov numbers, NCT01553591 and NCT01553747, respectively.)

► Irritable bowel syndrome (IBS) is one of the most common gastrointestinal disorders, but despite this, effective therapies are limited. This article reports the outcomes of 2 large trials looking at eluxadoline (100 or 75 mg daily vs placebo) in the treatment of IBS patients with diarrhea (IBS-D). This agent works through interactions with opioid receptors in the gastrointestinal tract. Eluxadoline (particularly at the 100-mg dose) was superior but the gain over placebo was somewhat modest (around 10%). There were improvements in both pain and stool function. Nausea, abdominal pain, and constipation were the most common side effects. Pancreatitis developed in 0.3% of patients. The safety committee determined that these episodes, in addition to a few episodes of elevated liver tests with pain, were likely related to the agent's effects on the sphincter of Oddi. These appeared to be more likely in patients without a gallbladder and with the higher (100-mg dose). None of the cases developed severe disease and all resolved with supportive therapy.

Although a gain of 10% over placebo seems modest, the lack of effective agents makes this potentially more important. If one is planning on using this agent the first consideration is to make sure the patient actually has IBS-D. Eluxadoline should not be used in constipated patients or in patients with chronic abdominal pain syndromes without diarrhea. Given the expense and potential side effects, initial therapy of IBS-D should still include lifestyle and diet changes. Rifaxamin is another agent with similar efficacy and perhaps a better safety profile. When these agents fail, a trial of eluxadoline may well be reasonable. The indicated dose is 100-mg daily in those with a gallbladder and 75 mg daily in those who have had a cholecystectomy. The agent should be avoided in patients with a history of liver or pancreatic disease and in patients taking more than 3 alcohol drinks per day. Worsening pain while on this agent should be investigated quickly to exclude pancreatitis.

**K. R. DeVault, MD**

# 47 Colon

### Relationship Between Microbiota of the Colonic Mucosa vs Feces and Symptoms, Colonic Transit, and Methane Production in Female Patients with Chronic Constipation

Parthasarathy G, Chen J, Chen X, et al (Mayo Clinic, Rochester, MN; et al)
*Gastroenterology* 150:367-379.e1, 2016

*Background & Aims.*—In fecal samples from patients with chronic constipation, the microbiota differs from that of healthy subjects. However, the profiles of fecal microbiota only partially replicate those of the mucosal microbiota. It is not clear whether these differences are caused by variations in diet or colonic transit, or are associated with methane production (measured by breath tests). We compared the colonic mucosal and fecal microbiota in patients with chronic constipation and in healthy subjects to investigate the relationships between microbiota and other parameters.

*Methods.*—Sigmoid colonic mucosal and fecal microbiota samples were collected from 25 healthy women (controls) and 25 women with chronic constipation and evaluated by 16S ribosomal RNA gene sequencing (average, 49,186 reads/sample). We assessed associations between microbiota (overall composition and operational taxonomic units) and demographic variables, diet, constipation status, colonic transit, and methane production (measured in breath samples after oral lactulose intake).

*Results.*—Fourteen patients with chronic constipation had slow colonic transit. The profile of the colonic mucosal microbiota differed between constipated patients and controls ($P < .05$). The overall composition of the colonic mucosal microbiota was associated with constipation, independent of colonic transit ($P < .05$), and discriminated between patients with constipation and controls with 94% accuracy. Genera from *Bacteroidetes* were more abundant in the colonic mucosal microbiota of patients with constipation. The profile of the fecal microbiota was associated with colonic transit before adjusting for constipation, age, body mass index, and diet; genera from *Firmicutes* (*Faecalibacterium, Lactococcus*, and *Roseburia*) correlated with faster colonic transit. Methane production was associated with the composition of the fecal microbiota, but not with constipation or colonic transit.

*Conclusions.*—After adjusting for diet and colonic transit, the profile of the microbiota in the colonic mucosa could discriminate patients with constipation from healthy individuals. The profile of the fecal microbiota was associated with colonic transit and methane production (measured in breath), but not constipation.

▶ Irritable bowel syndrome (IBS) is a common yet poorly understood and treated condition. There have been several advances in the understanding of IBS that is allowing more targeted treatment. Alterations in fecal microbiota have been suggested to be an important part of IBS, and in the diarrhea form of IBS, a nonabsorbable antibiotic (xifaximin) has been approved as a therapeutic option. Attempts to alter that biota with probiotics have also been advocated. This article looks at a different group: women with chronic constipation. After they controlled for diet and colon transit, the microbiota in the colon mucosa could distinguish between constipated patients and healthy individuals. Although different bacteria were associated with methane production, they did not correlate with either constipation or colon transit. There were also a few specific bacterial species that correlated with constipation.

Where does this leave us? First, it may be reasonable to attempt to alter gut flora in chronic constipation in addition to IBS. This could be with targeted probiotics or perhaps with antibiotics followed by probiotics. Fecal transplantation is another interesting option that deserves study. It is also possible that the interaction between these micro-organisms and food can be manipulated to therapeutic gain, perhaps in both the area of methane production and colonic transit.

**K. R. DeVault, MD**

---

**Risks and Benefits of Colonoscopy in Patients 90 Years or Older, Compared With Younger Patients**

Cha JM, Kozarek RA, La Selva D, et al (Kyung Hee Univ School of Medicine, Seoul, South Korea; Virginia Mason Med Ctr, Seattle, WA)

*Clin Gastroenterol Hepatol* 14:80-86.e1, 2016

---

*Background & Aims.*—Although the numbers of medical procedures performed on extremely elderly patients (90 years or older, nonagenarians) are increasing, there are no data on the performance, diagnostic yield, or safety of colonoscopy for these patients. We compared the performance and safety of diagnostic colonoscopy, as well as lesions detected, in nonagenarians with patients who were 75 to 79 years old.

*Methods.*—In a retrospective study, we compared data from 76 extremely elderly patients (90 years or older) with data from 140 very elderly patients (75 to 79 years old, controls), all of whom underwent diagnostic colonoscopy from January 2010 through March 2013 at Virginia Mason Medical Center. All colonoscopies were performed by 15 endoscopists. We compared rates of colonoscopy completion, bowel preparation quality, diagnostic yield, and adverse events.

*Results.*—In extremely elderly patients, more colonoscopies were performed under general anesthesia, compared with controls ($P < .001$). When extremely elderly patients underwent colonoscopies with moderate sedation, lower doses of midazolam and fentanyl were given, compared with controls ($P < .001$). Colonoscopies were completed in a lower proportion of extremely elderly patients (88.2% vs 99.3% for controls, $P < .001$), and these patients had a higher incidence of inadequate bowel preparation (29.7% vs 15.0% for controls, $P = .011$). Colonoscopies were also associated with cardiopulmonary events in a higher proportion of extremely elderly patients ($P = .006$) as well as overall adverse events, compared with controls ($P = .002$). A higher proportion of extremely elderly patients were found to have advanced neoplasia (28.4% vs 6.4% of controls, $P < .001$) as well as any neoplasia ($P < .001$ vs controls). A greater percentage of extremely elderly patients also had large lesions ($P = .002$) and malignancies detected by histology ($P < .001$ vs controls). Eleven extremely elderly patients (14.9%) were found to have cancer or high-grade dysplasia by colonoscopy.

*Conclusions.*—In patients 90 years or older, diagnostic colonoscopy is associated with increased risk for incomplete procedure, inadequate bowel preparation, and adverse events. However, a large proportion of patients are found to have advanced neoplasia and cancer, compared with patients 75 to 79 years old.

▶ Current guidelines suggest stopping colonoscopy screening at age 75. Despite this, there are few data on the use of colonoscopy in very old patients. This study compared colonoscopy in patients over age 90 years to a control cohort between ages 75 to 79. The very old patients were more likely to have an incomplete procedure, inadequate bowel preparation, and adverse events, but a large proportion of patients were found to have advanced neoplasia and cancer. It is important to note that the higher yield in this study could be related to the fact that these were "diagnostic" and not "screening" colonoscopies, but screening procedures were excluded in both groups. The increased yield could be related to a higher pretest probability (perhaps the very old patients may have had more issues suggesting disease before a colonoscopy was ordered).

Understanding the adverse events is important, although the very old patients were by nature "sicker" because they had a higher American Society of Anesthesiologists score (although I suspect older patients may get a higher score based on age rather than other know comorbidities). They had more complications (9.2% vs 0.7%) and more serious complications (5.3% vs 0%), but the major events were all survivable (1 nonfatal myocardial infarction, 1 bradycardia, and 1 tachycardia). These data do not change the indication or lack of indication for screening colonoscopy in the elderly but do provide important data to consider. It would be reasonable to consider a more extensive preparation in very old patients (perhaps a day or two of liquid diet before starting the actual preparation), which might decrease some the issues noted in this study. In addition, careful cardiovascular monitoring may be of added importance.

**K. R. DeVault, MD**

**American Gastroenterological Association Institute Guideline on the Medical Management of Microscopic Colitis**

Nguyen GC, the Clinical Guidelines Committee (Univ of Toronto, Ontario, Canada; Vanderbilt Univ School of Medicine, Nashville, TN; Mayo Clinic, Rochester, MN; et al)

*Gastroenterology* 150:242-246, 2016

These actionable recommendations for the medical management of microscopic colitis were developed under the framework of the GRADE methodology and were consistent with the Institute of Medicine's Standards for Developing Trustworthy Clinical Practice Guidelines. This guideline is intended to reduce practice variation and promote high-value care. The weight of evidence supports the first-line use of budesonide for induction and, when appropriate, maintenance therapy. Because the technical review and guideline focused on treatments assessed in clinical trials, it did not address the full armamentarium of therapies currently used in practice. We would endorse clinical trials that more rigorously assess the effectiveness of lower-cost alternatives such as antidiarrheal agents (eg, loperamide) and cholestyramine monotherapy with accompanying cost-effective analyses. The role of combination therapies has yet to fully explored. Due to the absence of clinical trial data, this guideline did not address medical treatment of corticosteroid-refractory microscopic colitis. Very limited evidence from case series, however, suggests that immunosuppressants such as azathioprine and anti-tumor necrosis factor agents may benefit these patients. We encourage prospective clinical trials to further investigate these early findings.

▶ This guideline statement produced by the American Gastroenterological Association provides outstanding information for physicians treating the common problem of microscopic colitis. This disorder produces difficult to control, watery diarrhea. It is common in patients over age 60. The diagnosis is made based on histological examination of biopsies obtained during sigmoidoscopoy or colonoscopy. There are two histological subtypes (lymphocytic and collagenous), which respond similarly so they were grouped together. Major concepts include the following: (1) budesonide is the best treatment for most patients, for both acute disease and maintenance; (2) mesalamine and bismuth salicylate are secondary options that should be considered when budesonide cannot be used; (3) systemic steroids should be considered in certain patients in whom the preceding treatments are not effective or are unavailable; (4) the combination of cholestyramine and mesalamine is not superior to mesalamine alone; and (5) other nonsupported treatments include *Boswellia serrata* and probiotics. Antidiarrheal agents such as loperamide have not been well studied but are often used, even before diagnosis.

**K. R. DeVault, MD**

**Increased Risk of Functional Gastrointestinal Sequelae After *Clostridium difficile* Infection Among Active Duty United States Military Personnel (1998–2010)**

Gutiérrez RL, Riddle MS, Porter CK (Naval Med Res Ctr, Silver Spring, MD)

*Gastroenterology* 149:1408-1414, 2015

*Background & Aims.*—Some acute enteric infections are associated with the development of functional gastrointestinal disorders, most commonly irritable bowel syndrome but also other functional and organic gastrointestinal sequelae. *Clostridium difficile* infection has increased in incidence and severity, however, few studies have evaluated functional disorders after this infection.

*Methods.*—We evaluated the epidemiology and sequelae of C *difficile* in the US military population by using the US Department of Defense's Armed Forces Health Surveillance Center Defense Medical Ecounter Database. We then performed a retrospective cohort study of 891 active-duty US military personnel who developed C *difficile* from 1998 to 2010 and 3231 matched subjects who had not been exposed to C *difficile*. Subjects were identified based on International Classification of Diseases, 9th revision, Clinical Modification codes for C *difficile* disease.

*Results.*—C *difficile* was associated independently with increased rate ratios (RRs) for incident irritable bowel syndrome (RR, 6.1; 95% confidence interval [CI], 2.9–12.9), gastroesophageal reflux disease (GERD) (RR, 1.9; 95% CI, 1.4–2.6), dyspepsia (RR, 3.3; 95%, 1.4–7.7), and constipation (RR, 2.2; 95% CI, 1.3–3.7). Approximately 14.1% of subjects with C *difficile* later were identified with one of these functional gastrointestinal disorders (FGDs), compared with 6% of controls. Community- and health care–associated C *difficile* were associated at similar rates with these sequelae. Patients were at increased risk for FGDs within 3 months of a C *difficile* episode, with one additional case of FGD developing for every 12 diagnoses of C *difficile*.

*Conclusions.*—The incidence of community- and health care–associated C *difficile* has increased in the US military population from 1998 through 2010. As for other gastrointestinal infections, C *difficile* disease is associated with clinically relevant functional sequelae in this military population.

▶ Irritable bowel syndrome (IBS) and other "functional" disorders have been commonly reported after intestinal infections including *Clostridium difficile* infection (CDI). This large study of military personnel confirmed an increase in IBS, but also increases in gastroesophageal reflux symptoms, dyspepsia, and constipation. There was a doubling of these symptoms after CDI compared with a control population. CDI produces considerable acute morbidity, and this study confirms that 14.1% of patients will develop chronic functional symptoms following CDI, thus worsening the public health impact of this infection.

Avoiding CDI should be a major goal of all providers. Key factors include avoiding unnecessary antibiotics and careful control of exposure in hospitals and long-term care facilities (handwashing, contact isolation, appropriate cleaning of exposed rooms and equipment). It is important to know that some of the chemical agents used for hand hygiene do not control CDI; soap and water may be better. Avoiding PPI in patients who can avoid that class of medication may also decrease risk. There are mixed data on the use of probiotics to prevent CDI. The current American College of Gastroenterology guideline on this subject is referenced here.[1]

**K. R. DeVault, MD**

*Reference*

1. Surawicz CM, Brandt LJ, Binion DG, et al. Guidelines for diagnosis, treatment and prevention of *Clostridium difficile* infections. *Am J Gastroenterol.* 2013;108: 478-498.

---

**Impact of Single- vs. Split-Dose Low-Volume Bowel Preparations on Bowel Movement Kinetics, Patient Inconvenience, and Polyp Detection: A Prospective Trial**

Horton N, Garber A, Hasson H, et al (Cleveland Clinic, OH)
*Am J Gastroenterol* 2016 [Epub ahead of print]

---

*Objectives.*—There are little data on bowel movement (BM) kinetics induced by bowel preparation. Whether single-dose (SID) or split-dose (SPD) regimens differ in terms of patient convenience is unclear. We compared BM kinetics, sleep and travel disruptions, and polyp detection rates in patients undergoing colonoscopy assigned to SID vs. SPDs.

*Methods.*—Patients were randomly assigned to 2-L SID or SPD (SPD1 and SPD2) bowel preparations. Surveys were completed querying the onset, duration, cessation, and intensity of BMs, along with sleep and travel disruption en route to the endoscopy center. Colon cleansing quality and polyp histology were recorded.

*Results.*—A total of 341 patients were enrolled, 51% in SPD and 49% in SID. Over half of patients had their first BM within 60 min of starting the preparation. After dosing, 92% of SID and 66% of SPD1 patients achieved clear effluent ($P < 0.001$), whereas it was reported in 97% of SPD2 patients ($P = 0.028$ vs. SID). Total duration ($P = 0.041$) and intensity ($P < 0.001$) of BMs were greater in SID. More patients in SID woke up for BMs (65.9 vs. 48.8%, $P < 0.003$). No differences in the need to stop driving en route to colonoscopy were noted. Bowel prep quality was better in SPD ($P < 0.001$). Although no difference in the adenoma detection rate was noted, the sessile-serrated polyp detection rate was greater in SPD than in SID (9.9 vs. 2.4%, $P = 0.004$).

*Conclusions.*—Our data demonstrate that SPD bowel preparation results in decreased intensity and duration of BMs, less patient inconvenience, improved bowel preparation, and increased sessile-serrated polyp detection rates.

▶ Colonoscopy is an important tool in the prevention of colon cancer. To be effective, the patient's colon needs to be well prepared. This preparation is one of the most unpleasant parts of the experience, and even the thought of the preparation prevents some from undergoing this life-saving procedure. Taking part of the high volume preparation the night prior to and other half the morning of the examination has been advocated as both more effective and better tolerated. This prospective trial sought to evaluate that concept further (split dose vs single dose).

The split-dose bowel preparation was superior in most ways, particularly better preparation with less uncomfortable and disruptive bowel movements (including less awakening at night for a bowel movement). The adenoma detection rate was similar, but the more difficult to detect, flat sessile serrated polyp detection rate was higher with split dose. This and other studies confirm that split dosing should be considered standard of care in colonoscopy preparation. Even early morning patients should be encouraged to wake up early and take the second of the split dose. It is important to note that these were 2-liter preparations and despite the lower volume had outstanding results, especially with split dosing.

**K. R. DeVault, MD**

**Interval Colorectal Cancer After Colonoscopy: Exploring Explanations and Solutions**

Adler J, Robertson DJ (Dartmouth-Hitchcock Med Ctr, Lebanon, NH; VA Med Ctr, White River Junction, VT)

*Am J Gastroenterol* 110:1657-1664, 2015

There is good evidence that colorectal cancer (CRC) screening has been successful at reducing both CRC incidence and death. Colonoscopy, utilized as either a primary screening tool or a follow-up exam when other screening tests are positive, has significantly contributed to these encouraging trends. However, it is well recognized that colonoscopy is not perfectly sensitive for the detection of neoplasia and that CRC can be diagnosed within a short interval following a colonoscopy that did not detect one. The literature surrounding these cases has rapidly expanded over the last decade. Specifically, studies aimed at understanding the frequency of these events and the likely explanations for their occurrence have been performed. This review will highlight current knowledge around the epidemiology of interval post colonoscopy CRC (PCCRC). The common explanations for these cancers including missed lesions, new lesions, and incompletely resected lesions will be reviewed and their contribution to interval PCCRC estimated. Finally, the relationship of these putative explanations to potential opportunities to prevent interval PCCRC will be explored. Current approaches to prevention largely center on consistent adherence to quality colonoscopy standards. Future approaches include advances in technology to better visualize the colon and adequately resect detected neoplasia. Finally, improvement in training as well as development of a culture of continuous quality improvement will be essential to maximize the benefits of colonoscopy in daily clinical practice.

▶ This review paper looks at the important issue of colon cancer occurring in patients who have been following colonoscopy-based screening guidelines. This is particularly important because screening guideline intervals of up to 10 years are now suggested, and screening more frequently may be flagged as a negative quality index. Important concepts brought out in this thoughtful review include the following:

1. Although defining the risk of developing a cancer after a screening colonoscopy in the period before the next suggested exam is difficult, a number of about 1:1000 would be a fair risk to include in the consenting of patients for screening colonoscopy.
2. Advanced adenomas and small cancers may be missed during screening colonoscopy. Rates around 5% have been suggested, but many think that is a high number with modern colonoscopy equipment and careful examinations that have been advocated across the colonoscopy practice. The authors estimate that missed lesions could account for up to 50% of the interval cancers.
3. Incompletely resected lesions are another potential cause. Adenomatous tissue is left behind in 10% or more of polyps thought to be completely resected. Larger polyps and those removed in a piecemeal fashion are at higher risk of incomplete resection.
4. It is clear that new lesions can appear in an appropriately screened colon where all lesions were removed, but they are likely the cause of a minority of interval cancers, and the rate is nearly impossible to define.
5. Adequate bowel preparation, documentation of cecal intubation, an adequate adenoma detection rate, and slow withdrawal of the colonoscope are all methods suggested to decrease the incidence of interval cancers. There are limited data to support each, and practitioners who fail in 1 or more of these metrics are more likely to have interval cancers.

The bottom line is that colonoscopy is currently an imperfect test but is the best we have currently. Improvements in colonoscopy equipment, resection devices, and perhaps most important, endoscopy training may eventually decrease the risk of missed lesions.

**K. R. DeVault, MD**

**Risks Associated With Anesthesia Services During Colonoscopy**

Wernli KJ, Brenner AT, Rutter CM, et al (Group Health Res Inst, Seattle, WA; Univ of Washington, Seattle; et al)

*Gastroenterology* 150:888-894, 2016

*Background & Aims.*—We aimed to quantify the difference in complications from colonoscopy with vs without anesthesia services.

*Methods.*—We conducted a prospective cohort study and analyzed administrative claims data from Truven Health Analytics MarketScan Research Databases from 2008 through 2011. We identified 3,168,228 colonoscopy procedures in men and women, aged 40–64 years old. Colonoscopy complications were measured within 30 days, including colonic (ie, perforation, hemorrhage, abdominal pain), anesthesia-associated (ie, pneumonia, infection, complications secondary to anesthesia), and cardiopulmonary outcomes (ie, hypotension, myocardial infarction, stroke), adjusted for age, sex, polypectomy status, Charlson comorbidity score, region, and calendar year.

*Results.*—Nationwide, 34.4% of colonoscopies were conducted with anesthesia services. Rates of use varied significantly by region (53% in the Northeast vs 8% in the West; $P < .0001$). Use of anesthesia service was associated with a 13% increase in the risk of any complication within 30 days (95% confidence interval [CI], 1.12–1.14), and was associated specifically with an increased risk of perforation (odds ratio [OR], 1.07; 95% CI, 1.00–1.15), hemorrhage (OR, 1.28; 95% CI, 1.27–1.30), abdominal pain (OR, 1.07; 95% CI, 1.05–1.08), complications secondary to anesthesia (OR, 1.15; 95% CI, 1.05–1.28), and stroke (OR, 1.04; 95% CI, 1.00–1.08). For most outcomes, there were no differences in risk with anesthesia services by polypectomy status. However, the risk of perforation associated with anesthesia services was increased only in patients with a polypectomy (OR, 1.26; 95% CI, 1.09–1.52). In the Northeast, use of anesthesia services was associated with a 12% increase in risk of any complication; among colonoscopies performed in the West, use of anesthesia services was associated with a 60% increase in risk.

*Conclusions.*—The overall risk of complications after colonoscopy increases when individuals receive anesthesia services. The widespread adoption of anesthesia services with colonoscopy should be considered within the context of all potential risks.

▶ This article reports the risk of complications in patients undergoing colonoscopy, comparing those who have sedation delivered by an anesthesia professional with those receiving anesthesia delivered by a gastroenterologist. They found an increased risk of perforation, bleeding, pain, anesthesia-related complications, and stroke in the anesthesia cohort. This is an important issue. For many years, sedation for endoscopic services was provided by gastroenterologists usually using a combination of a benzodiazepine and a narcotic. In the past decade more providers have gone to nurse aesthesis or anesthesiologist-administered propofol-based sedation. The argument is that patients prefer it and that it is "safer." In addition, in many settings, this can be a very financially advantageous arrangement. This and other articles call into question the safety side of the equation. Are the data from this study reasonable? I suspect they are indeed because the size of the study should have led to reasonable matching of the groups. Interestingly, the risk of complication was somewhat inversely related to the frequency of use (highest use in the Northeast with a 12% increased risk, and the lowest use in the West with a 60% increased risk). Perhaps "sicker" patients get anesthesia-based sedation in the West, or maybe they are less experienced in providing that service. That having been said, providers and patients should understand that using more expensive, anesthesia-based services is certainly not safer and in most studies less safe than gastroenterologist administered conscious sedation for routine endoscopic procedures.

**K. R. DeVault, MD**

---

### A Trial of Calcium and Vitamin D for the Prevention of Colorectal Adenomas

Baron JA, Barry EL, Mott LA, et al (Geisel School of Medicine at Dartmouth, Hanover, NH; et al)
*N Engl J Med* 373:1519-1530, 2015

---

*Background.*—Epidemiologic and preclinical data suggest that higher intake and serum levels of vitamin D and higher intake of calcium reduce the risk of colorectal neoplasia. To further study the chemopreventive potential of these nutrients, we conducted a randomized, double-blind, placebo-controlled trial of supplementation with vitamin D, calcium, or both for the prevention of colorectal adenomas.

*Methods.*—We recruited patients with recently diagnosed adenomas and no known colorectal polyps remaining after complete colonoscopy. We randomly assigned 2259 participants to receive daily vitamin $D_3$ (1000 IU), calcium as carbonate (1200 mg), both, or neither in a partial $2\times2$ factorial design. Women could elect to receive calcium plus random assignment to vitamin D or placebo. Follow-up colonoscopy was anticipated to be performed 3 or 5 years after the baseline examinations, according to the endoscopist's recommendation. The primary end point was adenomas diagnosed in the interval from randomization through the anticipated surveillance colonoscopy.

*Results.*—Participants who were randomly assigned to receive vitamin D had a mean net increase in serum 25-hydroxyvitamin D levels of 7.83 ng per milliliter, relative to participants given placebo. Overall, 43% of participants had one or more adenomas diagnosed during follow-up. The adjusted risk ratios for recurrent adenomas were 0.99 (95% confidence interval [CI], 0.89 to 1.09) with vitamin D versus no vitamin D, 0.95 (95% CI, 0.85 to 1.06) with calcium versus no calcium, and 0.93 (95% CI, 0.80 to 1.08) with both agents versus neither agent. The findings for advanced adenomas were similar. There were few serious adverse events.

*Conclusions.*—Daily supplementation with vitamin $D_3$ (1000 IU), calcium (1200 mg), or both after removal of colorectal adenomas did not significantly reduce the risk of recurrent colorectal adenomas over a period of 3 to 5 years. (Funded by the National Cancer Institute; ClinicalTrials.gov number, NCT00153816.)

▶ The concept of chemoprevention of colorectal carcinoma (CR) and of adenomas, which are precursor lesion of colorectal cancer, continue to be studied. Some preliminary data suggested supplementation with calcium and vitamin D to be protective. This large, randomized trial found no difference in the occurrence of new adenomas when supplementation was compared with placebo.

There may be many reasons to take calcium and vitamin D, but prevention of colon cancer does not seem to be one of them. On the other hand, the US Preventative Services Task Force recently released recommendations on the use of aspirin for prevention of both cardiovascular disease and colorectal carcinoma.[1] Interestingly, the use of aspirin for both of the indications is based on estimated cardiovascular risk and age (recommended for adults aged 50–59 with a > 10% 10-year cardiovascular risk and for consideration in those age 60–69). Aspirin is not beneficial in individuals with increased risk of gastrointestinal bleeding and the benefit in those under age 50 and over age 70 is not well defined.

**K. R. DeVault, MD**

*Reference*

1. Bibbins-Domingo K, U.S. Preventive Services Task Force. Aspirin use for the primary prevention of cardiovascular disease and colorectal cancer: US Preventative Services Task Force recommendation statement. *Ann Intern Med.* 2016;164: 836-845.

---

## Screening for Colorectal Cancer US Preventive Services Task Force Recommendation Statement

US Preventive Services Task Force (Univ of California, San Francisco; Group Health Res Inst, Seattle, WA; Univ of Iowa; et al)
*JAMA* 315:2564-2575, 2016

---

*Importance.*—Colorectal cancer is the second leading cause of cancer death in the United States. In 2016, an estimated 134 000 persons will be diagnosed with the disease, and about 49 000 will die from it. Colorectal cancer is most frequently diagnosed among adults aged 65 to 74 years; the median age at death from colorectal cancer is 68 years.

*Objective.*—To update the 2008 US Preventive Services Task Force (USPSTF) recommendation on screening for colorectal cancer.

*Evidence Review.*—The USPSTF reviewed the evidence on the effectiveness of screening with colonoscopy, flexible sigmoidoscopy, computed tomography colonography, the guaiac-based fecal occult blood test, the fecal immunochemical test, the multitargeted stool DNA test, and the methylated *SEPT9* DNA test in reducing the incidence of and mortality from colorectal cancer or all-cause mortality; the harms of these screening tests; and the test performance characteristics of these tests for detecting adenomatous polyps, advanced adenomas based on size, or both, as well as colorectal cancer. The USPSTF also commissioned a comparative modeling study to provide information on optimal starting and stopping ages and screening intervals across the different available screening methods.

*Findings.*—The USPSTF concludes with high certainty that screening for colorectal cancer in average-risk, asymptomatic adults aged 50 to 75 years is of substantial net benefit. Multiple screening strategies are available to choose from, with different levels of evidence to support their effectiveness, as well as unique advantages and limitations, although there are no empirical data to demonstrate that any of the reviewed strategies provide a greater net benefit. Screening for colorectal cancer is a substantially underused preventive health strategy in the United States.

*Conclusions and Recommendations.*—The USPSTF recommends screening for colorectal cancer starting at age 50 years and continuing until age 75 years (A recommendation). The decision to screen for colorectal cancer in adults aged 76 to 85 years should be an individual one, taking into account the patient's overall health and prior screening history (C recommendation).

▶ The task force concluded that average-risk, asymptomatic adults between ages 50 and 75 will have substantial benefit from screening. Seventy-six to 85-year-olds should be screened based on the patient's overall health and prior screening history. They provided a menu of options but did not provide strong guidance toward a preferred strategy. Those options include (with come comments on each from the article) the following:

1. Colonoscopy every 10 years: Most life years saved and cancer deaths averted, but higher risk of screening-related complications and perhaps cost.
2. Flexible sigmoidoscopy every 5 years: Lower years saved and death prevention, but perhaps less complications and cost.
3. Computed tomography colonography every 5 years: Intermediate benefit and complication/cost (some of the complication/cost come from incidental, non—colon-related findings).
4. Guaiac-based fecal occult blood testing, fecal immunochemical team (FIT) testing, fecal FIT Multitargeted stool DNA testing and serum-based methylated SPET19 DNA testing: all are intermediate in both efficacy and complication/cost. Appropriate intervals have not been well defined.

Although the draft statement from the US Preventive Services Task Force segregated the strategies into "recommended" and "alternative, the task force elected to remove that distinction from their final recommendations after public comment. In the original draft, the recommended tests were colonoscopy, sigmoidoscopy combined with FIT, guaiac-based testing, and stool-FIT testing.

**K. R. DeVault, MD**

# 48 Pancreas/Biliary

**Association Between Advances in High-Resolution Cross-Section Imaging Technologies and Increase in Prevalence of Pancreatic Cysts From 2005 to 2014**

Moris M, Bridges MD, Pooley RA, et al (Mayo Clinic, Jacksonville, FL)

*Clin Gastroenterol Hepatol* 14:585-593.e3, 2016

*Background & Aims.*—Increasingly, pancreatic cysts are discovered incidentally in patients undergoing cross-sectional imaging for nonpancreatic reasons. It is unclear whether this increase is caused by improved detection by progressively more sophisticated cross-sectional imaging techniques or by a true increase in prevalence. We aimed to determine the prevalence of incidental pancreatic cysts in patients undergoing magnetic resonance imaging (MRI) for nonpancreatic indications on successive, increasingly sophisticated MRI systems. Also, we compared prevalence based on the demographic characteristics of the patients.

*Methods.*—We collected data from MRIs performed at the Mayo Clinic in Florida during the sample months of January and February, from 2005 to 2014. Each patient's clinical chart was reviewed in chronological order to include the first 50 MRIs of each year (500 total). Patients were excluded if they had pancreatic disease including cysts, pancreatic surgery, pancreatic symptoms, pancreatic indication for the imaging study, or previous abdominal MRIs. An expert pancreatic MRI radiologist reviewed each image, looking for incidental pancreatic cysts.

*Results.*—Of the 500 patients analyzed, 208 patients (41.6%) were found to have an incidental cyst. A significant relationship was observed between pancreatic cysts and patient age ($P < .0001$), diabetes mellitus ($P = .001$), and nonpancreatic cancer ($P = .01$), specifically nonmelanoma skin cancer ($P = .03$) or hepatocellular carcinoma ($P = .02$). The multivariable model showed a strong association between hardware and software versions and detection of cysts ($P < .0001$); the old hardware detected pancreatic cysts in 30.3% of patients, whereas the newest hardware detected cysts in 56.3% of patients.

*Conclusions.*—Based on an analysis of data collected from 2005 through 2014, newer versions of MRI hardware and software corresponded with higher numbers of pancreatic cysts detected. Older age, diabetes, and the presence of nonpancreatic cancer (specifically nonmelanoma skin cancer and hepatocarcinoma) were also associated with the presence of cysts.

▶ Incidentally discovered pancreatic cysts are common and create a good bit of anxiety in both patients and health care providers. This interesting study looked at a cross section of magnetic resonance imaging (MRI) studies performed at a tertiary center over a 10-year period form 2005 to 2014. Cysts were very common (41.6%), and they found that changes in hardware and software resulted in a near doubling of pancreatic cyst detection during the study (from 23% to 56%). It is important to remember that all of these studies were done for "nonpancreatic" indications and that most of them were found during re-review by the expert MRI reader and usually not seen in the initial clinical read. Patients with cysts were also more likely to be older, have diabetes, and have nonpancreatic malignancies elsewhere in their bodies.

This study highlights the facts that incidental pancreatic cysts are very common, becoming more common as technology advances, are frequently overlooked on initial read, and, as best we can tell, are most often benign. Because these are so common and pancreatic cancer is not proportionately that common, finding and following these cysts may well be futile. The same does not apply to similar cysts in symptomatic patients and larger cysts (incidental or otherwise).

**K. R. DeVault, MD**

---

**A Prediction Rule for Risk Stratification of Incidentally Discovered Gallstones: Results From a Large Cohort Study**

Shabanzadeh DM, Sørensen LT, Jørgensen T (Bispebjerg Univ Hosp, Copenhagen, Denmark; Res Centre for Prevention and Health, Centre for Health, Capital Region of Copenhagen, Denmark; et al)

*Gastroenterology* 150:156-167, 2016

---

*Background & Aims.*—No one knows exactly what proportion of gallstones cause clinical events among subjects unaware of their gallstone status. We investigated the long-term occurrence of clinical events of gallstones and associations between ultrasound observations and clinical events.

*Methods.*—We analyzed data from 3 randomly selected groups in the general population of urban Copenhagen (age, 30–70 y) participating in an international study of cardiovascular risk factors (the Multinational mONItoring of trends and determinants in CArdiovascular disease study). In this study, participants (n = 6037) were examined from 1982 through 1994, and underwent abdominal ultrasound examinations to detect gallstones. Our study population comprised 664 subjects with gallstones; subjects were not informed of their gallstone status. Participants were followed up for clinical events through central registers until December 31, 2011. Independent variables included ultrasound characteristics, age, sex, comorbidity, and female-associated factors, which were analyzed using Cox regression.

*Results.*—Study participants were followed up for a median of 17.4 years (range, 0.1–29.1 y); 99.7% of participants completed the study. A total of 19.6% participants developed events (8.0% complicated and 11.6% uncomplicated). Ten percent had awareness of their gallstones; awareness was associated with uncomplicated and complicated events. Stones larger than 10 mm were associated with all events (hazard ratio [HR], 2.31; 95% confidence interval [CI], 1.45–3.69), acute cholecystitis (HR, 9.49; 95% CI, 2.05–43.92), and uncomplicated events (HR, 2.55; 95% CI, 1.38–4.71), including cholecystectomy (HR, 2.69; 95% CI, 1.29–5.60). Multiple stones were associated with all events (HR, 1.68; 95% CI, 1.00–2.81), complicated events (HR, 2.52; 95% CI, 1.05–6.04), and common bile duct stones (HR, 11.83; 95% CI, 1.54–91). There was an association between gallstones more than 5 years old and acute cholecystitis. Female sex was associated with all and uncomplicated events. We found a negative association between participant age and all events, uncomplicated events, and acute cholecystitis. Comorbidities and female-associated factors (intake of birth control pills or estrogens and number of births) were not associated with events. Compared with men with a single stone of 10 mm or smaller (reference), women with multiple stones greater than 10 mm had the highest risk for events (HR, 11.05; 95% CI, 3.76–32.44; unadjusted absolute risk, 0.0235 events/person-years).

*Conclusions.*—Fewer than 20% of subjects with gallstones develop clinical events. Larger, multiple, and older gallstones are associated with events. Further studies are needed to confirm the prediction rules.

▶ Gallstones are often discovered when imaging is performed of the upper abdominal region. The debate on what to do with these incidentally discovered stones has been going on for many years. This article attempts to better risk stratify the approach. The 664 patients were followed for a median of 17 years, and 130 (19.6%) developed a gallstone event. Factors associated with events included multiple and larger stones. Women were also more likely to have events. A woman with multiple, large stones was 11 times more likely to have a complication compared with a man with a single small stone. Interestingly 90% of the subjects did not know about their gallstones, and the 10% who did know about the stones had increased risk of an event. The majority of events were uncomplicated, but complications occurred in 8% including common duct stones, pancreatitis, and cholecystitis.

Take-home messages from this study include the fact that 80% of the gallstones never caused significant symptoms or resulted in an event. The majority did well even in those identified as higher risk. This and other studies have suggested that simply knowing about the gallstones increases the risk of cholecystectomy. Although it is probably not ethical to withhold that knowledge, educating patients to the benign nature of incidentally discovered stones might decrease their "risk" of cholecystectomy. In the end, most stones will continue to be followed, but ongoing data collection and modeling might eventually sort out a group where a more aggressive approach is needed.

**K. R. DeVault, MD**

# 49 Liver

**ACG Clinical Guideline: Liver Disease and Pregnancy**

Tran TT, Ahn J, Reau NS (Cedars Sinai Med Ctr, Los Angeles, CA; Oregon Health & Science Univ, Portland; Rush Univ, Chicago, IL)

*Am J Gastroenterol* 111:176-194, 2016

Consultation for liver disease in pregnant women is a common and oftentimes vexing clinical consultation for the gastroenterologist. The challenge lies in the need to consider the safety of both the expectant mother and the unborn fetus in the clinical management decisions. This practice guideline provides an evidence-based approach to common diagnostic and treatment challenges of liver disease in pregnant women.

▶ Abnormal liver tests and liver disease associated with pregnancy are common and challenging to diagnose and manage. The American College of Gastroenterology has produced a guideline statement on this topic. Important or novel concepts from that guideline include the following:

1. The first step in a patient with abnormal liver tests is to exclude causes independent of pregnancy.
2. When there is need for liver imaging, ultrasound is always the safest alternative; magnetic resonance imaging without gadolinium is safe in the second and third trimester. Computed tomography should be avoided if possible.
3. Endoscopy is safe but should be deferred to second or third trimester if possible. Meperidine and propofol are the safest sedatives.
4. Endoscopic retrograde cholangiopancreatography is possible in pregnancy, but radiation exposure should be minimized.
5. Symptomatic cholecystitis can be managed surgically if indicated during pregnancy.
6. Most benign liver masses should be ignored during pregnancy except for large hepatic adenomas where resection should be considered prior to pregnancy if possible.
7. In hepatitis B virus (HBV) infection, efforts should be made to prevent transmission from a pregnant mother to her child (immunization at birth and treatment during pregnancy in those with high viral load).
8. Women with risk factors for hepatitis C virus (HCV) infection should be screened, but therapy should generally not be offered during pregnancy.

Invasive procedures should be minimalized during pregnancy to decrease the risk of fetal transmission.

9. Cesarian delivery is not mandatory and breastfeeding is allowed with either HCV or HBV infection.
10. There are many liver illnesses unique to pregnancy, and suggested approaches are in the full paper for intrahepatic cholestasis of pregnancy, preeclampsia and eclampsia, HELLP syndrome, and acute fatty liver of pregnancy.

**K. R. DeVault, MD**

---

**Prevalence and Severity of Nonalcoholic Fatty Liver Disease in Non-Obese Patients: A Population Study Using Proton-Magnetic Resonance Spectroscopy**

Wei JL, Leung JC-F, Loong TC-W, et al (Chinese Univ of Hong Kong)

*Am J Gastroenterol* 110:1306-1314, 2015

---

*Objectives.*—Some studies suggest that non-obese patients with nonalcoholic fatty liver disease (NAFLD) may have more severe disease. We aim to study the epidemiology and severity of non-obese NAFLD.

*Methods.*—A total of 911 community subjects were randomly recruited from the census database of the Hong Kong Government. Intrahepatic triglycerides (IHTG) and liver fibrosis were assessed by protonmagnetic resonance spectroscopy and transient elastography, respectively. The Asian body mass index cutoff of 25 $kg/m^2$ was used to define non-obese NAFLD.

*Results.*—The prevalence of NAFLD was 19.3% in non-obese subjects and 60.5% in obese subjects ($P < 0.001$). Compared with obese NAFLD patients, non-obese NAFLD patients had similar IHTG content (median 9.8% vs. 9.9%; $P = 0.100$) but lower cytokeratin-18 fragments (149 vs. 182 IU/l; $P = 0.019$) and liver stiffness (4.6 vs. 5.6 kPa; $P < 0.001$). The G allele at the patatin-like phospholipase domain-containing protein 3 gene (*PNPLA3* rs738409) was more common in nonobese than obese NAFLD patients (78.4% vs. 59.8%; $P = 0.001$). Obesity, high hemoglobin $A_{1c}$, insulin resistance, hyperferritinemia, and the *PNPLA3* G allele were independent factors associated with NAFLD in non-obese subjects. Even among non-obese subjects with normoglycemia, those with NAFLD were more insulin resistant (mean homeostasis model assessment of insulin resistance: 2.0 ± 1.0 vs. 1.1 ± 1.1; $P < 0.001$).

*Conclusions.*—One-fifth of the general non-obese Chinese population has NAFLD. Non-obese patients with NAFLD do not have a higher risk of steatohepatitis or advanced fibrosis. Patients with risk factors of advanced fibrosis such as metabolic syndrome and *PNPLA3* G allele carriage should be assessed for severe NAFLD.

▶ Nonalcoholic fatty liver disease (NAFLD) is one of the most common liver diseases, a substantial cause of end-stage liver disease and is one of the top

3 causes of liver transplantation. It is commonly associated with obesity, but this study of community control subjects in China found it to be common in the obese (60.5%) and also in those with normal weights (19.3%). Severe NAFLD was more common in those with metabolic syndrome and a particular genetic allele (PNPLA3-G), which was also common in the nonobese patients with NAFLD. The nonobese NAFLD subjects also had higher waist circumference, insulin resistance, ferritin levels, and hyperlipidemia that nonobese subjects without NAFLD. Overall, liver disease in the obese was more severe.

This study was in a Chinese population, so there could be genetic or environmental differences from other groups, which will need to be examined in future studies. Also, the proportion of obesity in the sample (22.8%) was lower than in many Western populations, although this would suggest that the study might well underestimate the overall prevalence of NAFLD. The genetic allele is an important and interesting part of the study. Were these subjects doomed to NAFLD or could some intervention (dietary or pharmacologic) be protective? This will be an important area of future investigation. In fact, it would seem a large, prospective study of intervention in nonobese NAFLD should be supported by funding agencies. All of that having been said, this and other studies suggest that NAFLD is yet another major public health consequence on the ever-increasing obesity rates throughout the world.

**K. R. DeVault, MD**

# 50 Obesity

**Weight Loss and Health Status 3 Years after Bariatric Surgery in Adolescents**

Inge TH, for the Teen-LABS Consortium (Cincinnati Children's Hosp Med Ctr, OH; et al)

*N Engl J Med* 374:113-123, 2016

*Background.*—Bariatric surgery is increasingly considered for the treatment of adolescents with severe obesity, but few prospective adolescent-specific studies examining the efficacy and safety of weight-loss surgery are available to support clinical decision making.

*Methods.*—We prospectively enrolled 242 adolescents undergoing weight-loss surgery at five U.S. centers. Patients undergoing Roux-en-Y gastric bypass (161 participants) or sleeve gastrectomy (67) were included in the analysis. Changes in body weight, coexisting conditions, cardiometabolic risk factors, and weight-related quality of life and postoperative complications were evaluated through 3 years after the procedure.

*Results.*—The mean (±SD) baseline age of the participants was 17 ± 1.6 years, and the mean bodymass index (the weight in kilograms divided by the square of the height in meters) was 53; 75% of the participants were female, and 72% were white. At 3 years after the procedure, the mean weight had decreased by 27% (95% confidence interval [CI], 25 to 29) in the total cohort, by 28% (95% CI, 25 to 30) among participants who underwent gastric bypass, and by 26% (95% CI, 22 to 30) among those who underwent sleeve gastrectomy. By 3 years after the procedure, remission of type 2 diabetes occurred in 95% (95% CI, 85 to 100) of participants who had had the condition at baseline, remission of abnormal kidney function occurred in 86% (95% CI, 72 to 100), remission of prediabetes in 76% (95% CI, 56 to 97), remission of elevated blood pressure in 74% (95% CI, 64 to 84), and remission of dyslipidemia in 66% (95% CI, 57 to 74). Weight-related quality of life also improved significantly. However, at 3 years after the bariatric procedure, hypoferritinemia was found in 57% (95% CI, 50 to 65) of the participants, and 13% (95% CI, 9 to 18) of the participants had undergone one or more additional intraabdominal procedures.

*Conclusions.*—In this multicenter, prospective study of bariatric surgery in adolescents, we found significant improvements in weight, cardiometabolic health, and weight-related quality of life at 3 years after the procedure. Risks associated with surgery included specific micronutrient deficiencies and the need for additional abdominal procedures. (Funded by the National Institute of Diabetes and Digestive and Kidney Diseases and others; Teen-LABS ClinicalTrials.gov number, NCT00474318.)

▶ Obesity is a major public health issue in the Western world and affects both the young and old alike. Some younger patients with morbid obesity undergo bariatric surgery to control both obesity and its complications. In fact, the incidence of weight loss surgery more than doubled in young patients between 2003 and 2009. This study reports the 3-year outcome of patients under age 18 undergoing that surgery. They found impressive weight loss and improvement in many of the obesity-related complications. It seems that the younger patients have an even more impressive reversal of complications compared with older patients. The patients undergoing Roux-en-Y gastric bypass and those undergoing sleeve resection had similar outcomes. There were some complications including nutrient deficiency (low iron and a downward trend of several other nutrients). There was an intraabdominal reoperation in 13% with some having more than 1 procedure. Cholecystectomy was the most common operation. A similar percent had at least 1 endoscopy during the 3 years of the study.

It is clear that some patients with obesity will benefit from surgery. It is also clear that there are costs associated with surgery including the need for frequent monitoring of nutrients, frequent endoscopies, and need for revision and other surgical procedures directly related to the original surgery. Cholecystectomy is an interesting complication because obese patients have a high rate of cholelithiasis, which seems to commonly become symptomatic after rapid weight loss independent of bariatric surgery. This article provides data that allow young patients and their families to better understand the risk and potential benefits of bariatric surgery.

**K. R. DeVault, MD**

---

**Effect of morbid obesity, gastric banding and gastric bypass on esophageal symptoms, mucosa and function**

Borovicka J, Krieger-Grübel C, van der Weg B, et al (Kantonsspital St. Gallen, Switzerland; et al)

*Surg Endosc* 2016 [Epub ahead of print]

---

*Background.*—Obesity and gastroesophageal reflux disease (GERD) are commonly associated diseases. Bariatric surgery has been shown to have various impacts on esophageal function and GERD. Our aim was to evaluate changes in symptoms, endoscopic findings, bolus passage and esophageal function in patients after primary gastric bypass surgery as compared to patients converted from gastric banding to gastric bypass.

*Methods.*—Obese patients scheduled for laparoscopic Rouxen-Y gastric bypass (naïve-to-bypass) and patients who previously underwent gastric banding and were considered for conversion from gastric banding to gastric bypass (band-to-bypass) were included. Patients rated esophageal and epigastric symptoms (100 point VAS) and underwent upper endoscopy, impedance—manometry, and modified "timed barium swallow" before/after surgery.

*Results.*—Data from 66 naïve-to-bypass patients (51/66, 77 % females, mean age 41.2 ± 11.1 years) and 68 band-to-bypass patients (53/68, 78 % females, mean age 43.8 ± 10.0 years) were available for analysis. Esophageal symptoms, esophagitis, esophageal motility abnormalities and impaired esophageal bolus transit were more common in patients that underwent gastric banding compared to those that underwent gastric bypass. The majority of symptoms, lesions and abnormalities induced by gastric banding were decreased by conversion to gastric bypass. Esophagitis was present in 28/68 (41 %) and 13/47 (28 %) patients in the band-to-bypass group, pre- versus postoperatively, respectively, ($p < 0.05$). The percentage of swallows with normal bolus transit increased following transformation from gastric band to gastric bypass (57.9 ± 4.1 and 83.6 ± 3.4 %, respectively, $p < 0.01$).

*Conclusions.*—From an esophageal perspective, gastric bypass surgery induces less motility disorders and esophageal symptoms and should be therefore favored over gastric banding in difficult to treat obese patients at risk of repeated bariatric surgery.

▶ Obesity continues to be a major public health problem in the Western World. This has led to an increase in the number of patients undergoing bariatric surgery. A number of patients who have had bariatric surgery develop unacceptable swallowing problems. In addition, patients who have undergone gastric banding fail at times and require conversion to a Roux-en-Y gastric bypass. This study compared esophageal physiology in patients who had a primary bypass to a group who were being converted from banding to bypass (either because of unacceptable symptoms or insufficient weight loss). The major findings were less esophageal symptoms and better physiology in the bypass group and improvement in both with the conversion.

The choices for bariatric surgery have expanded over the past several years as has our understanding of esophageal issues related to both obesity and obesity surgery. Obese patients frequently have reflux and, depending on procedure, can continue to suffer from reflux and even have a worsening of esophageal symptoms after surgery. In the extreme, an achalasia-like pattern has been noted in some patients after banding. Because the bypass patients in this study were "failing," it is not surprising that they had more esophageal symptoms than the naïve group, but those symptoms did show improve after the revision. This study provides more data to question the use of gastric banding. Many centers have abandoned or limited banding and offer bypass or sleeve gastrectomy as the surgery of choice.[1]

**K. R. DeVault, MD**

*Reference*

1. Abraham A, Ikramuddin S, Jahansouz C, et al. Trends in bariatric surgery: procedure selection, revisional surgeries, and readmissions. *Obesity Surg.* 2016;26: 1371-1377.

# 51 Miscellaneous

---

**Centrally Mediated Disorders of Gastrointestinal Pain**

Keefer L, Drossman DA, Guthrie E, et al (Icahn School of Medicine at Mount Sinai, NY; Univ of North Carolina and Ctr for Education and Practice of Biopsychosocial Care LLC, Chapel Hill; Manchester Royal Infirmary, UK; et al)

*Gastroenterology* 150:1408-1419, 2016

---

Centrally mediated abdominal pain syndrome, formerly known as functional abdominal pain syndrome, can be distinguished from other functional gastrointestinal disorders by its strong central component and relative independence from motility disturbances. Centrally mediated abdominal pain syndrome is a result of central sensitization with disinhibition of pain signals rather than increased peripheral afferent excitability. A newly described condition, narcotic bowel syndrome/opioid-induced gastrointestinal hyperalgesia, is characterized by the paradoxical development of, or increases in, abdominal pain associated with continuous or increasing dosages of opioids. Patients only have relief when opioids are withdrawn. We define both conditions in the context of epidemiology, pathophysiology, clinical evaluation, and treatment, emphasizing the importance of a physician–patient relationship in all aspects of care.

▶ This is a consensus statement on a common clinical problem. Centrally mediated abdominal pain syndrome (CAPS) was formerly described as functional abdominal pain syndrome. This name change emphasizes the fact that these patients have pain that is mostly independent of gut function (not regularly related to either meals or bowel function) compared with irritable bowel syndrome (IBS) and dyspepsia, which are bowel- and meal-related, respectively. Some patients will evolve from IBS or dyspepsia to CAPS as pain becomes the predominant and sometimes only symptom. The pain in CAPS is constant, nearly constant, or frequently recurring, with pain occurring more or less every day. These are often challenging patients who frequently request additional diagnostic studies, lack the ability to take responsibility for managing their disease, minimize or resist the possibility of a psychosocial component, and often make request for narcotic analgesics. Treatment surrounds a supportive, but not enabling, health care team. Low-dose antidepressant therapy that can be titrated upward to effect is appropriate. Severe cases should be referred to a team-based program that may include cognitive behavioral therapy and perhaps other alternative methods of pain control. Narcotics should be avoided.

A second form of CAPs is narcotic bowel syndrome/opiate-induced gastrointestinal hyperalgesia. This is often an extension of the CAPS illness that worsens rather than improves with often escalating doses of narcotics. Aggressive, multidisciplinary approaches have been developed by several centers and perhaps offer the best approach to this challenging population. It is important to recognize that some of these patients also use and at times abuse other agents, such as cannabis.

**K. R. DeVault, MD**

---

**Association of Proton Pump Inhibitors With Risk of Dementia: A Pharmacoepidemiological Claims Data Analysis**

Gomm W, von Holt K, Thomé F, et al (German Ctr for Neurodegenerative Diseases, Bonn, Germany; et al)

*JAMA Neurol* 73:410-416, 2016

---

*Importance.*—Medications that influence the risk of dementia in the elderly can be relevant for dementia prevention. Proton pump inhibitors (PPIs) are widely used for the treatment of gastrointestinal diseases but have also been shown to be potentially involved in cognitive decline.

*Objective.*—To examine the association between the use of PPIs and the risk of incident dementia in the elderly.

*Design, Setting, and Participants.*—We conducted a prospective cohort study using observational data from 2004 to 2011, derived from the largest German statutory health insurer, Allgemeine Ortskrankenkassen (AOK). Data on inpatient and outpatient diagnoses (coded by the German modification of the *International Statistical Classification of Diseases and Related Health Problems, Tenth Revision*) and drug prescriptions (categorized according to the Anatomical Therapeutic Chemical Classification System) were available on a quarterly basis. Data analysis was performed from August to November 2015.

*Exposures.*—Prescription of omeprazole, pantoprazole, lansoprazole, esomeprazole, or rabeprazole.

*Main Outcomes and Measures.*—The main outcome was a diagnosis of incident dementia coded by the German modification of the *International Statistical Classification of Diseases and Related Health Problems, Tenth Revision*. The association between PPI use and dementia was analyzed using time-dependent Cox regression. The model was adjusted for potential confounding factors, including age, sex, comorbidities, and polypharmacy.

*Results.*—A total of 73 679 participants 75 years of age or older and free of dementia at baseline were analyzed. The patients receiving regular PPI medication (n = 2950; mean [SD] age, 83.8 [5.4] years; 77.9% female) had a significantly increased risk of incident dementia compared with the patients not receiving PPI medication (n = 70 729; mean [SD] age, 83.0 [5.6] years; 73.6% female) (hazard ratio, 1.44 [95% CI, 1.36-1.52]; $P < .001$).

*Conclusions and Relevance.*—The avoidance of PPI medication may prevent the development of dementia. This finding is supported by recent pharmacoepidemiological analyses on primary data and is in line with mouse models in which the use of PPIs increased the levels of β-amyloid in the brains of mice. Randomized, prospective clinical trials are needed to examine this connection in more detail.

▶ Proton pump inhibitors (PPI) are highly effective in the control of acid-related symptoms and mucosal disease of the upper gastrointestinal tract. They have recently been associated with several complications in large observational data sets including pneumonia, *Clostridium difficile* infection, and several nutritional deficiencies. One of the most recent studies associated PPI with an increased risk of dementia. In this study of almost 74 000 patients, those on regular PPI medication were at increased risk of developing dementia.

As with many studies of this type, the data are obtained from administrative databases (similar to insurance claim data in the United States). These data are certainly not precise, but the hope is that with a large enough sample size those issues can be minimized. PPI use was defined as filling a prescription at least once every 3 months. They controlled covariates as much as possible but, the PPI use group were slightly older, more likely to be female, taking more medications, and more likely to have depression, stroke, or ischemic heart disease. Where does that leave us? Given this and the numerous other complications, prudence would lead one toward the following approach:

1. Face up to the possibility that some of the associations may be true.
2. Know why the patient is on the medication. Some may not need it.
3. For reflux patients, emphasize lifestyle changes, particularly diet and weight loss.
4. Practice step-down therapy seeking the lowest form of acid suppression that provides adequate symptom relief.
5. Make sure patients understand that fear of these rare complications is not a reason to choose reflux surgery.

**K. R. DeVault, MD**

PART SEVEN

# ENDOCRINOLOGY, DIABETES, AND METABOLISM

DEREK LEROITH, MD, PhD

# Introduction

As is customary, the Endocrinology chapter of the YEAR BOOK provides the reader with commentaries on recent articles covering diabetes, obesity, lipid disorders, thyroid diseases, bone disorders, pediatric endocrinology and others.

The articles chosen range from basic and clinical science with a translational aspect that hopefully will afford the physician to keep abreast of the latest clinical-relevant research and therapeutic approaches in these common endocrine diseases.

**Derek LeRoith, MD, PhD**

# 52 Diabetes Mellitus

**Preexisting Insulin Autoantibodies Predict Efficacy of Otelixizumab in Preserving Residual β-Cell Function in Recent-Onset Type 1 Diabetes**

Demeester S, Keymeulen B, Kaufman L, et al (Vrije Universiteit Brussel, Belgium; et al)

*Diabetes Care* 38:644-651, 2015

*Objective.*—Immune intervention trials in recent-onset type 1 diabetes would benefit from biomarkers associated with good therapeutic response. In the previously reported randomized placebo-controlled anti-CD3 study (otelixizumab; GlaxoSmithKline), we tested the hypothesis that specific diabetes autoantibodies might serve this purpose.

*Research Design and Methods.*—In the included patients (n = 40 otelixizumab, n = 40 placebo), β-cell function was assessed as area under the curve (AUC) C-peptide release during a hyperglycemic glucose clamp at baseline (median duration of insulin treatment: 6 days) and every 6 months until 18 months after randomization. (Auto)antibodies against insulin (I[A]A), GAD (GADA), IA-2 (IA-2A), and ZnT8 (ZnT8A) were determined on stored sera by liquid-phase radiobinding assay.

*Results.*—At baseline, only better preserved AUC C-peptide release and higher levels of IAA were associated with better preservation of β-cell function and lower insulin needs under anti-CD3 treatment. In multivariate analysis, IAA ($P = 0.022$) or the interaction of IAA and C-peptide ($P = 0.013$) independently predicted outcome together with treatment. During follow-up, good responders to anti-CD3 treatment (i.e., $IAA^+$ participants with relatively preserved β-cell function [≥25% of healthy control subjects]) experienced a less pronounced insulin-induced rise in I(A)A and lower insulin needs. GADA, IA-2A, and ZnT8A levels were not influenced by anti-CD3 treatment, and their changes showed no relation to functional outcome.

*Conclusions.*—There is important specificity of IAA among other diabetes autoantibodies to predict good therapeutic response of recent-onset type 1 diabetic patients to anti-CD3 treatment. If confirmed, future immune intervention trials in type 1 diabetes should consider both relatively preserved functional β-cell mass and presence of IAA as inclusion criteria.

▶ Type 1 diabetes is an autoimmune disease in which T cells induce destruction of the insulin-producing beta cells of the islets in the pancreas. Various trials have used antibodies to reduce the impact of the T-cell-induced destruction and have been partially successful in those type 1 diabetic individuals who maintain some function of the beta cell as determined by continued C-peptide secretion. Because a number of type 1 diabetic individuals are nonresponders, it is important to identify these patients using appropriate biomarkers to avoid using these immunomodulators with potential adverse effects in the nonresponders. In the trial that used the anti-CD3 antibody otelixizumab, the investigators measured antibodies to well-known beta-cell markers including insulin autoantibody (IAA), GAD antibody (GADA), insulinoma-associated protein-2 (IA-2A), and zinc transporter 8 (ZNT8A) at the clinical start of the study. The IAA was the autoantigen that predicted to best outcome in the trial with the better C-peptide levels seen on clamp studies. Although all the serum levels of the autoantibodies eventually declined, it was the initially IAA levels that predicted the improved outcome from the anti-CD3 therapeutic regimen. The possibility exists that the patients with the higher IAA were younger at onset and had more insulinitis, thus suggesting a greater degree of autoimmunity and therefore more likely to respond to the antibody-induced reductions in autoimmunity. Because anti-CD3 therapy has also been shown to have an effect on B cells as well as T cells, this may further explain the reduced autoimmunity and the positive outcome. Thus the measurements of IAA may prove useful in future trials using immunotherapy that are critical both for new-onset type 1 diabetes as well as for transplantations because the autoimmunity is often resurrected in patients with transplanted islets or pancreata.

**D. LeRoith, MD, PhD**

---

**Predictive Low-Glucose Insulin Suspension Reduces Duration of Nocturnal Hypoglycemia in Children Without Increasing Ketosis**

Buckingham BA, for the In Home Closed Loop Study Group (Stanford Univ, CA; et al)

*Diabetes Care* 38:1197-1204, 2015

---

*Objective.*—Nocturnal hypoglycemia can cause seizures and is a major impediment to tight glycemic control, especially in young children with type 1 diabetes. We conducted an in-home randomized trial to assess the efficacy and safety of a continuous glucose monitor–based overnight predictive low-glucose suspend (PLGS) system.

*Research Design and Methods.*—In two age-groups of children with type 1 diabetes (11–14 and 4–10 years of age), a 42-night trial for each child was conducted wherein each night was assigned randomly to either having the PLGS system active (intervention night) or inactive (control night). The primary outcome was percent time <70 mg/dL overnight.

*Results.*—Median time at <70 mg/dL was reduced by 54% from 10.1% on control nights to 4.6% on intervention nights ($P < 0.001$) in 11–14-year-olds ($n = 45$) and by 50% from 6.2% to 3.1% ($P < 0.001$) in 4–10-year-olds ($n = 36$). Mean overnight glucose was lower on control versus intervention nights in both age-groups (144 ± 18 vs. 152 ± 19 mg/dL [$P < 0.001$] and 153 ± 14 vs. 160 ± 16 mg/dL [$P = 0.004$], respectively).

Mean morning blood glucose was 159 ± 29 vs. 176 ± 28 mg/dL ($P < 0.001$) in the 11–14-year-olds and 154 ± 25 vs. 158 ± 22 mg/dL ($P = 0.11$) in the 4–10-year-olds, respectively. No differences were found between intervention and control in either age-group in morning blood ketosis.

*Conclusions.*—In 4–14-year-olds, use of a nocturnal PLGS system can substantially reduce overnight hypoglycemia without an increase in morning ketosis, although overnight mean glucose is slightly higher.

► Type 1 diabetics are now more commonly treated with insulin pumps for convenience and better glycemic control. However, they are often prone to nocturnal hypoglycemia and even seizures, making tight glycemic control difficult. Until recently, ascertainment or prediction of such events was limited, until the advent of continuous glucose monitoring (CGMS). Although CGMS may alarm patients to the impending hypoglycemic event, patients are often oblivious to the alarm, and a new system has been devised, namely, an overnight predictive low-glucose suspend (PLGS) system. The pump suspension system comprised a glucose sensor (Medtronic Diabetes) in which the CGM and pump communicated with a bedside laptop computer running the hypoglycemia prediction algorithm (referred to as "the system"). The system estimated the glucose level and rate of change and suspended basal insulin delivery if the current sensor glucose was predicted to fall to < 80 mg/dL in the next 30 minutes. Insulin was automatically suspended for sensor glucose values 70 mg/dL. Basal insulin was restored on the first CGM rise during insulin suspension. Thus, overnight excessive insulin delivery maybe avoided with this type of technique. One of the major concerns of interrupted insulin delivery that may occur with insulin pumps, especially at night, is morning hyperglycemia and ketosis. This has been seen commonly with mechanical problems and needle dislodging for example. With the current PLGS technology, this was avoided because of restoration of basal insulin in a timely fashion. The present trial studied type 1 patients in groups aged 4 to 11 years and 11 to 14 years and was shown to substantially reduce overnight hypoglycemia.

**D. LeRoith, MD, PhD**

---

### Therapies to Preserve β-Cell Function in Type 1 Diabetes

Ludvigsson J (Linköping Univ, Sweden)

*Drugs* 76:169-185, 2016

---

In spite of modern techniques, the burden for patients with type 1 diabetes mellitus will not disappear, and type 1 diabetes will remain a life-threatening disease causing severe complications and increased mortality. We have to learn of ways to stop the destructive process, preserve residual insulin secretion or even improve the disease via β-cell regeneration. This will give a milder disease, a more stable metabolism, simpler treatment and perhaps even cure. Therapies based on single drugs have not shown sufficient efficacy; however, there are several treatments with encouraging efficacy and no apparent, or rather mild, adverse events. As the disease process is heterogeneous, treatments have to be chosen to fit relevant subgroups of patients, and step by step efficacy can possibly be improved by the use of combination therapies. Thus immunosuppressive therapies like anti-CD3 and anti-CD20 monoclonal antibodies might be combined with fusion proteins such as etanercept [tumor necrosis factor (TNF)-α inhibitor] and/or abatacept (CTLA4-Ig) early after onset to stop the destructive process, supported by β-cell protective agents. The effect may be prolonged by using autoantigen therapy [glutamate decarboxylase (GAD) proinsulin], and by adding agents facilitating β-cell regeneration [e.g. glucagon-like peptide-1 (GLP-1)] there should be a good chance to make the disease milder, perhaps leading to cure in some patients.

▶ Destruction of the beta cells of the islet of the pancreas by autoimmune disease is the basis for type 1 diabetes, however, it is now evident that individuals with type 2 diabetes also show reduced function and in many cases reductions in the mass of the beta cells. In type 2 diabetes, the effect of insulin resistance and its consequences places enormous pressure on the beta cells, and if the individual is genetically predisposed to the disease, the beta cell fails. Preservation of beta cell function is therefore important in both type 1 and type 2 diabetes.

One therapeutic regime that has been hypothesized to reduce the impact on the beta cell is the reduction of glucotoxicity (and lipotoxicity), using insulin for example to correct the metabolic conditions, so called "beta cell rest." Another would be the use of insulin sensitizers. Attempts to directly reduce beta cell stress have used nicotinamide, omega-3 fatty acids, and vitamin D, mostly without significant success. In type 1 diabetes, immunosuppression using cyclosporine, azathioprine, and antilymphocytic globulin have similarly had partial success, but all at the expense of severe adverse effects. Immunomodulators include anti-CD3, large-dose immunoglobulin G, plasma and photophoresis, and tumor necrosis factor-alpha inhibitors, among others. One of the reasons for the slow progress in the treatment of the B-cell disorder in type 1 diabetes maybe the reluctance to use combined therapy. Furthermore, conceptually it is believed that type 1 diabetes is a homogenous disease and therefore no selections are made before introducing a new form of therapy into the trials. Biomarkers may certainly improve the selection before instituting a trial. Finally, one should ask the ethical question as to whether the adverse events occurring with certain drugs outweigh the excellent therapy we now have for patients with type 1 diabetes and the excellent future we can offer the patients.

**D. LeRoith, MD, PhD**

**Two treatment approaches for human regular U-500 insulin in patients with type 2 diabetes not achieving adequate glycemic control on high-dose U-100 insulin therapy with or without oral agents: a randomized, titration-to-target clinical trial**

Hood RC, Arakaki RF, Wysham C, et al (Endocrine Clinic of Southeast Texas, Beaumont, TX; Univ of Hawaii at Manoa, Honolulu; Rockwood Clinic, Spokane, WA; et al)

*Endocr Pract* 21:782-793, 2015

*Objective.*—To compare the efficacy and safety of 2 dosing regimens for human regular U-500 insulin (U-500R, 500 units/mL) replacing high-dose U-100 insulins with or without oral antihyperglycemic drugs in patients with inadequately controlled type 2 diabetes (T2D).

*Methods.*—We conducted a 24-week, open-label, parallel trial in 325 patients (demographics [means]: age, 55.4 years; diabetes duration, 15.2 years; body mass index, 41.9 kg/m$^2$; glycated hemoglobin [$HbA_{1c}$], 8.7%; U-100 insulin dose, 287.5 units administered in 5 injections/day [median; range, 2 to 10]). Patients were randomized to thrice-daily (TID, n = 162) or twice-daily (BID, n = 163) U-500R after a 4-week lead-in period. The primary outcome was $HbA_{1c}$ change from baseline.

*Results.*—After 24 weeks, both treatments demonstrated significant $HbA_{1c}$ reductions (TID, −1.12%; BID, −1.22%; both, $P < .001$) and clinical equivalence (difference, −0.10%; 95% confidence interval, −0.33 to 0.12%; noninferiority margin, 0.4%). Comparable increases in total daily U-500R dose (TID, 242.7 to 343.1 units; BID, 249.0 to 335.0 units) were observed. Incidence and rate of documented symptomatic hypoglycemia (≤70 mg/dL) were lower for TID versus BID ($P = .003$ and $P = .02$, respectively); severe hypoglycemia was similar between treatments. Weight gain was similar in both groups (TID, 5.4 kg; BID, 4.9 kg).

*Conclusion.*—Initiation and titration of U-500R using either algorithm (TID or BID) improves glycemic control effectively and safely with fewer injections in patients with T2D treated with high-dose/high-volume U-100 insulin. These results provide clinicians with a practical framework for using U-500R in severely insulin-resistant patients with suboptimally controlled T2D.

► A number of patients with type 2 diabetes require more than 200 units of insulin daily for adequate diabetes control. Most of these patients demonstrate long-standing diabetes, overweight or obesity, and insulin resistance as the major reasons for the inability of large doses of insulin to control their blood glucose levels adequately. For these patients, human regular U-500 insulin is available and has been available, but perhaps underused for many years. The current study was undertaken to determine whether there was an appropriate paradigm for the use of human regular U-100 insulin in these patients. Patients were chosen who were receiving large doses of insulin (U-100 between 200 to 600 units per day) often in 5 divided doses. The patients were administered the insulin injections either twice daily (BID) or 3 times daily (TID). Dose escalation was performed according to self-monitoring of plasma glucose (SMPG) and using a classic "treat-to-target" methodology, that is, small gradual increments. Both groups had significant reductions in $HbA_{1c}$ and 7-point blood glucose measurements over a 24-week period, with little difference between the groups. However, documented symptomatic hypoglycemia was lower in the TID versus the BID group. Severe hypoglycemia and weight gain was similar between groups. The major impact this study will have on health care providers is to educate us regarding the value of a concentrated insulin (U-500) that contains 500 units per milliliter and makes large insulin requirements much more easily injectable and necessary only twice a day. Thus one would predict that compliance in these patients may make better glucose control achievable.

**D. LeRoith, MD, PhD**

---

**Patients achieving good glycemic control ($HbA_{1c}$ <7%) experience a lower rate of hypoglycemia with insulin degludec than with insulin glargine: a meta-analysis of phase 3a trials**

Einhorn D, Handelsman Y, Bode BW, et al (Scripps Whittier Diabetes Inst, La Jolla, CA; Metabolic Inst of America, Tarzana, CA; Atlanta Diabetes Associates, GA; et al)

*Endocr Pract* 21:917-926, 2015

---

*Objective.*—Meta-analysis to compare hypoglycemia rates of basal insulin degludec (IDeg) with insulin glargine (IGlar) in patients with diabetes achieving good glycemic control (hemoglobin $A_{1c}$ [$HbA_{1c}$] <7% at end of trial).

*Methods.*—In a preplanned meta-analysis, patient data from 7 randomized, treat-to-target, 26- or 52-week trials in patients with type 1 diabetes mellitus (T1DM) or type 2 diabetes mellitus (T2DM) who administered IDeg (n = 2,899) or IGlar (n = 1,431) once daily were analyzed. Using a negative binomial regression model, this meta-analysis compared hypoglycemia rates in patients achieving $HbA_{1c}$ <7% at end of trial with IDeg (n = 1,347) and IGlar (n = 697).

*Results.*—In all trials, IDeg was noninferior to IGlar in $HbA_{1c}$ reduction from baseline. At end of trial, 2,044 patients (T2DM, n = 1,661; T1DM, n = 383) achieved $HbA_{1c}$ <7%. The overall confirmed hypoglycemia rate, defined as plasma glucose <56 mg/dL or severe hypoglycemia if requiring assistance, was significantly lower with IDeg versus IGlar (estimated rate ratio [ERR] IDeg:IGlar, 0.86; 95% confidence interval [CI], 0.76 to 0.98). The nocturnal confirmed hypoglycemia rate, defined as occurring between midnight and 6:00 AM, was significantly lower with IDeg (ERR, 0.63; 95% CI, 0.52 to 0.77). In the maintenance period (16 weeks onward when average insulin dose and glycemic levels stabilized), the overall confirmed hypoglycemia rate was significantly lower (ERR, 0.79; 95% CI, 0.68 to 0.92) and the nocturnal confirmed hypoglycemia rate was significantly lower (ERR, 0.57; 95% CI, 0.45 to 0.72) with IDeg versus IGlar.

*Conclusion.*—Patients with T1DM and T2DM achieved $HbA_{1c}$ <7% with significantly lower rates of overall and nocturnal confirmed hypoglycemia with IDeg versus IGlar. The lower hypoglycemia rate with IDeg was more pronounced in the maintenance period.

▶ The major concerns of diabetic patients, whether type 1 or type 2 diabetes, in regard to insulin therapy is hypoglycemia and weight increase. The fear of hypoglycemia is particularly problematic because the symptoms are often quiet disconcerting and has traditional affected adherence and the maintenance of glycemic control. Nocturnal hypoglycemia is of particular clinical concern because many episodes are asymptomatic, and mild episodes can easily become severe. Repeated hypoglycemia, even when mild, may impair the counterregulatory responses and lead to "hypoglycemic unawareness." With the introduction of long-acting basal insulin analogues, the problem with hypoglycemia was markedly reduced; however, both Glargine (IGlar) and Determir insulin (IDet) are not peakless and have been associated with hypoglycemia. Thus newer, longer-acting insulins have been developed, such as insulin Degludec (IDeg), which has a longer half-life and is expected to have fewer hypoglycemic attacks. A meta-analysis was performed to compare the rates of hypoglycemia between IDeg and IGlar, in patients, both type and type 2, that reached HbA1c levels of < 7% at the completion of the trials. The meta-analysis demonstrated that in the trials, IDeg was noninferior to IGlar in obtaining the target glycemic control, namely, an HbA1c less than 7%. Furthermore, in these patients with good glycemic control, there was a significant reduction hypoglycemic events including nocturnal hypoglycemia. Although the exact mechanism(s) involved in this improvement in hypoglycemia has yet to be determined, it is postulated that 1 factor maybe the flat pharmacodynamic profile of IDeg versus IGlar. Nevertheless, it behoves the health care provider to ensure that insulin-taking diabetes have a minimal amount of hypoglycemia.

**D. LeRoith, MD, PhD**

---

**Glucagon secretion is increased in patients with Type 2 diabetic nephropathy**

Wang X, Yang J, Chang B, et al (Tianjin Med Univ, China)

*J Diabetes Complications* 30:488-493, 2016

---

*Aims.*—Currently little is known about the relationship between renal function, albuminuria and glucagon; we analyzed the secretion of glucagon (GLA) and C-peptide in Type 2 diabetic patients with different degrees of nephropathy.

*Methods.*—357 patients with Type 2 diabetes including 119 cases without nephropathy and 238 cases with nephropathy were divided into four groups according to the stages of diabetic nephropathy. Patients with diabetic nephropathy were further classified according to the level of estimated glomerular filtration rate (eGFR). OGTT and insulin, C-peptide, glucagon releasing tests were performed in all patients. Characteristics of glucagon and C-peptide secretion in different groups were compared. Glucagon/glucose ratio (GLA/GLU) and glucagon/insulin ratio (GLA/INS) were used to represent the inhibition of glucose or insulin on glucagon secretion, respectively.

*Results.*—With the progress of diabetic nephropathy, glucagon level increased significantly; the glucagon peak after glucose load delayed from 60 min to 120 min, whereas C-peptide level decreased significantly. Related factors analysis suggested that glucagon was independently correlated with eGFR. Further analysis showed that glucagon level was higher in group with eGFR < 60 ml/min compared with that in group with eGFR ≥ 60 ml/min. In addition, both GLA/INS and GLA/GLU were higher in group with eGFR < 60 ml/min compared with those in group with eGFR ≥ 60 ml/min.

*Conclusions.*—Patients with Type 2 diabetic nephropathy have worsened islet alpha and beta cell function. Therefore medications based on the regulation of glucagon secretion may improve glycemic control and also be beneficial for delaying the progress of diabetic nephropathy.

▶ Diabetic vascular complications are either microvascular or macrovascular in origin. Microvascular complications are more common in type 1 diabetes and include nephropathy, retinopathy and neuropathy. Macrovascular disease occurs more commonly in type 2 diabetes. However, with long-standing disease, type 1 diabetics develop macrovascular complications and, vice versa, Type 2 diabetics develop microvascular disease. Of the microvascular complications occurring in type 2 diabetes, nephropathy is the more common and should be screened for annually in these patients starting immediately following clinical diagnosis. Serum creatinine and albuminuria as well as estimated glomerular filtration rate (GFR) are used for following the deterioration in renal function, which is important for both altering various medications to accommodate the reduced renal function as well as the introduction of specific medications that may help retard the deteriorating renal function such as angiotensinogen-converting enzyme inhibitors and angiotensin receptor blocking agents. New evidence suggests that there is an association between serum glucagon levels and nephropathy with a rise in fasting glucagon levels paralleling the reduction in GFR. Glucagon elevations in diabetes are commonly seen and possibly represent a reduction in pancreatic beta-cell insulin secretion or insulin resistance, thereby reducing the effect of insulin on the pancreatic glucagon-secreting alpha cell. In turn, glucagon increases hepatic glucose production that may affect the circulating glucose levels and harm the kidney. Thus far, the mechanism through which glucagon levels relate to the deterioration of the kidney is as yet undefined; the question remains as to whether its causative or merely a biomarker requires further research.

**D. LeRoith, MD, PhD**

**Long-term Glycemic Variability and Risk of Adverse Outcomes: A Systematic Review and Meta-analysis**

Gorst C, Kwok CS, Aslam S, et al (Univ of Manchester, UK; Univ Hosps of North Midlands, Stoke-on-Trent, UK; Manchester Academic Health Science Centre, UK; et al)

*Diabetes Care* 38:2354-2369, 2015

*Objective.*—Glycemic variability is emerging as a measure of glycemic control, which may be a reliable predictor of complications. This systematic review and meta-analysis evaluates the association between $HbA_{1c}$ variability and micro- and macrovascular complications and mortality in type 1 and type 2 diabetes.

*Research Design and Methods.*—Medline and Embase were searched (2004–2015) for studies describing associations between $HbA_{1c}$ variability and adverse outcomes in patients with type 1 and type 2 diabetes. Data extraction was performed independently by two reviewers. Random-effects meta-analysis was performed with stratification according to the measure of $HbA_{1c}$ variability, method of analysis, and diabetes type.

*Results.*—Seven studies evaluated $HbA_{1c}$ variability among patients with type 1 diabetes and showed an association of $HbA_{1c}$ variability with renal disease (risk ratio 1.56 [95% CI 1.08–2.25], two studies), cardiovascular events (1.98 [1.39–2.82]), and retinopathy (2.11 [1.54–2.89]). Thirteen studies evaluated $HbA_{1c}$ variability among patients with type 2 diabetes. Higher $HbA_{1c}$ variability was associated with higher risk of renal disease (1.34 [1.15–1.57], two studies), macrovascular events (1.21 [1.06–1.38]), ulceration/gangrene (1.50 [1.06–2.12]), cardiovascular disease (1.27 [1.15–1.40]), and mortality (1.34 [1.18–1.53]). Most studies were retrospective with lack of adjustment for potential confounders, and inconsistency existed in the definition of $HbA_{1c}$ variability.

*Conclusions.*—$HbA_{1c}$ variability was positively associated with micro- and macrovascular complications and mortality independently of the $HbA_{1c}$ level and might play a future role in clinical risk assessment.

▶ Microvascular and macrovascular complications of both type 1 and type 2 diabetes is associated with poor glycemic control. Most studies have suggested that elevated hyperglycemia as measured by HbA1c is causative, in addition to other factors including poor lipid and blood pressure control. In a meta-analysis, the authors describe the effect of glycemic variability on adverse outcomes, including all-cause mortality, renal disease, retinopathy, and cardiovascular disease. There are a number of postulates to explain effects of short glycemic variability, such as postprandial increases in inflammatory cytokines, oxidative stress, and endothelial damage. On the other hand, long-term variability effects may require a further explanation. One possibility is that long-term variability has an effect via "metabolic memory" or the so-called legacy effect. An example of this is the effect of early well-controlled type 1 diabetics in the DCCT trial, for a period of 7 years and then over the subsequent 15 or more years had similar HbA1c levels as the control group. Nevertheless, in the long-term the original well-controlled group showed a reduction in cardiovascular disease, despite having similar levels of glycemic control compared with the control group, in the period after the trial. To date there is no good explanation for the legacy effect because most of the mechanisms described may vary over time. One explanation that requires investigation is the effect on gene expression and the epigenome; epigenetic effects can affect gene expression and be long lasting. The take-home message is keeping the HbA1c as close to normal as can be achieved safely in individual patients and reducing the glycemic variability, achieveable by multiple measurements and careful attention to medications.

**D. LeRoith, MD, PhD**

---

**Effect of Calorie Restriction on Mood, Quality of Life, Sleep, and Sexual Function in Healthy Nonobese Adults: The CALERIE 2 Randomized Clinical Trial**

Martin CK, for the Comprehensive Assessment of Long-term Effects of Reducing Intake of Energy (CALERIE) Phase 2 Study Group (Pennington Biomedical Res Ctr, Baton Rouge, Louisiana; et al)

*JAMA Intern Med* 176:743-752, 2016

---

*Importance.*—Calorie restriction (CR) increases longevity in many species and reduces risk factors for chronic diseases. In humans, CR may improve health span, yet concerns remain about potential negative effects of CR.

*Objective.*—To test the effect of CR on mood, quality of life (QOL), sleep, and sexual function in healthy nonobese adults.

*Design, Setting, and Participants.*—A multisite randomized clinical trial (Comprehensive Assessment of Long-term Effects of Reducing Intake of Energy Phase 2 [CALERIE 2]) was conducted at 3 academic research institutions. Adult men and women (N = 220) with body mass index (BMI; calculated as weight in kilograms divided by height in meters squared) of 22.0 to 28.0 were randomized to 2 years of 25% CR or an ad libitum (AL) control group in a 2:1 ratio favoring CR. Data were collected at baseline, 12 months, and 24 months and examined using intent-to-treat analysis. The study was conducted from January 22, 2007, to March 6, 2012. Data analysis was performed from July 18, 2012, to October 27, 2015.

*Interventions.*—Two years of 25% CR or AL.

*Main Outcomes and Measures.*—Self-report questionnaires were administered to measure mood (Beck Depression Inventory-II [BDI-II], score range 0-63, higher scores indicating worse mood, and Profile of Mood States [POMS], with a total mood disturbance score range of −32 to 200 and higher scores indicating higher levels of the constructs measured), QOL (Rand 36-Item Short Form, score range 0-100, higher scores reflecting better QOL, and Perceived Stress Scale, score range 0-40, higher scores indicating higher levels of stress), sleep (Pittsburgh Sleep Quality Index [PSQI], total score range 0-21, higher scores reflecting worse sleep quality), and sexual function (Derogatis Interview for Sexual Function-Self-report, total score range 24-188, higher scores indicating better sexual functioning).

*Results.*—In all, 218 participants (152 women [69.7%]; mean [SD] age, 37.9 (7.2) years; mean [SD] BMI, 25.1 [1.6]) were included in the analyses. The CR and AL groups lost a mean (SE) of 7.6 (0.3) kg and 0.4 (0.5) kg, respectively, at month 24 ($P < .001$). Compared with the AL group, the CR group had significantly improved mood (BDI-II: between-group difference [BGD], −0.76; 95% CI, −1.41 to −0.11; effect size [ES], −0.35), reduced tension (POMS: BGD, −0.79; 95% CI, −1.38 to −0.19; ES, −0.39), and improved general health (BGD, 6.45; 95% CI, 3.93 to 8.98; ES, 0.75) and sexual drive and relationship (BGD, 1.06; 95% CI, 0.11 to 2.01; ES, 0.35) at month 24 as well as improved sleep duration at month 12 (BGD, −0.26; 95% CI, −0.49 to −0.02; ES, −0.32) (all $P < .05$). Greater percent weight loss in the CR group at month 24 was associated with increased vigor (Spearman correlation coefficient, $\rho = -0.30$) and less mood disturbance ($\rho = 0.27$) measured with the POMS, improved general health ($\rho = -0.27$) measured with the SF-36, and better sleep quality per the PSQI total score ($\rho = 0.28$) (all $P < .01$).

*Conclusions and Relevance.*—In nonobese adults, CR had some positive effects and no negative effects on health-related QOL.

*Trial Registration.*—clinicaltrials.gov Identifier: NCT00427193.

► Obesity and the metabolic syndrome are well known to be associated with risk factors for cardiovascular disease as well as an increased incidence of type 2 diabetes. Furthermore, there is a relationship between obesity and an increased risk for cancer and cancer-related mortality. Thus, not surprisingly, obesity and the metabolic syndrome are associated with a shortened life span. Most of these complications have been shown to be reduced in animal models that were fed a low-calorie diet and have led to the hypothesis that calorie restriction may increase longevity in humans. Because long-term studies on calorie restriction are difficult in humans for periods longer than a few years, investigators have compromised with the length of the studies. The Comprehensive Assessment of Long-term Effects of Reducing Intake of Energy Phase 2 (CALERIE 2) examined the effect of calorie restriction (CR) on disease risk factors and predictors of longevity in nonobese individuals. The CR was a reduction in approximately 25% of calories over a 2-year period and compared with a control group. The CR group lost 8 kg of body weight and experienced improvement in mood, sleep, sexual drive, and general quality of life. This study is an example of how calorie restriction even for shorter periods may have positive effects, and although longevity cannot be affected by a 2-year study, nor can the potential reduction in type 2 diabetes or cancer be determined, the positive effects on quality of life as shown by assessing improvements in sleep, sexual function, and mood, for example, certainly suggest that calorie restriction is beneficial.

**D. LeRoith, MD, PhD**

## Empagliflozin, Cardiovascular Outcomes, and Mortality in Type 2 Diabetes

Zinman B, for the EMPA-REG OUTCOME Investigators (Mount Sinai Hosp, Toronto, Ontario, Canada)

*N Engl J Med* 373:2117-2128, 2015

*Background.*—The effects of empagliflozin, an inhibitor of sodium–glucose cotransporter 2, in addition to standard care, on cardiovascular morbidity and mortality in patients with type 2 diabetes at high cardiovascular risk are not known.

*Methods.*—We randomly assigned patients to receive 10 mg or 25 mg of empagliflozin or placebo once daily. The primary composite outcome was death from cardiovascular causes, nonfatal myocardial infarction, or nonfatal stroke, as analyzed in the pooled empagliflozin group versus the placebo group. The key secondary composite outcome was the primary outcome plus hospitalization for unstable angina.

*Results.*—A total of 7020 patients were treated (median observation time, 3.1 years). The primary outcome occurred in 490 of 4687 patients (10.5%) in the pooled empagliflozin group and in 282 of 2333 patients (12.1%) in the placebo group (hazard ratio in the empagliflozin group, 0.86; 95.02% confidence interval, 0.74 to 0.99; $P = 0.04$ for superiority). There were no significant between-group differences in the rates of myocardial infarction or stroke, but in the empagliflozin group there were significantly lower rates of death from cardiovascular causes (3.7%, vs. 5.9% in the placebo group; 38% relative risk reduction), hospitalization for heart failure (2.7% and 4.1%, respectively; 35% relative risk reduction), and death from any cause (5.7% and 8.3%, respectively; 32% relative risk reduction). There was no significant between-group difference in the key secondary outcome ($P = 0.08$ for superiority). Among patients receiving empagliflozin, there was an increased rate of genital infection but no increase in other adverse events.

*Conclusions.*—Patients with type 2 diabetes at high risk for cardiovascular events who received empagliflozin, as compared with placebo, had a lower rate of the primary composite cardiovascular outcome and of death from any cause when the study drug was added to standard care. (Funded by Boehringer Ingelheim and Eli Lilly; EMPA-REG OUTCOME ClinicalTrials.gov number, NCT01131676.)

▶ A large number of new antidiabetic medications have been developed recently for use in treating type 1 and type 2 diabetics. The latest class of oral agents is the sodium-glucose cotransporter-2 inhibitors (SGLT2-i). These agents block the reabsorption of glucose from the renal tubule leading a loss of glucose in the urine. The effect of SGLT inhibition leads to loss of calories and weight reduction, reductions in blood pressure, and reductions in HbA1c. The most common side effects are urinary and genital infections. This family of compounds has therefore become an important addition to our armamentarium for treating diabetic patients, particularly as add-on therapies to established oral agents. Good glucose control has repeatedly been shown to prevent progression of microvascular complications in both type 1 and type 2 diabetics, particularly retinopathy and nephropathy. However, demonstrating an effect of tight control on macrovascular complications has been extremely difficult. This can be explained by the use of statin therapy to control hypercholesterolemia and the use of successful antihypertensive therapies, both of which have major effects on the macrovascular system. The latest SGLT inhibitor, empagliflozin, was tested in thousands of type 2 diabetic high-risk patients and shown to lower the cardiovascular event rate, heart failure, and death from any cardiovascular cause. Previously the only effects of antidiabetic therapy on the cardiovascular system have been the "legacy" effects seen with the DCCT (use of insulin in type 1 diabetics) and similar trials in which, many years after the trial, a reduction in cardiovascular disease has been shown. The empagliflozin trial is the first to demonstrate an early effect of the drug on cardiovascular system outcomes.

**D. LeRoith, MD, PhD**

---

### No Effect of High-Dose Vitamin D Treatment on β-cell Function, Insulin Sensitivity, or Glucose Homeostasis in Subjects With Abnormal Glucose Tolerance: A Randomized Clinical Trial

Wagner H, Alvarsson M, Mannheimer B, et al (Karolinska Institutet, Stockholm, Sweden)

*Diabetes Care* 39:345-352, 2016

---

*Objective.*—There has been conflicting evidence regarding the potential role of vitamin D in glucose homeostasis. This study was designed to investigate the effect of high-dose vitamin D3 treatment on β-cell function, insulin sensitivity, and glucose tolerance in subjects with prediabetes or diet-treated type 2 diabetes.

*Research Design and Methods.*—Subjects ($n = 44$) were randomized to 30,000 IU vitamin D3 once weekly or placebo for 8 weeks. Hyperglycemic clamp assessed first-phase (0–12 min) and second phase (12–120 min) insulin response, insulin sensitivity, and disposition index (DI). An oral glucose tolerance test assessed glucose tolerance and glycosylated hemoglobin assessed glycemic control.

*Results.*—A total of 21 (vitamin D) and 22 (placebo) subjects completed the study, respectively. Season-adjusted 25-OH-vitamin D [25(OH)D] levels were doubled in the active treated group (43–82 nmol/L). No effect of vitamin D treatment, compared with placebo, was seen on first-phase or second-phase insulin secretion. There were no group differences in insulin sensitivity, DI, or any measures of glycemic control. No hypercalcemia or other adverse effects of vitamin D treatment were seen compared with placebo. Subgroup analyses of those with the lowest basal and greatest increase in 25(OH)D levels did not change these results.

*Conclusions.*—This study gives no support for any substantial effect of high-dose vitamin D treatment for 8 weeks in prediabetes or diet-treated type 2 diabetes on β-cell function, insulin sensitivity, or glycemic control.

▶ In addition to its established effects on bone metabolism, vitamin D has been proposed as having other important roles in disease states including diabetes. Whether these effects are relevant to type 1 diabetes and/or type 2 diabetes has not been established. Serum levels of 25 hydroxyvitamin D have been associated with the development of type 2 diabetes in individuals with prediabetes. However, randomized controlled trials are required to demonstrate causality. A few trials have shown contradictory results, and most used less direct measurements; none used the clamp technology, which has higher precision value. In the current 8-week-long controlled trial, high-dose vitamin D (30 000 IU given once weekly) was administered to individuals with prediabetes or diabetics managed on diet alone. The primary end point was the measurement of beta-cell function (first phase insulin secretion using a hyperglycemia clamp). Secondary end points included insulin sensitivity, altered fasting glucose and/or oral glucose tolerance test, HbA1c, and lipid profiles. The results of the study failed to show any effect on β-cell function, insulin sensitivity or any of the parameters studied. Furthermore, there was no effect on these parameters even when analyzing those individuals who had the highest rise in serum 25 hydroxyvitamin D while on the high-dose therapeutic arm of the study. Thus, one may conclude from these studies that there is little value to the use of vitamin D in attempting to affect glucose homeostasis, and the use of vitamin D should remain as indicated for bone metabolism, where its value has been definitively demonstrated.

**D. LeRoith, MD, PhD**

---

**Diabetic Retinopathy in Newly Diagnosed Subjects With Type 2 Diabetes Mellitus: Contribution of β-Cell Function**

Roy Chowdhury S, Thomas RL, Dunseath GJ, et al (Univ Hosp of Wales, Cardiff, UK; Swansea Univ, UK; et al)

*J Clin Endocrinol Metab* 101:572-580, 2016

---

*Purpose.*—The association of hyperglycemia and diabetic retinopathy (DR) in established type 2 diabetes mellitus (T2DM) subjects is well accepted. However, the association between β-Cell responsiveness and insulin sensitivity leading to fasting and postprandial hyperglycemia with DR in newly diagnosed treatment-naïve T2DM subjects remain unreported.

*Methods.*—A total of 544 newly diagnosed treatment-naïve T2DM subjects were screened for DR (digital photography) and underwent a standardized meal tolerance test. Serial plasma glucose and insulin levels were measured, and fasting ($M_0$) and postprandial β-Cell responsiveness calculated Calculating Pancreatic Response Program along with homeostasis model assessment β-Cell function (HOMA-B) and HOMA-Insulin Sensitivity. A subgroup of 201 subjects also underwent a frequently sampled

IV glucose tolerance test and the acute insulin response to glucose, insulin sensitivity, and glucose effectiveness ($S_G$) estimated (MINMOD model).

*Results.*—A total of 16.5% (90) subjects had DR at diagnosis. Subjects with DR had significantly reduced $M_0$, HOMA-B and $S_G$ leading to higher fasting and postprandial (2 hour) glucose and significantly lower fasting and postprandial (2 hour) insulin. Factors independently associated with DR in multivariate logistic regression analysis were $M_0$, HOMA-B, and $S_G$ with fasting and postprandial (2 hour) glucose and insulin. There was no statistical difference in glycated hemoglobin, systolic blood pressure, acute insulin response to glucose, and insulin sensitivity between those with or without DR.

*Principal Conclusions.*—In this cohort of newly diagnosed T2DM subjects, DR is associated with reduced β-Cell responsiveness, resulting from β-Cell failure rather than insulin resistance, leading to fasting and postprandial hyperglycemia and hypoinsulinemia.

▶ Diabetes is now considered a worldwide epidemic, with almost one-third demonstrating diabetic retinopathy and ~10% with vision-threatening diabetic retinopathy. Risk factors involved in the development and progression of diabetic retinopathy include hyperglycemia, duration of diabetes, hypertension, and dyslipidemia. Intensive glucose and lipid lowering in trials such as the Diabetes Control and Complications Trial, UK Prospective Diabetes Study, and Accord have clearly demonstrated a risk reduction; for every 1% reduction in HbA1c, there is a 37% risk reduction. There have been contradictory reports regarding the role of the beta cell and insulin resistance as causative factors in the relationship between type 2 diabetes and retinopathy, and the present study identified more than 500 patients with recent diagnosis of diabetes. They used the frequent sampled intravenous glucose tolerance test and a meal tolerance test that are well described test for beta cell function and insulin sensitivity. (0 patients (16.5%) had diabetic retinopathy at the onset of diabetes. The metabolic studies demonstrated a reduction in beta-cell function with reduced fasting and postprandial insulin levels, associated with higher fasting and postprandial glucose levels. The measurements of insulin resistance were not associated with the diabetic retinopathy. A number of studies have relied on the HbA1c as a measure glucose control and related the HbA1c to complications. However, more recently, there is growing evidence that glucose variability maybe more important in determining the risk for complications such as microangiopathy. Similarly, postprandial hyperglycemia may be an important factor; neither of these variables necessarily show in the HbA1c levels. Thus, understanding the basic pathophysiology is important in determining the factors involved in dysglycemia and its effect on complications, with the idea of preventing diabetic complications.

**D. LeRoith, MD, PhD**

**Optimized human regular U-500 insulin treatment improves β-cell function in severely insulin-resistant patients with long-standing type 2 diabetes and high insulin requirements**

Mari A, Rosenstock J, Ma X, et al (CNR Inst of Neuroscience, Padova, Italy; Diabetes and Endocrine Ctr, Dallas, TX; Eli Lilly and Company, Indianapolis, IN; et al)

*Endocr Pract* 21:1344-1352, 2015

*Objective.*—To assess β-cell function and insulin sensitivity following improvement in glycemic control in severely insulin-resistant patients with poorly controlled type 2 diabetes (T2D).

*Methods.*—A subset of patients in a 24-week, openlabel, randomized trial comparing thrice-daily (n = 14/162) versus twice-daily (n = 11/163) human regular U-500 insulin (U-500R) underwent mixed meal tolerance testing at baseline and endpoint. Baseline characteristics were similar between treatment groups (combined means: age, 54.0 years; diabetes duration, 13.6 years; body mass index, 38.8 kg/m$^2$; glycated hemoglobin [$HbA_{1c}$], 8.3%; U-100 insulin dose, 287.6 units/day, 2.6 units/kg/day). Primary outcome measure was ratio of area under the curve (AUC) for C-peptide to glucose ($AUC_{C\text{-peptide}}/AUC_{glucose}$) at 24-week endpoint.

*Results.*—Change from baseline $HbA_{1c}$, daily U-500R dose, and weight were −1.17% ($P$ = .0002), +80.8 units ($P$ = .0003), and +5.9 kg ($P$ = .33), respectively. β-Cell function significantly improved after 24 weeks of U-500R therapy in combined treatment groups. The $AUC_{C\text{-peptide}}/AUC_{glucose}$ increased 34.0% (ratio of least-squares geometric mean, 1.34; 95% confidence interval, 1.18 to 1.52; $P$ = .0001). Integral of total insulin secretion rate increased from 27.0 to 33.7 nmol/m$^2$, and glucose sensitivity improved from 18.3 to 24.0 pmol/min/m$^2$/mM (both, $P$ = .02). Matsuda index improved from 0.8 to 1.3 ($P$ = .008).

*Conclusion.*—Despite long-standing diabetes and poor glycemic control at baseline, functional recovery of β-cells was observed with improved glycemic control in these severely insulin-resistant patients with T2D, possibly due to alleviation of glucotoxicity.

▶ The natural history of type 2 diabetes involves deterioration of beta-cell function. Before the clinical detection of diabetes, patients often go through a phase of prediabetes or glucose intolerance that is usually not detected clinically. During the phase of preclinical and early diabetes, the beta cell of the pancreas usually increases production of and secretion of insulin in an attempt to overcome the peripheral insulin resistance that is associated with obesity and type 2 diabetes. During the subsequent years of overt type 2 diabetes, the beta cell becomes progressively dysfunction, leading to a worsening of the diabetes condition. On of the important aspects of research in type 2 diabetes is how to prevention this progressive deterioration. Both glucotoxicity (chronic hyperglycemia) and lipotoxicity (chronic elevations of plasma free fatty acids) and the combination (glucolipitoxicity) are well-described factors involved in beta-cell dysfunction. Indeed, correction of these factors has been demonstrated to prevent or reverse to some degree the deterioration in beta-cell function. In the present study, patients with severe insulin resistance were treated with human regular U-500 insulin either 2 or 3 times daily. $HbA_{1c}$ levels reduced over the 24-week trial and measurements of beta-cell function were performed. C-peptide is an indirect measurement of insulin secretory ability of the beta cell and improved significantly, as did glucose sensitivity. Thus, it is apparent that one can reverse beta-cell dysfunction, even in severely insulin resistant overweight/obese type 2 patients by improved glucose control; in this case using U-500 insulin.

**D. LeRoith, MD, PhD**

**Metformin use and mortality in patients with advanced chronic kidney disease: national, retrospective, observational, cohort study**

Hung S-C, Chang Y-K, Liu J-S, et al (Tzu Chi Univ, Hualien, Taiwan; Natl Health Res Insts, Zhunan, Taiwan; et al)

*Lancet Diabetes Endocrinol* 3:605-614, 2015

*Background.*—Metformin is recommended as a first-line treatment for patients with type 2 diabetes. However, use of this drug has been contraindicated in individuals with impaired kidney function because of the perceived risk of lactic acidosis. Evidence now supports cautious use of metformin in people with mild-to-moderate chronic kidney disease. However, studies examining the use of metformin in patients with advanced chronic kidney disease are lacking. We aimed to assess the safety of metformin in patients with type 2 diabetes and advanced (approximately stage 5) chronic kidney disease.

*Methods.*—We did a retrospective, observational, cohort study of patients with type 2 diabetes who were enrolled prospectively in Taiwan's national health insurance research database between Jan 1, 2000, and June 30, 2009, and had follow-up data until Dec 31, 2009. We included individuals with a serum creatinine concentration greater than 530 μmol/L, which is approximately equivalent to stage 5 chronic kidney disease. From a consecutive sample of 12 350 patients with type 2 diabetes and chronic kidney disease, 1005 used metformin and 11 345 were non-users. We matched users and non-users of metformin by propensity score in a 1:3 ratio. Our primary outcome was all-cause mortality.

*Findings.*—813 metformin users were matched by propensity score to 2439 non-users. The two groups of patients did not differ significantly by 30 baseline clinical and socioeconomic variables. Median follow-up in the matched cohort was 2·1 years (range 0·3–9·8). All-cause mortality was reported in 434 (53%) of 813 metformin users and in 1012 (41%) of 2439 non-users. After multivariate adjustment, metformin use was an independent risk factor for mortality (adjusted hazard ratio 1·35, 95% CI 1·20–1·51; $p < 0·0001$). The increased mortality risk was dose-dependent and was consistent across all subgroup analyses. However, metformin use compared with no use was associated with a higher but non-significant risk of metabolic acidosis (1·6 vs 1·3 events per 100 patient-years; adjusted hazard ratio 1·30, 95% CI 0·88–1·93; $p = 0·19$).

*Interpretation.*—Use of metformin in people with type 2 diabetes and a serum creatinine concentration greater than 530 µmol/L is associated with a significantly increased risk of all-cause mortality compared with non-users. Metformin use should not be encouraged in this patient group.

▶ Metformin is widely used as the first-line antidiabetic agent after recommended lifestyle change has failed to affect metabolic control in new-onset mild type 2 diabetes. Other than mild to moderate gastrointestinal side effects, metformin is generally well tolerated. An important, although extremely rare, side effect is lactic acidosis, which is seen in severe renal disease, due to the accumulation of lactic acid. Serum creatinine levels above 1.4 mg/dL and 1.5 mg/dL in women and men, respectively, have traditionally been used as indications for cessation of use of metformin. More recently, the American Diabetes Association of the European Association for the Study of Diabetes have suggested that metformin maybe safe unless the estimated glomerular filtration rate (eGFR) falls to < 30 mL/min per 1.73 $m^2$. In this retrospective, observational study, 12 350 patients with stage 5 renal disease were followed for a decade. Approximately 1000 were treated with metformin, and the rest were nonusers of metformin. Not surprisingly metabolic acidosis was more common in the metformin group. In addition, all cause mortality was also significantly increased by 35% in those patients using metformin compared with the nonuser patients, and the primary cause was cardiovascular disease. Previous studies have noted that eGFR of between 30 and 45 mL/min 1.73 $m^2$ are not associated with metabolic acidosis. Thus although practice guidelines have been "loosened" of late in regard to the use of metformin in mild renal disease, the use of metformin in more advanced renal disease remains dangerous and to be avoided. Given that the health care provider has many alternative medications including insulin, cases of metformin-induced lactic/metabolic acidosis should remain a remnant of the past.

**D. LeRoith, MD, PhD**

# 53 Obesity

## Circadian Clock Control of Liver Metabolic Functions

Reinke H, Asher G (Univ of Düsseldorf, Germany; Weizmann Inst of Science, Rehovot, Israel)

*Gastroenterology* 150:574-580, 2016

The circadian clock is an endogenous biological timekeeping system that synchronizes physiology and behavior to day/ night cycles. A wide variety of processes throughout the entire gastrointestinal tract and notably the liver appear to be under circadian control. These include various metabolic functions such as nutrient uptake, processing, and detoxification, which align organ function to cycle with nutrient supply and demand. Remarkably, genetic or environmental disruption of the circadian clock can cause metabolic diseases or exacerbate pathological states. In addition, modern lifestyles force more and more people worldwide into asynchrony between the external time and their circadian clock, resulting in a constant state of social jetlag. Recent evidence indicates that interactions between altered energy metabolism and disruptions in the circadian clock create a downward spiral that can lead to diabetes and other metabolic diseases. In this review, we provide an overview of rhythmic processes in the liver and highlight the functions of circadian clock genes under physiological and pathological conditions; we focus on their roles in regulation of hepatic glucose as well as lipid and bile acid metabolism and detoxification and their potential effects on the development of fatty liver and nonalcoholic steatohepatitis.

▶ The circadian clock is a cell-autonomous molecular system that independently leads to rhythmic oscillations in the expression of various genes. The genes in turn lead to considerable changes in the physiology and behavior of the organ and the organism. The central or "master clock" resides in the hypothalamus and sets the time for all the body clocks by sending neuronal and hormonal transmission signals. The central clock is affected by light, whereas as the peripheral clocks are more affected by cell metabolism, the physiological and metabolic state of the surrounding tissues, and serum-borne signals. The signals are transmitted to transcriptional signals to control rhythmic outputs. Nutrient signaling is critical for determining glucose uptake and glucose production. However, the circadian clock provides the rhythmic baseline regulation of many functions, including insulin and glucagon release that affect glucose uptake and production. Similarly, hepatic lipid metabolism is regulated by the circadian clock and like glucose, lipids are potential regulators of circadian rhythmicity. Most important, there is accumulating evidence that circadian misalignment maybe a risk factor metabolic disease and in the liver particularly, nonalcoholic fatty liver disease and hepatic steatohepatitis. This type of disorder can be seen in shift workers, and behavioral modifications could be a powerful tool in these cases as well as the jetlag effects on liver disorders. Finally, there is increasing evidence that the microbiome plays a role in inducing or worsening metabolic disorders, particularly gastrointestinal metabolism. Thus feeding time often affects the gut microbiome composition, perhaps secondary to bile acid synthesis. Disruptions of the intestinal microbiome have been associated with diet, obesity, and even diabetes. The circadian control of the microbiome is an interesting area of translational research.

**D. LeRoith, MD, PhD**

## Body-Mass Index in 2.3 Million Adolescents and Cardiovascular Death in Adulthood

Twig G, Yaniv G, Levine H, et al (Sheba Med Ctr, Tel Hashomer, Israel; Hebrew Univ—Hadassah School of Public Health and Community Medicine, Jerusalem, Israel; et al)

*N Engl J Med* 374:2430-2440, 2016

*Background.*—In light of the worldwide increase in childhood obesity, we examined the association between body-mass index (BMI) in late adolescence and death from cardiovascular causes in adulthood.

*Methods.*—We grouped data on BMI, as measured from 1967 through 2010 in 2.3 million Israeli adolescents (mean age, 17.3 ± 0.4 years), according to age- and sex-specific percentiles from the U.S. Centers for Disease Control and Prevention. Primary outcomes were the number of deaths attributed to coronary heart disease, stroke, sudden death from an unknown cause, or a combination of all three categories (total cardiovascular causes) by mid-2011. Cox proportional-hazards models were used.

*Results.*—During 42,297,007 person-years of follow-up, 2918 of 32,127 deaths (9.1%) were from cardiovascular causes, including 1497 from coronary heart disease, 528 from stroke, and 893 from sudden death. On multivariable analysis, there was a graded increase in the risk of death from cardiovascular causes and all causes that started among participants in the group that was in the 50th to 74th percentiles of BMI (i.e., within the accepted normal range). Hazard ratios in the obese group (≥95th percentile for BMI), as compared with the reference group in the 5th to 24th percentiles, were 4.9 (95% confidence interval [CI], 3.9 to 6.1) for death from coronary heart disease, 2.6 (95% CI, 1.7 to 4.1) for death from stroke, 2.1 (95% CI, 1.5 to 2.9) for sudden death, and 3.5 (95% CI, 2.9 to 4.1) for death from total cardiovascular causes, after adjustment for sex, age, birth year, sociodemographic characteristics, and height. Hazard ratios for death from cardiovascular causes in the same percentile groups increased from 2.0 (95% CI, 1.1 to 3.9) during follow-up for 0 to 10 years to 4.1 (95% CI, 3.1 to 5.4) during follow-up for 30 to 40 years; during both periods, hazard ratios were consistently high for death from coronary heart disease. Findings persisted in extensive sensitivity analyses.

*Conclusions.*—A BMI in the 50th to 74th percentiles, within the accepted normal range, during adolescence was associated with increased cardiovascular and all-cause mortality during 40 years of follow-up. Overweight and obesity were strongly associated with increased cardiovascular mortality in adulthood. (Funded by the Environment and Health Fund.)

▶ The obesity epidemic is occurring worldwide, and more importantly, it is seen not just in adults but more recently also in children and adolescents. Whereas in Western societies the obesity is seen as an increase in body mass index (BMI) 30, in Asian populations, it is often visceral adiposity in the absence of increased BMI. Obesity is generally associated with the metabolic syndrome that includes insulin resistance, hypertension, hyperlipidemia, and borderline hyperglycemia or frank diabetes and often results in atherosclerotic cardiovascular disease. A small proportion of obese individuals remain "healthy obese" without the manifestations of the metabolic syndrome, although this may be only a temporary phenomenon.

In this study, more than 2 million adolescents were examined and then followed from age 16 to 19 years—in some cases, for about 40 years. Overall increased cardiovascular death in middle age was seen with BMI percentiles in the upper range (over 85% percentile of BMI ranges) during adolescence. What was important in this study was the graded response. Thus even between the 50th and 75th percentiles of BMI ranges, there was an increase in cardiovascular mortality. Thus, overweight children and adolescents should be screened for relevant risk factors that make up the metabolic syndrome, including blood pressure levels, lipid levels, and serum glucose levels. In many cases, these risk factors are mildly abnormal in overweight or obese children, and it behoves the practicing clinician to consider intervention, whether to stress lifestyle changes or even intervene with appropriate medications. The findings are applicable to the worldwide childhood obesity epidemic, even though in this study it focused on men more than women.

**D. LeRoith, MD, PhD**

---

**Insights Into the Role of the Microbiome in Obesity and Type 2 Diabetes**

Hartstra AV, Bouter KEC, Bäckhed F, et al (Univ of Amsterdam, the Netherlands; Univ of Göteborg, Sweden; et al)

*Diabetes Care* 38:159-165, 2015

---

The worldwide prevalence of obesity and type 2 diabetes mellitus (T2DM) continues to rise at an alarming pace. Recently the potential role of the gut microbiome in these metabolic disorders has been identified. Obesity isassociated with changes in the composition of the intestinal microbiota, and the obese microbiome seems to be more efficient in harvesting energy from the diet. Lean male donor fecal microbiota transplantation (FMT) in males with metabolic syndrome resulted in a significant improvement in insulin sensitivity in conjunction with an increased intestinal microbial diversity, including a distinct increase in butyrate-producing bacterial strains. Such differences in gut microbiota composition might function as early diagnostic markers for the development of T2DM in high-risk patients. Products of intestinal microbes such as butyrate may induce beneficial metabolic effects through enhancement of mitochondrial activity, prevention of metabolic endotoxemia, and activation of intestinal gluconeogenesis via different routes of gene expression and hormone regulation. Future research should focus on whether bacterial products (like butyrate) have the same effects as the intestinal bacteria that produce it, in order to ultimately pave the way for more successful interventions for obesity and T2DM. The rapid development of the currently available techniques, including use of fecal transplantations, has already shown promising results, so there is hope for novel therapies based on the microbiota in the future.

▶ Obesity is commonly associated with the metabolic syndrome that includes insulin resistance, hyperlipidemia, hypertension, and glucose intolerance. Most patients with type 2 diabetes are overweight and have elements of the metabolic syndrome. There numerous organs involved in these disorders, ranging from liver, adipose, muscle, beta cell, the central nervous system and the gastrointestinal (GI) tract. The GI tract has recently gained attention due to the numerous gut hormones that are released and affect appetite and various organs involved in glucose homeostasis, such as the beta cell. More recently, the microbiome has become of tremendous interest to biologist as a system that maybe involved in numerous disease, among them obesity, diabetes and even cancer. Studies in both mice and humans have shown that gut microbiota differ in composition between obese and lean subjects. Germ-free mice were leaner despite increased food intake and when intestinal bacteria were transferred from normal mice to GF mice, the latter increased their body weight substantially within a short period. Thus there maybe "lean" microbiota and "obese" microbiota and this has led to an interest in fecal microbiota transplantation in humans; some recent small trials showing some promise. One of the mechanisms through which microbiota may enhance insulin sensitivity is the release of butyrate, a short-chain fatty acid produced by fermentation of dietary fiber. One area of recent is the effect of bariatric surgery on weight reduction and the early improvement of type 2 diabetes even before the weight reduction can be see. Roux-en-Y gastric bypass surgery affects the microbiota almost immediately and could be 1 contributor to the effect on insulin resistance.

**D. LeRoith, MD, PhD**

# 54 Lipoproteins, Atherosclerosis, and Cardiovascular Risk

**Changes in lipid and carbohydrate metabolism under mTOR- and calcineurin-based immunosuppressive regimen in adult patients after liver transplantation**

Zimmermann A, Zobeley C, Weber MM, et al (Univ Med Ctr, Mainz, Germany)
*Eur J Intern Med* 29:104-109, 2016

*Background.*—Cardiovascular disease is a leading cause of long-term mortality after liver transplantation (LT). Life long immunosuppression harbors the risk of metabolic alterations. We aimed to analyze the impact of calcineurin (CNI)-only containing regimen (group A) compared to mTOR-containing regimen (group B) on lipid and carbohydrate metabolism.

*Patients/Methods.*—92 adult patients after LT, University of Mainz (group A—78 patients, group B—14 patients; 65 M/27 F; mean age 59 +/− 10.2 years; mean time from LT 5.8 +/− 5 years). Clinical data, comorbidities, and medication were assessed. Fasting lipid profile including small dense LDLs (sdLDL) and oral glucose tolerance tests were performed.

*Results.*—Group B had significantly higher levels of total cholesterol (TC), LDL-cholesterol (LDL-C), triglycerides (TG) and sdLDL, with persistence of higher TC, TG, sdLDLs (mg/dl) after exclusion of patients under lipid lowering medication. Concentrations above the upper limits of normal were found: for LDL-C in 9% of group A/35.7% of group B ($p = 0.016$); for TG: in 32.1% of group A/92.9% in group B ($p = 0.0001$). A positive correlation between time since LT (years) and sdLDL (mg/dl) was found in group B ($p = 0.018$). In patients without previously known diabetes, NODAT and impaired glucose tolerance developed in 27.9% of group A/44.4% of group B (n.s.).

*Conclusion.*—Patients under mTOR-containing regimen are at higher risk to develop dyslipidemia with increased atherogenic sdLDLs compared to patients under CNI-only-containing regimen and display more frequently a dysglycemic status, with uncertain relevance for long-term cardiovascular risk. A careful monitoring after LT is needed to identify early metabolic risk and manage this appropriately.

▶ Organ transplantation generally requires immunosuppressive therapies to prevent the rejection of the donor organ by the host. Complications of liver transplantation include cardiovascular events, which represent the commonest cause of death in these patients. Unfortunately one of the major side effects of the immunosuppressive therapies is a significant alteration in lipid levels. Mammalian target of rapamycin (mTOR)-inhibitors have profound effects on the dyslipidemia, whereas calcineurin-inhibitors (CNI) are less of a problem regarding dyslipidemia. Thus mTOR inhibitors raise the circulating total, low-density lipoprotein (LDL), and small dense LDL cholesterol as well as triglycerides. However, there is evidence that mTOR inhibitors have direct cardioprotective effects and that certain CNIs such as cyclosporine increase the levels of total, LDL cholesterol, high-density lipoprotein cholesterol and serum triglycerides. Of importance is that in addition to changes in lipids by mTOR inhibitors, there are additional effects on carbohydrate metabolism; this is less obvious with calcineurin inhibitor regimen. The significance of these findings is that immunosuppressive therapies are now widely used in autoimmune disorders and patients undergoing transplantation. These immunosuppressive therapies have significant effects on the lipid profiles, and some affect carbohydrate metabolism. Although the exact mechanism of these adverse effects are not yet defined, it behoves us to identify patients who are prone to a worsening of lipid and glucose levels even before the transplantation and to continue to monitor all patients posttransplantation and of course treat expediently and appropriately to prevent the cardiovascular complications that occur secondary to the alterations in lipid and glucose changes.

**D. LeRoith, MD, PhD**

---

**Fresh Fruit Consumption and Major Cardiovascular Disease in China**

Du H, for the China Kadoorie Biobank Study (Univ of Oxford, UK; et al)

*N Engl J Med* 374:1332-1343, 2016

---

*Background.*—In Western populations, a higher level of fruit consumption has been associated with a lower risk of cardiovascular disease, but little is known about such associations in China, where the consumption level is low and rates of stroke are high.

*Methods.*—Between 2004 and 2008, we recruited 512,891 adults, 30 to 79 years of age, from 10 diverse localities in China. During 3.2 million person-years of follow-up, 5173 deaths from cardiovascular disease, 2551 incident major coronary events (fatal or nonfatal), 14,579 ischemic strokes, and 3523 intracerebral hemorrhages were recorded among the 451,665 participants who did not have a history of cardiovascular disease or antihypertensive treatments at baseline. Cox regression yielded adjusted hazard ratios relating fresh fruit consumption to disease rates.

*Results.*—Overall, 18.0% of participants reported consuming fresh fruit daily. As compared with participants who never or rarely consumed fresh fruit (the "nonconsumption" category), those who ate fresh fruit daily had lower systolic blood pressure (by 4.0 mm Hg) and blood glucose levels (by 0.5 mmol per liter [9.0 mg per deciliter]) ($P < 0.001$ for trend for both comparisons). The adjusted hazard ratios for daily consumption versus nonconsumption were 0.60 (95% confidence interval [CI], 0.54 to 0.67) for cardiovascular death, and 0.66 (95% CI, 0.58 to 0.75), 0.75 (95% CI, 0.72 to 0.79), and 0.64 (95% CI, 0.56 to 0.74), respectively, for incident major coronary events, ischemic stroke, and hemorrhagic stroke. There was a strong log-linear dose–response relationship between the incidence of each outcome and the amount of fresh fruit consumed. These associations were similar across the 10 study regions and in subgroups of participants defined by baseline characteristics.

*Conclusions.*—Among Chinese adults, a higher level of fruit consumption was associated with lower blood pressure and blood glucose levels and, largely independent of these and other dietary and nondietary factors, with significantly lower risks of major cardiovascular diseases. (Funded by the Wellcome Trust and others.)

▶ Cardiovascular disease is a leading cause of early death and morbidity worldwide, irrespective of the economic status of that country. The risk factors include obesity, diabetes, hyperlipidemia, and hypertension. Dietary patterns play a major role in this disease process, and one aspect that has been well established is the intake of fresh fruit and vegetables. In this study of more than half a million Chinese from 10 separate regions, fresh fruit intake was assessed and found to be inadequate. Only about 18% of the population studied actually reported a daily intake of some fresh fruit. Interestingly there was a direct correlation between the amount of daily fresh fruit intake and cardiovascular disease including myocardial infarction, ischemic stroke, and hemorrhagic stroke. Not surprisingly, in this group of nonobese individuals, blood pressure was lower, as was blood glucose. Reduced levels of both of these potential risk factors could explain the differences in cardiovascular events because together with hyperlipidemia they are well-known risk factors for cardiovascular complications. The greater daily intake of fresh fruit was noted to be in women who were better educated and had a higher household income. The unanswered question from the study is how is fresh fruit causally associated with the improved outcome. These individuals were not leaner as measured by body mass index or waist circumference. Because fresh fruit is a rich source of certain minerals such as potassium, folate, antioxidants, and phytochemicals and is low in sodium and fats, there remain multiple possibilities to explain the results. In any case, the study strongly supports the hypothesis that fresh fruits and vegetables are important for our diet.

**D. LeRoith, MD, PhD**

**Beta-cell function is associated with carotid intima-media thickness independently of insulin resistance in healthy individuals**

Roussel R, Natali A, Balkau B, et al (Centre de Recherche des Cordeliers, Paris, France; Univ of Pisa, Italy; UVSQ-UPS, Villejuif, France; et al)

*J Hypertens* 34:685-691, 2016

*Objective.*—It is a common belief that early atherosclerosis in prediabetes is causally linked to endothelial insulin resistance. Another condition, a low insulin secretion, may be associated with insufficient insulin action on the vascular wall and consequently favor atherosclerosis. Our aim was to test this hypothesis in people without diabetes, taking into account the gold-standard measurement of insulin sensitivity, a major confounder in the relationship between insulin secretion and atherosclerosis.

*Methods.*—We studied the European Relationship between Insulin Sensitivity and Cardiovascular Risk cohort of 451 men and 593 women (44 ± 8 years, mean ± SD) who were free of diabetes, hypertension, dyslipidemia, and other known chronic or acute conditions. All underwent an oral glucose tolerance test, a euglycemic-hyperinsulinemic clamp (M/I measured insulin sensitivity), and B-mode carotid ultrasound.

*Results.*—Intima–media thickness (IMT) in the common carotid artery was negatively associated with insulin secretion indexes, with Spearman partial correlation coefficients: −0.09, −0.08, −0.06 for respectively, the disposition index, the early insulin response and the beta cell glucose sensitivity, after adjusting for established factors, including clamp-measured insulin sensitivity (all $P < 0.05$). For quartiles 1 (lowest) to 4 of the disposition index, the covariate-adjusted geometric means of IMT (mm) were 0.605 (95% confidence interval: 0.596–0.614), 0.596 (0.587–0.605), 0.597 (0.587–0.606), and 0.586 (0.577–0.596) ($P_{trend} = 0.004$). Similar results were found for the two other surrogate measures of insulin secretion. No interaction with sex was observed.

*Conclusion.*—Insulin secretion was associated with early carotid atherosclerosis in nondiabetic individuals, independently of other risk factors, including insulin sensitivity measured by the gold-standard method.

▶ Atherosclerotic cardiovascular disease is a common complication of type 2 diabetes. Type 2 diabetes and the metabolic syndrome are associated with insulin resistance, hyperinsulinemia at early stages, hypertension, hyperlipidemia, and impaired glucose tolerance—all risk factors for the vascular complications that include myocardial disease and stroke. An indicator of atherosclerosis is the measurement of intima-media thickness (IMT) using the B-mode carotid ultrasound technology. IMT reflects subclinical atherosclerosis and is a marker for cardiovascular risk even in nondiabetic patients. The present study used individuals in the Relationship between Insulin Sensitivity and Cardiovascular Risk (RISC) cohort. Only "healthy" individuals were studied: those not on therapy for hypertension, hyperlipidemia, or hyperglycemia and of normal weight. All individuals underwent oral glucose tolerance test and euglycemia-hyperinsulinemic clamps. Interestingly, there was a relationship between the increase in IMT and the defect in beta function as measured by the insulin secretory response to glucose. This relationship was independent of the insulin sensitivity index. Previously it was shown that IMT was related to insulin resistance and the risk factors associated with insulin resistance. This relatively unique finding suggests that insulin deficiency may somehow predispose the vessel wall to alterations that could lead to atherosclerosis. Indeed, an ancillary study of the ORIGIN trial showed that insulin use reduced IMT in a subset of patients. One may therefore conclude that insulinopenia is potentially deleterious to the vasculature and that insulin therapy may indeed be advantageous to the diabetic patients and not harmful to diabetic patients as many have believed over the years.

**D. LeRoith, MD, PhD**

---

**A Multicenter Observational Study of Incretin-based Drugs and Heart Failure**

Filion KB, for the CNODES Investigators (Jewish General Hosp, Montreal, Quebec, Canada; et al)

*N Engl J Med* 374:1145-1154, 2016

---

*Background.*—There is concern that antidiabetic incretin-based drugs, including dipeptidyl peptidase 4 (DPP-4) inhibitors and glucagon-like peptide 1 (GLP-1) analogues, can increase the risk of heart failure. Ongoing clinical trials may not have large enough samples to effectively address this issue.

*Methods.*—We applied a common protocol in the analysis of multiple cohorts of patients with diabetes. We used health care data from four Canadian provinces, the United States, and the United Kingdom. With the use of a nested case–control analysis, we matched each patient who was hospitalized for heart failure with up to 20 controls from the same cohort; matching was based on sex, age, cohort-entry date, duration of treated diabetes, and follow-up time. Cohort-specific hazard ratios for hospitalization due to heart failure among patients receiving incretin-based drugs, as compared with those receiving oral antidiabetic-drug combinations, were estimated by means of conditional logistic regression and pooled across cohorts with the use of random-effects models.

*Results.*—The cohorts included a total of 1,499,650 patients, with 29,741 hospitalized for heart failure (incidence rate, 9.2 events per 1000 persons per year). The rate of hospitalization for heart failure did not increase with the use of incretin-based drugs as compared with oral antidiabetic-drug combinations among patients with a history of heart failure (hazard ratio, 0.86; 95% confidence interval [CI], 0.62 to 1.19) or among those without a history of heart failure (hazard ratio, 0.82; 95% CI, 0.67 to 1.00). The results were similar for DPP-4 inhibitors and GLP-1 analogues.

*Conclusions.*—In this analysis of data from large cohorts of patients with diabetes, incretin-based drugs were not associated with an increased risk of hospitalization for heart failure, as compared with commonly used combinations of oral antidiabetic drugs. (Funded by the Canadian Institutes of Health Research; ClinicalTrials.gov number, NCT02456428.)

▶ Initially there was concern regarding the safety of incretin therapy and possible increased risk of pancreatitis and pancreatic cancer. Although these concerns have been reduced with the long-term postmarketing data, physicians are aware that any untoward abdominal pain should be an indication for cessation of the use of incretin therapy until fully evaluated to exclude pancreatitis. Previous pancreatitis remains an absolute contraindication for the use of these therapies, and although nausea and vomiting may result from the incretin-mimetic injectable use, abdominal pain is a possible indication of pancreatitis. More recent outcome trials initially suggested a 27% increase in hospitalization for heart failure in the SAVOR-TIMI trial using Saxagliptin, the oral DPP-IV inhibitor. More than a million patients from Canada, the United Kingdom, and the United States were included in the present analysis, comprising diabetic patients with a history of heart failure and those without a history of heart failure. The patients all had type 2 diabetes and were seen in routine clinical practice. Overall there was no increase incidence of hospitalization for heart failure, whether they were patients with or without a history of heat heart failure. Furthermore, there was not difference when separately analyzing those on DPP-IV inhibitors or those receiving incretin-mimetic agents by injection. Although this is a retrospective analyses and therefore has its inherent issues compared with randomized controlled trials, the large number of individuals included gives one confidence in the results and allows health care providers to use these agents comfortably, while still remaining vigilant, as with all new antidiabetic drugs that are introduced into this growing market.

**D. LeRoith, MD, PhD**

---

## Pioglitazone after Ischemic Stroke or Transient Ischemic Attack

Kernan WN, for the IRIS Trial Investigators (Yale Univ, New Haven, CT)
*N Engl J Med* 374:1321-1331, 2016

---

*Background.*—Patients with ischemic stroke or transient ischemic attack (TIA) are at increased risk for future cardiovascular events despite current preventive therapies. The identification of insulin resistance as a risk factor for stroke and myocardial infarction raised the possibility that pioglitazone, which improves insulin sensitivity, might benefit patients with cerebrovascular disease.

*Methods.*—In this multicenter, double-blind trial, we randomly assigned 3876 patients who had had a recent ischemic stroke or TIA to receive either pioglitazone (target dose, 45 mg daily) or placebo. Eligible patients did not have diabetes but were found to have insulin resistance on the basis of a score of more than 3.0 on the homeostasis model assessment of insulin resistance (HOMA-IR) index. The primary outcome was fatal or nonfatal stroke or myocardial infarction.

*Results.*—By 4.8 years, a primary outcome had occurred in 175 of 1939 patients (9.0%) in the pioglitazone group and in 228 of 1937 (11.8%) in the placebo group (hazard ratio in the pioglitazone group, 0.76; 95% confidence interval [CI], 0.62 to 0.93; $P = 0.007$). Diabetes developed in 73 patients (3.8%) and 149 patients (7.7%), respectively (hazard ratio, 0.48; 95% CI, 0.33 to 0.69; $P < 0.001$). There was no significant between-group difference in all-cause mortality (hazard ratio, 0.93; 95% CI, 0.73 to 1.17; $P = 0.52$). Pioglitazone was associated with a greater frequency of weight gain exceeding 4.5 kg than was placebo (52.2% vs. 33.7%, $P < 0.001$), edema (35.6% vs. 24.9%, $P < 0.001$), and bone fracture requiring surgery or hospitalization (5.1% vs. 3.2%, $P = 0.003$).

*Conclusions.*—In this trial involving patients without diabetes who had insulin resistance along with a recent history of ischemic stroke or TIA, the risk of stroke or myocardial infarction was lower among patients who received pioglitazone than among those who received placebo. Pioglitazone was also associated with a lower risk of diabetes but with higher risks of weight gain, edema, and fracture. (Funded by the National Institute of Neurological Disorders and Stroke; ClinicalTrials.gov number, NCT00091949.)

▶ Pioglitazone is a thiazolidinedione that has important antidiabetic effects. The most prominent effect is on adipocyte storage of fat, thereby removing unwanted triglyceride from liver and muscle and markedly improving insulin resistance. Improved lipid profiles and effects on arterial wall macrophages are added benefits. It has been used successfully in conjunction with other oral antidiabetic agents and with insulin, reducing the dosage of insulin required. However, its side effect profile and the introduction of newer agents have reduced its desirability. These include increased weight, water retention, and precipitation of heart failure and increased risk for fragility bone fractures. Suggestions of increased bladder cancer were not borne out in long-term studies.

The results of a recent trial in patients without diabetes but with insulin resistance with a recent history of transient ischemic attack or stroke showed a significant reduction in myocardial infarction and stroke. The patients were classified using the Homeostatic Model Assessment—Insulin Resistance index, which basically measures fasting insulin and glucose; it is a rather crude measure of insulin resistance although useful in large population studies. The results support the secondary outcomes seen in the PROactive trial, but the mechanisms are unclear. They could include the lipid changes, the antiinflammatory effects of the drug, or the reduction in insulin resistance. Pioglitazone is known to activate the PPARgamma protein that apparently mediates the increase in adipogenesis and triglyceride storage and in addition activates the PPAR-alpha protein, which may be responsible for the reductions in lipid profiles through increased fatty acid oxidation. Whatever the mechanisms, the results could suggest a new paradigm in the prevention of these cardiovascular system complications, although potential side effects should be kept in mind.

**D. LeRoith, MD, PhD**

**Randomized Controlled Trial of Intensive Versus Conservative Glucose Control in Patients Undergoing Coronary Artery Bypass Graft Surgery: GLUCOCABG trial**

Umpierrez G, Cardona S, Pasquel F, et al (Emory Univ, Atlanta, GA)

*Diabetes Care* 38:1665-1672, 2015

*Objective.*—The optimal level of glycemic control needed to improve outcomes in cardiac surgery patients remains controversial.

*Research Design and Methods.*—We randomized patients with diabetes ($n = 152$) and without diabetes ($n = 150$) with hyperglycemia to an intensive glucose target of 100–140 mg/dL ($n = 151$) or to a conservative target of 141–180 mg/dL ($n = 151$) after coronary artery bypass surgery (CABG) surgery. After the intensive care unit (ICU), patients received a single treatment regimen in the hospital and 90 days postdischarge. Primary outcome was differences in a composite of complications, including mortality, wound infection, pneumonia, bacteremia, respiratory failure, acute kidney injury, and major cardiovascular events.

*Results.*—Mean glucose in the ICU was 132 ± 14 mg/dL (interquartile range [IQR] 124–139) in the intensive and 154 ± 17 mg/dL (IQR 142–164) in the conservative group ($P < 0.001$). There were no significant differences in the composite of complications between intensive and conservative groups (42 vs. 52%, $P = 0.08$). We observed heterogeneity in treatment effect according to diabetes status, with no differences in complications among patients with diabetes treated with intensive or conservative regimens (49 vs. 48%, $P = 0.87$), but a significant lower rate of complications in patients without diabetes treated with intensive compared with conservative treatment regimen (34 vs. 55%, $P = 0.008$).

*Conclusions.*—Intensive insulin therapy to target glucose of 100 and 140 mg/dL in the ICU did not significantly reduce perioperative complications compared with target glucose of 141 and 180 mg/dL after CABG surgery. Subgroup analysis showed a lower number of complications in patients without diabetes, but not in patients with diabetes treated with the intensive regimen. Large prospective randomized studies are needed to confirm these findings.

▶ Patients undergoing cardiac surgery as well as others in the intensive care units (ICUs) have been shown to be hyperglycemic. More than two-thirds of diabetes patients and about half of those without a known history of diabetes have hyperglycemia, which has been shown to an independent risk factor of morbidity and mortality after cardiac surgery. In addition, they are prone to wound infections, renal failure, postoperative stroke, longer hospital stays, and reduced long-term survival. Initial studies show an improvement in outcomes with good metabolic control (blood glucose levels <110 mg/dL) using intensive insulin therapy in the ICU, whereas more recent studies have shown an increase in hypoglycemia, leading the major organizations recommending blood glucose levels between 140 and 180 md/dL. In the present controlled trial, intensive care patients (equal numbers of nondiabetics and diabetics) who had undergone coronary artery bypass surgery (CABG) were maintained with blood glucose levels of 100 to 140 mg/dL or 140 to 180 md/dL. Interestingly, the effect of intensive control of blood glucose levels with regard to reducing complications was not detected overall, but specifically in the nondiabetic population. Diabetics did not show a decrease in complications when tight metabolic control was achieved. Although the trial involved a relatively small population, it did confirm the value of tight control between 100 and 140 mg/dL. One important feature to consider is that because of the concern of hypoglycemia resulting for very tight metabolic control the comparison was between 100 and 140 mg/dL or 140 and 180 md/dL, whereas the original trials that had major effects had a tight control target of $<110$ mg/dL. This may explain the absence of overall improvement, especially in the patients with diagnosed diabetes before hospitalization and surgery.

**D. LeRoith, MD, PhD**

# 55 Thyroid

---

**Update on the treatment of hypothyroidism**

Jonklaas J (Georgetown Univ, Washington, DC)

*Curr Opin Oncol* 28:18-25, 2016

---

*Purpose of Review.*—Differentiated thyroid cancer is a malignancy that is rapidly increasing in frequency. As thyroidectomy plays a central role in the treatment of thyroid cancer, it is incumbent on physicians treating this patient group to be well versed in the intricacies of treating hypothyroidism.

*Recent Findings.*—Treatment of hypothyroidism may be refined by careful attention to dose selection, monitoring of therapy and achievement of thyrotropin goals that are specific to the individual patient's overall clinical situation. These goals are common not only to patients with a sole diagnosis of hypothyroidism, as discussed in the recent American Thyroid Association Guidelines, but also to patients with hypothyroidism in the setting of thyroid cancer. Several recent studies have illuminated our understanding of the benefits and risks of thyrotropin suppression therapy in patients with differentiated thyroid cancer. Multiple studies of combination therapy with levothyroxine and liothyronine for treating hypothyroidism have not led to a clear conclusion about its benefits over levothyroxine monotherapy. Animal studies have advanced our understanding of the altered serum and tissue milieu that characterizes levothyroxine monotherapy. Crossing the bridge from this translational research into clinical research using sustained release triiodothyronine preparations may ultimately enhance the health of our patients.

*Summary.*—Continued refinement of our understanding of thyroid status and our ability to flawlessly implement thyroid hormone replacement is an active area of research.

▶ Hypothyroidism is a lifelong disorder and requires replacement using levothyroxine (LT4). On the other hand, LT4 is also used in thyroid cancer patients postsurgical removal of the gland to suppress the TSH levels because TSH a growth factor for thyroid tissue. In athyreotic patients, the approximate dosage of LT4 is 1.8 mcg/kg/day, but this can vary due to many factors, including age and body weight. It is appropriate to adjust the dosage according to relevant TSH levels as well as any symptoms the patients may volunteer or comorbidities in that particular patient. The TSH levels vary with age, for example, the upper limit was slightly raised with age. Patients with differentiated thyroid cancer (DTC), on the other hand, should have lower levels of TSH (TSH suppression). These suppressed levels resulted in better long-term prognosis for the patients.

Unfortunately, prolonged suppression of TSH has been associated with increased osteoporosis, reduced bone mineral density in both hip and spine, and increased fracture risk. Another possible effect is on cognition, with a reduction in those with suppressed TSH. Although these complications are unfortunate, they should not mitigate against suppression of TSH in cases of DTC. LT4 administration is very dependent on gastrointestinal absorption, and food, beverages, and other medications may interfere and should be avoided; their consumption is often an explanation for reduced efficacy. Some new formulations are being developed, such as a liquid formulation that may be more convenient for patients. Finally, there are some patients who have problems with deiodinase enzymes and are less able to convert LT4 to T3. There are now combinations therapies utilizing LT4 and LT3 or liothyronine.

**D. LeRoith, MD, PhD**

---

**Lenvatinib: Role in thyroid cancer and other solid tumors**

Cabanillas ME, Habra MA (The Univ of Texas MD Anderson Cancer Ctr, Houston)

*Cancer Treat Rev* 42:47-55, 2016

---

Despite recent breakthroughs in treatment of advanced thyroid cancers, prognoses remain poor. Treatment of advanced, progressive disease remains challenging, with limited treatment options. Small-molecule tyrosine kinase inhibitors, including vandetanib, cabozantinib, sorafenib, and lenvatinib, which are now FDA-approved for thyroid cancer, have shown clinical benefit in advanced thyroid cancer. Lenvatinib is approved for treatment of locally recurrent or metastatic, progressive, radioactive iodine (RAI)-refractory differentiated thyroid cancer (DTC). It has been studied in phase II and III trials for treatment of advanced RAI-refractory DTC, and in a phase II trial for medullary thyroid cancer (MTC). Lenvatinib targets vascular endothelial growth factor receptors 1–3 (VEGFR1–3), fibroblast growth factor receptors 1–4 (FGFR-1–4), RET, c-kit, and platelet-derived growth factor receptor a (PDGFR$\alpha$). Its antitumor activity may be due to antiangiogenic properties and direct antitumor effects. Lenvatinib has demonstrated antitumor activity in a variety of solid tumors, including MTC, in phase I and II clinical trials. In a phase II study in advanced RAI-refractory DTC, lenvatinib-treated patients achieved a 50% response rate (RR), with median progression-free survival (PFS) of 12.6 months. In a phase III trial in RAI-refractory DTC, median PFS in lenvatinib-treated patients was 18.3 months, with a 65% overall RR, versus 3.6 months in placebo-treated patients, with a 2% RR. Adverse events occurring in >50% of patients included hypertension, diarrhea, fatigue/asthenia, and decreased appetite. Lenvatinib is a promising new agent for treatment of patients with advanced thyroid cancer.

► Thyroid cancer in the United States and elsewhere is increasing, possibly in part because of increased awareness. Differentiated thyroid cancer (DTC) accounts for about 95% of cases, comprising papillary and follicular thyroid carcinomas. Medullary thyroid cancer (MTC) is about 4%, and the rest are anaplastic. Although the primary form of therapy for DTC is surgical removal, recurrences are often treated with radioactive iodine (RAI); however, RAI is not always tolerated or sufficient. There are a number of Food and Drug Administration—approved small molecule inhibitors used for DTC and others for MTC. Most these small molecules are kinase inhibitors. One of the more recent additions is Lenvatinib, which targets vascular endothelial growth factor receptors 1-3 (VEGFR1-3), fibroblast growth factor receptors 1-4 (FGFR1-4), RET oncogene, c-kit, platelet derived growth factor receptor α (PDGFRα), and mast/stem cell growth factor receptor; this broad spectrum effect is the main reason for its efficacy in DTC and MTC. The results of a phase III trial (SELECT) were recently published. Patients with RAI-refractory DTC were randomized, double-blinded in a placebo-controlled study, and 392 patients received the active drug. Progression-free survival was prolonged by Levantinib from 3.6 months in patients receiving placebo to 18.3 months. The most common side effects included hypertension (68%), diarrhea (59%), fatigue/asthenia (59%), and decreased appetite (50%). &1 patients (27%) died during the trial in the Levantinib group due to pulmonary embolism, hemorrhagic stroke, and other causes. The efficacy of the drug is apparently due to its antiangiogenic properties through inhibition of vascular endothelial growth factor receptors and fibroblast growth factor receptors, as well as its effects as a direct antitumor drug, and it certainly holds promise for these patients.

**D. LeRoith, MD, PhD**

---

**Thyroid disorders in pregnancy**

Yalamanchi S, Cooper DS (The Johns Hopkins Univ, Baltimore, MD)

*Curr Opin Obstet Gynecol* 27:406-415, 2015

---

*Purpose of Review.*—Recognition and management of thyroid disease during pregnancy is challenging with conflicting recommendations from various professional organizations.

*Recent Findings.*—We review the literature related to the diagnosis and management of gestational hypothyroidism and hyperthyroidism. We also discuss postpartum thyroiditis, thyroid nodules and thyroid cancer. The evidence clearly demonstrates that both overt hypothyroidism and hyperthyroidism should be treated, but controversy exists regarding the treatment of subclinical hypothyroidism and thyroid antibody positive euthyroidism, and whether pregnant women should be screened for thyroid disease.

*Summary.*—Appropriate management of thyroid disease during pregnancy is important for maternal and fetal health, particularly the recognition and management of hypothyroidism and thyrotoxicosis.

▶ There are conflicting recommendations from various organizations and societies regarding the screening and management of thyroid disorders in pregnancy.

The physiologic changes explain the altered thyroid function tests, and it is important to understand these so that health care providers do not over- or underdiagnose or inappropriately treat pregnant women. Pregnant women maybe taking insufficient iodine in their diet and in supplements. Thyroxine-binding globulin (TBG) is the major carrier of T3 and T4. TBG is increased by estrogen, especially in the first trimester, thereby increasing total T3 and T4; however, they should not be greater than 150% of the normal range. During the second trimester in particular, human chorionic gonadotropin rises, and, because it binds to the thyroid-stimulating hormone (TSH) receptor, may cause a slight rise in T4 with a fall in TSH. This corrects during the third trimester. Therefore, the normal range of thyroid function test needs to accommodate these physiologic changes. Hashimoto thyroiditis is the commonest cause of hypothyroidism in pregnancy. Overt hypothyroidism affects the mother resulting in hypertension, preeclampsia, and anemia. Fetal abnormalities, miscarriages, and other pregnancy-related problems are also increased. There is a controversy on whether subclinical hypothyroidism carries similar risks of miscarriage. Neurocognition in the offspring may occur as well. Pregnancy increases the requirements for replacement therapy in preexisting hypothyroidism, and all patients should be treated with levothyroxine with the aim of keeping the TSH in the normal pregnancy, trimester-appropriate range. Graves disease is the commonest cause of pregnancy-related hyperthyroidism. Diagnosis is often difficult because of the effect of pregnancy-related hormonal changes on the TSH and T4 levels. Free T4 should be normal. Thyroid antibody testing is important in both Hashimoto and Graves diagnoses. During pregnancy, radioactive iodine is contraindicated, and antithyroid drugs are used, keeping surgery for only the nonresponders or those with compression symptoms. Postpartum one should screen the neonate for hypothyroidism secondary to the antithyroid drugs used in the mother. Postpartum thyroiditis occurs during the first year and includes thyrotoxicosis, hypothyroidism alone, or thyrotoxicosis followed by hypothyroidism. Finally, if a thyroid nodule is discovered during pregnancy, fine-needle biopsy should be performed and treatment may include following the nodule clinically, or, if appropriate, surgery may safely be performed during the second trimester.

**D. LeRoith, MD, PhD**

# 56 Osteoporosis

**The effect of 8 or 5 years of denosumab treatment in postmenopausal women with osteoporosis: results from the FREEDOM Extension study**

Papapoulos S, Lippuner K, Roux C, et al (Leiden Univ Med Ctr, The Netherlands; Berne Univ Hosp and Univ, Switzerland; Paris Descartes Univ, France; et al)

*Osteoporos Int* 26:2773-2783, 2015

*Summary.*—The FREEDOM study and its Extension provide long-term information about the effects of denosumab for the treatment of postmenopausal osteoporosis. Treatment for up to 8 years was associated with persistent reduction of bone turnover, continued increases in bone mineral density, low fracture incidence, and a favorable benefit/risk profile.

*Introduction.*—This study aims to report the results through year 5 of the FREEDOM Extension study, representing up to 8 years of continued denosumab treatment in postmenopausal women with osteoporosis.

*Methods.*—Women who completed the 3-year FREEDOM study were eligible to enter the 7-year open-label FREEDOM Extension in which all participants are scheduled to receive denosumab, since placebo assignment was discontinued for ethical reasons. A total of 4550 women enrolled in the Extension (2343 long-term; 2207 cross-over). In this analysis, women in the long-term and cross-over groups received denosumab for up to 8 and 5 years, respectively.

*Results.*—Throughout the Extension, sustained reduction of bone turnover markers (BTMs) was observed in both groups. In the long-term group, mean bone mineral density (BMD) continued to increase significantly at each time point measured, for cumulative 8-year gains of 18.4 and 8.3 % at the lumbar spine and total hip, respectively. In the cross-over group, mean BMD increased significantly from the Extension baseline for 5-year cumulative gains of 13.1 and 6.2 % at the lumbar spine and total hip, respectively. The yearly incidence of new vertebral and nonvertebral fractures remained low in both groups. The incidence of adverse and serious adverse events did not increase over time. Through Extension year 5, eight events of osteonecrosis of the jaw and two events of atypical femoral fracture were confirmed.

*Conclusions.*—Denosumab treatment for up to 8 years was associated with persistent reductions of BTMs, continued BMD gains, low fracture incidence, and a consistent safety profile.

▶ There are numerous drugs used in the prevention and treatment of postmenopausal osteoporosis. Vitamin D (~600 IU) and ~1000 mg of calcium per day are recommended supplementation. Estrogen and selective estrogen receptor modulators (SERMs) inhibit bone resorption and reduce fracture risk. Bisphosphonates, given orally or intravenously, reduce bone turnover and fractures. The first biologic therapy approved for treating osteoporosis was denosumab. It has a distinct mechanism of action; it inhibits bone resorption by binding to the receptor activator of nuclear factor-κβligand (RANKL), thereby decreasing the differentiation of osteoclasts, bone cells involved in bone resorption. Teriparatide is an anabolic agent that, in contrast to those inhibiting bone resorption, actually increases bone formation.

Initial studies with denosumab were promising and led to approval by the Food and Drug Administration, both in regard to efficacy and minimal side effects. The present data describe the long-term follow-up in postmenopausal women on the drug for up to 8 years. Both C-terminal telopeptide of type 1 collagen (CTx) and procollagen type 1 N-terminal propeptide (P1NP), measures of bone resorption remained reduced, whereas as bone mineral density remained elevated. Both vertebral and nonvertebral fractures were reduced and continued to be reduced even after 8 years of therapy. Adverse and severe adverse event were minimal as in the initial study.

Denosumab has thus become an effective alternative and often the drug of choice in postmenopausal women with osteoporosis especially given that bisphosphonates have side effects that are often unacceptable. The convenience of denosumab includes the requirement for a single injection twice a year.

**D. LeRoith, MD, PhD**

---

**Higher Dietary Calcium Intakes Are Associated With Reduced Risks of Fractures, Cardiovascular Events, and Mortality: A Prospective Cohort Study of Older Men and Women**

Khan B, Nowson CA, Daly RM, et al (The Univ of Melbourne, St Albans, Australia; Deakin Univ, Burwood, Australia; et al)

*J Bone Miner Res* 30:1758-1766, 2015

---

The aim of this population-based, prospective cohort study was to investigate long-term associations between dietary calcium intake and fractures, non-fatal cardiovascular disease (CVD), and death from all causes. Participants were from the Melbourne Collaborative Cohort Study, which was established in 1990 to 1994. A total of 41,514 men and women (~99% aged 40 to 69 years at baseline) were followed up for a mean (SD) of 12 (1.5) years. Primary outcome measures were time to death from all causes (n = 2855), CVD-related deaths ($n = 557$), cerebrovascular disease-related deaths ($n = 139$), incident non-fatal CVD ($n = 1827$), incident stroke events ($n = 537$), and incident fractures ($n = 788$). A total of 12,097 participants (aged ≥50 years) were eligible for fracture analysis and 34,468 for non-fatal CVD and mortality analyses. Mortality was ascertained by record linkage to registries. Fractures and CVD were ascertained from interview ~13 years after baseline. Quartiles of baseline energy-adjusted calcium intake from food were estimated using a food-frequency questionnaire. Hazard ratios (HR) and odds ratios (OR) were calculated for quartiles of dietary calcium intake. Highest and lowest quartiles of energy-adjusted dietary calcium intakes represented unadjusted means (SD) of 1348 (316) mg/d and 473 (91) mg/d, respectively. Overall, there were 788 (10.3%) incident fractures, 1827 (9.0%) incident CVD, and 2855 people (8.6%) died. Comparing the highest with the lowest quartile of calcium intake, for all-cause mortality, the HR was 0.86 (95% confidence interval [CI] 0.76–0.98, $p_{trend} = 0.01$); for non-fatal CVD and stroke, the OR was 0.84 (95% CI 0.70–0.99, $p_{trend} = 0.04$) and 0.69 (95% CI 0.51–0.93, $p_{trend} = 0.02$), respectively; and the OR for fracture was 0.70 (95% CI 0.54–0.92, $p_{trend} = 0.004$). In summary, for older men and women, calcium intakes of up to 1348 (316) mg/d from food were associated with decreased risks for fracture, non-fatal CVD, stroke, and all-cause mortality.

▶ There have been multiple studies on the effect of calcium supplementation with or without vitamin D on the risk of various cardiovascular events and mortality. These studies have often demonstrated conflicting results, some suggesting improvements and others suggesting an increased risk of cardiovascular events including stroke, myocardial infarction, and death. Because vitamin D and calcium supplementation has been proven to be most beneficial for adults and aging individuals in regard to bone health, such confusion about cardiovascular system outcomes is problematic. This study from Australia involved a large cohort of older men and women followed for more than 12 years. Calcium intake was more than 1000 mg/dL per day obtained from dietary sources. The reduction in fractures and cardiovascular events and mortality was very reassuring. What has not been clear is the mechanism involved in calcium's effects on the cardiovascular system. A number of possibilities have been identified. Calcium affects the lipid profile and hypertension and may even affect the degree of obesity. Hypertension is a risk factor for stroke, and in this study in older men and women, the presence of hypertension affected the results; the positive effects of calcium supplementation on the cardiovascular system was particularly prominent in those without hypertension. Because elderly individuals are often calcium-deficient, mild secondary hyperparathyroidism may be present and corrected by an adequate calcium intake. Parathyroid hormone is well known to adversely affect the cardiovascular system. Finally, it is important to be careful not to overdose with calcium supplementation; the recommended supplemental dose of calcium should be between 1000 and 13000 mg/dL daily, thereby avoiding any untoward effects.

**D. LeRoith, MD, PhD**

### Hyponatremia Is Associated With Increased Osteoporosis and Bone Fractures in a Large US Health System Population

Usala RL, Fernandez SJ, Mete M, et al (Georgetown Univ Med Ctr, Washington, DC; MedStar Health Res Inst, Washington, DC)
*J Clin Endocrinol Metab* 100:3021-3031, 2015

*Context.*—The significance of studies suggesting an increased risk of bone fragility fractures with hyponatremia through mechanisms of induced bone loss and increased falls has not been demonstrated in large patient populations with different types of hyponatremia.

*Objective.*—This matched case-control study evaluated the effect of hyponatremia on osteoporosis and fragility fractures in a patient population of more than 2.9 million.

*Design, Setting, and Participants.*—Osteoporosis (n = 30 517) and fragility fracture (n = 46 256) cases from the MedStar Health database were matched on age, sex, race, and patient record length with controls without osteoporosis (n = 30 517) and without fragility fractures (n = 46 256), respectively. Cases without matched controls or serum sodium ($Na^+$) data or with $Na^+$ with a same-day blood glucose greater than 200 mg/dL were excluded.

*Main Outcome Measures.*—Incidence of diagnosis of osteoporosis and fragility fractures of the upper or lower extremity, pelvis, and vertebrae were the outcome measures.

*Results.*—Multivariate conditional logistic regression models demonstrated that hyponatremia was associated with osteoporosis and/or fragility fractures, including chronic [osteoporosis: odds ratio (OR) 3.97, 95% confidence interval (CI) 3.59−4.39; fracture: OR 4.61, 95% CI 4.15−5.11], recent (osteoporosis: OR 3.06, 95% CI 2.81−3.33; fracture: OR 3.05, 95% CI 2.83−3.29), and combined chronic and recent hyponatremia (osteoporosis: OR 12.09, 95% CI 9.34−15.66; fracture: OR 11.21, 95% CI 8.81−14.26). Odds of osteoporosis or fragility fracture increased incrementally with categorical decrease in median serum $Na^+$.

*Conclusions.*—These analyses support the hypothesis that hyponatremia is a risk factor for osteoporosis and fracture. Additional studies are required to evaluate whether correction of hyponatremia will improve patient outcomes.

▶ Hyponatremia is the most common electrolyte disorder and may be induced by commonly used therapeutic agents. Even mild hyponatremia has been associated with increased morbidity and mortality. Because bone is a major reservoir of sodium and may release large amounts during stressful situations, it has been proposed that there maybe an association of hyponatremia and osteoporosis. Two groups of patients were studied: one with classic osteoporosis and the other with fragility fractures. Most patients were in the older age groups aged 50 years and older, with a significant number over 80 years of age. Those with fragility fractures included a larger proportion even below 30 years of age. Unlike previous studies, the present study showed that chronic hyponatremia was associated with a 4-fold increase in osteoporosis. Furthermore, there was a dose-dependent relationship and a time-dependent relationship: the more recent the hyponatremia, the higher the risk. This also suggested that the hyponatremic-induced osteoporosis is reversible. In regard to fragility fractures, there was a similar association with increased risk of fracture with the presence of hyponatremia. Of particular note was the increased fracture risk despite the absence of osteoporosis. Interestingly, recent hyponatremia and chronic hyponatremia both increased the risk of fracture independently, but the risk was even further increased when both were present, suggesting independent causality mechanisms. Although the exact mechanism through which hyponatremia causes osteoporosis and an increased fracture risk is unknown, it behoves the clinician to pay particular attention to electrolyte balance, especially serum sodium levels, because of the risk of fractures that severely affect the lives of the aging population.

**D. LeRoith, MD, PhD**

# 57 Pituitary

**Osilodrostat, a potent oral 11β-hydroxylase inhibitor: 22-week, prospective, Phase II study in Cushing's disease**

Fleseriu M, Pivonello R, Young J, et al (Oregon Health and Science Univ, Portland; Università Federico II di Napoli, Naples, Italy; Université Paris-Sud, France; et al)

*Pituitary* 19:138-148, 2016

*Purpose.*—In a 10-week proof-of-concept study (LINC 1), the potent oral 11β-hydroxylase inhibitor osilodrostat (LCI699) normalized urinary free cortisol (UFC) in 11/12 patients with Cushing's disease. The current 22-week study (LINC 2; NCT01331239) further evaluated osilodrostat in patients with Cushing's disease.

*Methods.*—Phase II, open-label, prospective study of two patient cohorts. Follow-up cohort: 4/12 patients previously enrolled in LINC 1, offered re-enrollment if baseline mean UFC was above ULN. Expansion cohort: 15 newly enrolled patients with baseline UFC > 1.5 × ULN. In the follow- up cohort, patients initiated osilodrostat twice daily at the penultimate efficacious/tolerable dose in LINC 1; dose was adjusted as needed. In the expansion cohort, osilodrostat was initiated at 4 mg/day (10 mg/day if baseline UFC > 3 × ULN), with dose escalated every 2 weeks to 10, 20, 40, and 60 mg/day until UFC ≤ ULN. Main efficacy endpoint was the proportion of responders (UFC ≤ ULN or ≥50 % decrease from baseline) at weeks 10 and 22.

*Results.*—Overall response rate was 89.5 % (n/N = 17/19) at 10 weeks and 78.9 % (n/N = 15/19) at 22 weeks; at week 22, all responding patients had UFC ≤ ULN. The most common AEs observed during osilodrostat treatment were nausea, diarrhea, asthenia, and adrenal insufficiency (n = 6 for each). New or worsening hirsutism (n = 2) and/or acne (n = 3) were reported among four female patients, all of whom had increased testosterone levels.

*Conclusions.*—Osilodrostat treatment reduced UFC in all patients; 78.9% (n/N = 15/19) had normal UFC at week 22. Treatment with osilodrostat was generally well tolerated.

► Cushing disease is associated with significant morbidity and mortality. Transphenoidal surgery is successful in almost 90% of microadenomas but less than 65% of macroadenomas. Radiotherapy is an additional treatment modality as is bilateral adrenalectomy; these latter therapies being associated with major disadvantages. Medical therapy has therefore been an important sought-after alternative or additional form of therapy. Two major groups of therapeutic agents are aimed at the pituitary gland. One group is dopamine agonists, such bromocriptine or a more efficient dopamine agonist, cabergoline. The dopamine agonists are capable of significantly reducing urinary cortisol levels and may affect the progression of the pituitary tumor. They are not without side effects. Because corticope adenomas do not express significant levels of somatostatin receptor subtype, they are not readily responsive to octreotide and lanreotide, but do respond to pasireotide because they express the subtype 2 receptor. Other peripherally acting agents include metyrapone and ketoconazole (adrenal steroidogenesis inhibitors), mitotane (adrenolytic agent), and mifepristone (glucocorticoid receptor antagonist). A newer potentially useful agent is osilodrostat, which is an oral inhibitor of 11β-hydroxylase, that catalyzes the final step of cortisol synthesis. Although similar to the action of metyrapone, it is longer acting and more potent. The current study was performed in a small number of patients with Cushing disease and for a limited period of time. However, the results suggest that the new agent is efficacious and has potential as a therapeutic agent. Its safety profile was considered satisfactory, with the major concern being changes in the size of the pituitary adenoma/gland in a few of the cases. This is due to loss of negative feedback to the hypothalamus/pituitary leading to enlargement of the pituitary and development of Nelson's syndrome, a complication to beware of with all peripheral therapeutic agents as opposed to treatments directed directly at the pituitary adenoma itself.

**D. LeRoith, MD, PhD**

---

**Safety and Efficacy of Oral Octreotide in Acromegaly: Results of a Multicenter Phase III Trial**

Melmed S, Popovic V, Bidlingmaier M, et al (Cedars-Sinai Med Ctr, Los Angeles, CA; Clinical Ctr of Serbia, Belgrade, Serbia; Medizinische Klinik IV, Munich, Germany; et al)

*J Clin Endocrinol Metab* 100:1699-1708, 2015

---

*Background.*—A novel oral octreotide formulation was tested for efficacy and safety in a phase III, multicenter, open-label, dose-titration, baseline-controlled study in patients with acromegaly.

*Methods.*—We enrolled 155 complete or partially controlled patients (IGF-1 <1.3 × upper limit of normal [ULN], and 2-h integrated GH <2.5 ng/mL) receiving injectable somatostatin receptor ligand (SRL) for ≥ 3 months. Subjects were switched to 40 mg/d oral octreotide capsules (OOCs), and the dose escalated to 60 and then up to 80 mg/d to control IGF-1. Subsequent fixed doses were maintained for a 7-month core treatment, followed by a voluntary 6-month extension.

*Results.*—Of 151 evaluable subjects initiating OOCs, 65% maintained response and achieved the primary endpoint of IGF-1 <1.3 × ULN and mean integrated GH <2.5 ng/mL at the end of the core treatment period and 62% at the end of treatment (up to 13 mo). The effect was durable, and 85 % of subjects initially controlled on OOCs maintained this response up to 13 months. When controlled on OOCs, GH levels were reduced compared to baseline, and acromegaly-related symptoms improved. Of 102 subjects completing the core treatment, 86% elected to enroll in the 6-month extension. Twenty-six subjects who were considered treatment failures (IGF-1 ≥ 1.3 × ULN) terminated early, and 23 withdrew for adverse events, consistent with those known foroctreotide or disease related.

*Conclusions.*—OOC, an oral therapeutic peptide, achieves efficacy in controlling IGF-1 and GH after switching from injectable SRLs for up to 13 months, with a safety profile consistent with approved SRLs. OOC appears to be effective and safe as an acromegaly monotherapy.

▶ Acromegaly is associated with considerable morbidity. Removal of the pituitary tumor, commonly by transsphenoidal surgery, is often incomplete, and continued excess of growth hormone (GH) and insulin-like growth factor-1 (IGF-1) levels are associated with hypertension, cardiovascular, and cerebrovascular disease. Until recently, the most effective chronic form of therapy to maintain normal GH and IGF-1 levels in these patients has been somatostatin analogs, octreotide and lanreotide by injection often daily or less often once slow-release formulations were developed. The availability of oral medications has been sought after to replace the injectables for many diseases given the inconvenience experienced by patients using injectables. A new formulation has been developed and tested for the use of octreotide in cases of acromegaly. Oral octreotide capsules were developed that contained octreotide acetate and a novel transient permeability enhancer (TPE). The TPE enabled the octreotide to pass via paracellular tight junctions that were reversibly permeabilized, allowing on small molecules to pass. Luminal pathogens and endobacterial toxins were excluded in this process. More than 150 patients were included in the trial and tested for more than a year. Patients well controlled on somatostatin receptor ligands were switched to the oral formulation and then after 1 month started on the oral octreotide. In most patients, the levels of GH returned basal levels. Acromegaly symptoms included headache, perspiration, asthenia, swelling of extremities, and joint pain when they were untreated, and the patients on the oral octreotide soon noticed marked improvement in these acromegaly-associated symptoms. Thus oral octreotide is a viable form of anti-acromegaly medication, allowing patients to avoid the injections that are uncomfortable and problematic.

**D. LeRoith, MD, PhD**

# Article Index

## Chapter 1: Systemic Lupus Erythematosus



## Chapter 2: Rheumatoid Arthritis



## Chapter 3: Seronegative Spondyloarthropathies



## Chapter 4: Osteoarthritis

## Chapter 5: Gout



## Chapter 6: Scleroderma



## Chapter 7: Sjogren's Syndrome



## Chapter 8: Vasculitis



## Chapter 9: Idiopathic Inflammatory Myopathy



## Chapter 10: Polymyalgia Rheumatica



## Chapter 11: Chronic Juvenile Arthritis



## Chapter 12: Fibromyalgia



## Chapter 13: Drug Toxicity

## Chapter 14: Miscellaneous Rheumatic Diseases and Therapies



## Chapter 15: Bacterial Infections



## Chapter 16: Viral Infections



## Chapter 17: Fungal Infections



## Chapter 18: Tuberculosis



## Chapter 19: Vaccines

## Chapter 20: Clinical Diagnostics



## Chapter 21: Health Care Associated Infections



## Chapter 22: Miscellaneous



## Chapter 23: New Antibiotics



## Chapter 24: Mediators and Modifiers of Kidney Disease

## Chapter 25: Acute Kidney Injury



## Chapter 26: Selected Topics in Clinical Nephrology



## Chapter 27: Chronic Kidney Disease

## Chapter 36: Critical Care Medicine



## Chapter 37: Arrhythmias



## Chapter 38: Cardiomyopathy



## Chapter 39: Chronic Coronary Artery Disease

## Chapter 48: Pancreas/Biliary



## Chapter 49: Liver



## Chapter 50: Obesity



## Chapter 51: Miscellaneous



## Chapter 52: Diabetes Mellitus

## Chapter 57: Pituitary

# Author Index

## A



## B



## C



## D



## E



## F

## M



## N



## O



## P



## Q



## R



## S

Kolibri 360 GmbH
Ferdinand-Jühlke-Straße 7
99095 Erfurt, Deutschland
produktsicherheit@kolibri360.de